PROBLEMS AND SOLUTIONS IN HUMAN ASSESSMENT
Honoring Douglas N. Jackson at Seventy

PROBLEMS AND SOLUTIONS IN HUMAN ASSESSMENT
Honoring Douglas N. Jackson at Seventy

edited by

Richard D. Goffin
University of Western Ontario

Edward Helmes
Edith Cowan University

KLUWER ACADEMIC PUBLISHERS
Boston / Dordrecht / London

Distributors for North, Central and South America:
Kluwer Academic Publishers
101 Philip Drive
Assinippi Park
Norwell, Massachusetts 02061 USA
Telephone (781) 871-6600
Fax (781) 871-6528
E-Mail <kluwer@wkap.com>

Distributors for all other countries:
Kluwer Academic Publishers Group
Distribution Centre
Post Office Box 322
3300 AH Dordrecht, THE NETHERLANDS
Telephone 31 78 6392 392
Fax 31 78 6546 474
E-Mail <services@wkap.nl>

 Electronic Services <http://www.wkap.nl>

Library of Congress Cataloging-in-Publication Data
Problems and solutions in human assessment: honoring Douglas N. Jackson at seventy/
edited by Richard D. Goffin, Edward Helmes.
    p. cm.
  Includes bibliographical references and indexes.
  ISBN 0-7923-7768-0 (alk. paper)
    1. Personality assessment. I. Jackson, Douglas Northrop, 1929- II. Goffin, Richard D.,
1956- III. Helmes, Edward, 1949-

  BF'698.4 .P666 2000
  155.2'8--dc21
                                                                    00-022209

Printed on acid-free paper.

Printed in the United States of America

CONTENTS

List of Figures   ix

List of Tables   xi

Authors   xiii

Foreword   xix

Preface   xxi

**SECTION I. Conceptual and Methodological Influences in the
Assessment of Individual Differences**   1

1.   **Consequences of Test Interpretation and Use: The Fusion of
      Validity and Values in Psychological Assessment**   3

      Samuel Messick
      Educational Testing Service

2.   **The Role of Social Desirability in the Assessment of Personality
      Constructs**   21

      Edward Helmes
      Edith Cowan University

3.   **Construct Explication through Factor or Component Analysis:
      A Review and Evaluation of Alternative Procedures for
      Determining the Number of Factors or Components**   41

      Wayne F. Velicer, Cheryl A. Eaton, and Joseph L. Fava
      University of Rhode Island

4.   **Improved Standard Errors of Standardized Parameters in
      Covariance Structure Models: Implications for Construct
      Explication.**   73

      Mortaza Jamshidian
      University of Central Florida
      and Peter M. Bentler
      University of California, Los Angeles

SECTION II. Construct-Oriented Assessment Within the Domain of Personality   95

5.   **Application of the Construct Heuristic to the Screening of Psychopathology: The Holden Psychological Screening Inventory (HPSI)**   97

      Ronald R. Holden
      Queen's University

6.   **Construct Validity and the Search for Cross-Cultural Consistencies in Personality**   123

      Sampo V. Paunonen
      The University of Western Ontario

7.   **The Challenge of Construct Validity in the Assessment of Psychopathology**   141

      Leslie C. Morey
      Texas A&M University

8.   **Individual Differences and Scientific Productivity**   173

      J. Philippe Rushton
      The University of Western Ontario

9.   **Recent Studies of Intelligence and Personality using Jackson's Multidimensional Aptitude Battery and Personality Research Form**   195

      Philip A. Vernon
      The University of Western Ontario

SECTION III. Construct-Oriented Assessment of Individual Differences in Industrial/ Organizational Psychology   213

10.   The Assessment of Personality Constructs in Industrial-Organizational Psychology   215

Mitchell G. Rothstein and Richard D. Goffin
The University of Western Ontario

11.   Predicting Job Performance using Personality Constructs: Are Personality Tests Created Equal?   249

Richard D. Goffin, Mitchell G. Rothstein
The University of Western Ontario
and Norman G. Johnston
Private Practice, Toronto

12.   What Constructs Underlie Measures of Honesty or Integrity?   265

Kevin R. Murphy
Colorado State University

13.   Construct Validation in Organizational Behavior Research: The Case of Organizational Commitment   285

Natalie J. Allen and John P. Meyer
The University of Western Ontario

14.   The Construct of Goal Commitment: Measurement and Relationships with Task Performance   315

Gerard H. Seijts
University of Manitoba,
and Gary P. Latham
University of Toronto

15.   A Perspective   333

Douglas N. Jackson
The University of Western Ontario

Author and Subject Index   345

LIST OF FIGURES

Chapter 3
1. An illustration of the Parallel Analysis Procedure (Random Generation, 100 Matrices; M = 3, P = 24, N = 75, CS = .60).   50
2. An Illustration of the MAP Procedure (Trace of the Squared Partial Correlation Matrix; M = 3, P = 24, N = 75, CS = .60).   54
3. The number of cases (out of a possible 270) where each of the ten methods produced a legitimate estimate of M.   63
4. The mean deviation from the correct value of M for each of the ten methods.   64
5. The percent of cases where each of the ten methods produced an exactly accurate estimate of M.   64
6. The standard deviation of the estimates produced by each of the ten methods.   65

Chapter 4
1. Absolute relative bias for the delta (D) method, and quadratic approximation (Q) method for Examples 1, 2, and 3 with sample sizes N = 75, 150, and 500.   84
2. Absolute relative bias for the ordinary bootstrap (B), bootstrap with delta control function (BD), and bootstrap with regression control function (BR) for Examples 1, 2, and 3 with sample sized N = 75, 150, and 500. The size of the bootstrap sample in each case is b = 250.   86
3. Log$_{10}$ efficiencies of the bootstrap-delta (BD) method, and the bootstrap-regression (BR) method relative to the ordinary bootstrap (B) for Examples 1, 2, and 3 with sample sizes N = 75, 150, and 500. The size of the bootstrap sample in each case is b = 250.   88
4. Absolute relative bias for the ordinary bootstrap (B), bootstrap with delta control function (BD), and bootstrap with regression control function (BR) for examples 1, 2, and 3 with sample sizes N = 75, 150, and 500. The size of the bootstrap sample in each case is b = 50.   90

Chapter 5
1. Domain of psychopathology based on factor analysis of Jackson's Basic Personlity Inventory.   103
2. Varimax-rotated canonical loadings of HPSI and Q-SAD scales.   116
3. Varimax-rotated canonical loadings of HPSI and BSI scales.   118

Chapter 6
1. A hierarchical model of personality organization.   124

Chapter 7
1. An example of the relationship between the severity of psychopathology represented by an item and its utility in making different diagnostic distinctions.   153

Chapter 8
1. Plot of mean factor pattern coefficients of personality traits on dimensions of research productivity and teaching effectiveness, averaged across two studies. Only those traits with absolute values of >0.30 on either factor in both studies are shown (Based on data in Rushton, Murray & Paunonen, 1983).   182
2. Factor plot of dimensions derived from multimethod factor analysis: Factor I – Technically-Oriented Achievement versus Social Recognition, and Factor IV – Practical (Based on data in Seiss & Jackson, 1970).   184
3. Jackson Vocational Interest Survey profile of 276 male chemists.   185
4. Second-order achievement factors: Competitive acquisitiveness and concern for excellence. (After Jackson, Ahmed, & Heapy, 1976)   189

LIST OF TABLES

Chapter 2
1. Examples of Items from Jackson's Social Desirability Scale Item Pool   30

Chapter 3
1. A Comparison of Nine Alternative Methods on Three Evaluative Criteria   43
2. Summary of Alternative Procedures for Implementing the MAP Procedure   58

Chapter 5
1. Steps in the Construction of the Holden Psychological Screening Inventory (HPSI)   104
2. HPSI Scale Internal Consistency Reliability (Coefficient Alpha)   109
3. Congruence of HPSI Item Factor Loading Matrices Orthogonally Rotated to Target Matrix Based on Scoring Key   110
4. Convergent Validities (Zero-order Correlations) for the HPSI Scale of Psychiatric Symptomatology   111
5. Convergent Validities (Zero-order Correlations) for the HPSI Scale of Social Symptomatology   112
6. Convergent Validities (Zero-order Correlations) for the HPSI Scale of Depression   113
7. Varimax-Rotated Factor Loadings for HPSI, MMPI-2, and BPI Scales   114
8. Varimax-Rotated Factor Loadings for HPSI and BPI Scales   115

Chapter 7
1. The 22 Full Scales of the PAI.   146
2. PAI Subscales and their Descriptions.   148
3. A Sample of Instruments Used in the Validation of the PAI to Date.   166

Chapter 8
1. Frequencies and Cumulative Percentage for the Distribution of Citations of and Publications by Faculty Members at the Top 100 British, Canadian, and American Graduate Department of Psychology   175
2. Split-half reliabilities of peer and student ratings of personality computed across professor targets for each of 29 personality traits (decimals omitted).   179
3. Weber's Types of Leadership Styles   187

Chapter 11
1. Convergence of PRF and 16PF Scales   258
2. Hierarchical Regressions   259

Chapter 12
1. Dimensions Often Reported in Analyses of Integrity Tests   269
2. Examples of Integrity Tests   270

Chapter 14
1. Hollenbeck, Williams and Klein's (1989) goal commitment items.   319

THE AUTHORS

NATALIE J. ALLEN received her Ph.D. (Psychology) in 1985 from the University of Western Ontario where she is an Associate Professor in the Department of Psychology. For several years, her research has dealt with the conceptualization and measurement of employee commitment to organizations, the development of employee commitment, and its behavioral consequences. More recent research focuses on work teams and, in particular, the composition of teams and issues of alignment between organizations and their teams. Her work appears in the *Journal of Applied Psychology*, *Evaluation and Program Planning*, the *Journal of Vocational Behavior*, and the *Academy of Management Journal*. She is the co-author, with John Meyer, of a recently published book entitled *Commitment in the Workplace: Theory, Research and Application* (Sage, 1997).

PETER M. BENTLER, working under Douglas Jackson, received his Ph.D. in Clinical Psychology from Stanford University in 1964. He spent a postdoctoral year at the Educational Testing Service, working under Samuel Messick. Since that time he has been at the University of California, Los Angeles, where he is now Professor and Chair of Psychology as well as Professor of Statistics. He has published widely in personality and applied social psychology, especially on drug use and abuse, and on psychometrics and multivariate analysis, especially on structural equation modeling. He is author of the EQS Structural Equations Program. He has been an elected president of the Society of Multivariate Experimental Psychology, the Psychometric Society, and the Division of Evaluation, Measurement and Statistics of the American Psychological Association. He also received the latter's Distinguished Scientific Contributions Award.

CHERYL A. EATON is currently a data analyst at the Center for Alcohol and Addiction Studies at Brown University. She has provided the data management and statistical analysis support for numerous NIH funded grants on the assessment and treatment of addictive behaviors over the past 15 years. She earned her M. A. in Experimental Psychology at the University of Rhode Island.

JOSEPH L. FAVA is a Research Professor at the Cancer Prevention Research Center at the University of Rhode Island. He received his Ph.D. in Quantitative Psychology in 1990 from the University of Rhode Island. He specializes in applied measure development and multivariate statistical techniques used in measure development, including component analysis, factor analysis, and structural equation modeling. He is Co-principal Investigator on several National Cancer Institute research grants that intervene on behavioral risks for cancer. His publications have appeared in both methodological and health-oriented journals. He is a member of Divisions 5, 38, and 50 of the American Psychological Association, the Society of Behavioral Medicine, the American Statistical Association, the Psychometric Society, and the National Cancer Institute Information Associates Program.

RICHARD D. GOFFIN is Associate Professor of Psychology at The University of Western Ontario. He received his Ph.D. from the University of Western Ontario (1988). He is the author, or coauthor, of more than a dozen articles on assessment-related issues in a wide range of journals (e.g., *Journal of Applied Psychology*, *Multivariate Behavioral Research*, *Personnel Psychology*, and *Organizational Behavior and Human Decision Processes*). His areas of research include performance appraisal, personnel selection, and personality.

EDWARD HELMES obtained his Masters degree in physiological psychology and then his Ph.D. in 1978 in psychological measurement from the University of Western Ontario, with subsequent graduate training in neuropsychology and clinical psychology. His work has been a combination of clinical work in teaching hospitals and private practice, together with part-time academic teaching. His research has been in the areas of psychological assessment and ageing. He has worked clinically in the areas of chronic pain, both outpatient and chronic psychiatric disorders, and disability and physical rehabilitation. He moved to Perth in 1996 to coordinate the geropsychology program at Edith Cowan University.

RONALD R. HOLDEN is a Professor of Psychology at Queen's University, Kingston, Ontario, Canada. He received his undergraduate education at the University of Toronto and his graduate training, specializing in clinical psychology, at the University of Western Ontario. Dr. Holden's clinical training and research affiliations have included the Clarke Institute of Psychiatry, London Psychiatric Hospital, and Kingston Psychiatric Hospital. He has held academic appointments at the University of Western Ontario, Trent University, and Queen's University. Dr. Holden's primary research foci are the topics of test construction, psychometrics, assessment, and suicide.

DOUGLAS N. JACKSON is the author of a number of widely used psychological tests and questionnaires in personality, psychopathology, intellectual abilities, and vocational interests. His *Jackson Vocational Interest Survey* has influenced the career planning of more than half a million young people. His theoretical bases and methods for developing psychological tests have been influential in setting the standard for psychological tests in the latter half of the 20th century. Jackson's *Personality Research Form* has been acknowledged as one of the three most widely cited personality questionnaires in the psychological research literature. He has also published widely in psychology in a variety of areas, including applied multivariate analysis, psychometrics, computer assisted test administration and interpretation, response biases and distortions in personality assessment, personality scale construction, the nature of intelligence, sex difference in intellectual abilities, social conformity, personality and job performance, vocational interest measurement, job performance evaluation, cognitive styles and personality, and personality scale validation. He has published more than 150 articles in refereed journals, as well as several dozen book chapters. He has served on several boards of editors of psychological journals, and has co-edited two books.

MORTAZA JAMSHIDIAN recieved his Ph.D. in Applied Mathematics under Robert I. Jennrich from the University of California, Los Angeles in 1988. He worked at BMDP

Statistical Software from 1988 to 1990, and served as assistant professor in the mathematics department at Isfahan University of Technology in Iran between 1990 to 1994. During this period he made a number of visits to the Department of Psychology at UCLA where he collaborated with Peter Bentler on a number of computational methodologies related to structural equation models. He came back to work at BMDP in 1994 until 1996. He then secured a position at the Department of Statistics at University of Central Florida where he is now serving as Assistant Professor.

NORMAN G. JOHNSTON received his Ph.D. in Social Psychology from Wayne State University in 1975. He has held several teaching, administrative and consulting positions. Since 1989, he has maintained an independent   practice in I/O Psychology, consulting with a variety of private and   public sector organizations. His consulting practice is largely focussed on the assessment of managers and executives for selection or development, design and operation of assessment centers, design of test based selection systems, and program and evaluation research. His research and publications reflect his consulting interests and are an   integral part of his work with client organizations. He is based in   Toronto, Canada.

GARY P. LATHAM is formerly the Ford Motor Research Professor and Chairman of the Management and Organization Department of the Business School at the University of Washington. As of September, 1990 he accepted an endowed chair at the University of Toronto where he is currently the Secretary of State Professor of Organizational Effectiveness. Gary is a Fellow of both the American and Canadian Psychological Associations. He is a Fellow of the Academy of Management, he is a member of the Society of Organizational Behavior and a Fellow of the Royal Society of Canada. In 1997 he was the first recipient of the award for "Distinguished Contributions to Industrial-Organizational Psychology" from the Canadian Psychological Association. In 1998 he was awarded the "Distinguished Contributions to Psychology as A Profession" from the American Psychological Association. He is President of the Canadian Psychological Association. Gary consults widely in industry. Among his clients are Domtar, Stentor, and the Royal Bank of Canada.   Among Gary's creative accomplishments is the development of the situational interview for selecting employees and the development of behavioral observation scales for performance appraisal.   Gary's books include, "Increasing Productivity Through Performance Appraisal" (with Dr. K.N. Wexley), "A Theory of Goal Setting and Task Performance" (with Dr. E.A. Locke), "Developing and Training Human Resources in Organizations" (with Dr. K.N. Wexley), and "Goal Setting: A Motivational Technique That Works" (with Dr. E.A. Locke).

SAMUEL J. MESSICK had a long and distinguished career, characterized by the breadth of his vision and the diversity of his research and theorizing. Messick was associated with the Educational Testing Service for almost his entire career, beginning as a psychometric fellow in 1951, serving for many years as vice president for research, and concluding it as distinguished research scientist. He is known for his ground-breaking work in construct validation, which is the subject of his chapter, one of his last contributions. He also did important work in the theory and measurement of cognitive styles and abilities, personality assessment and theory, scaling, educational evaluation and policy, the effects of coaching on mental testing, creativity, and impression management and response styles, among other areas. He was an outstanding communicator in his multiple roles as an adjunct professor in the graduate division of the City University of New York, as an advisor to research fellows and staff at ETS, and as a member of professional, governmental, and public-interest policy committees. Samuel Messick and Douglas Jackson collaborated on a long list of publications and informally exchanged ideas for more than four decades.

JOHN P. MEYER received his Ph.D. in 1978 from The University of Western Ontario, where he is currently Professor and Chair of the Industrial and Organizational Psychology program. His research interests are in the areas of work motivation and work attitudes, with emphasis on the development and consequences of employee commitment. His research has been published in in leading journals in the field of I/O psychology (e.g., *Journal of Applied Psychology, Personnel Psychology*) and management (e.g., *Academy of Management Journal, Journal of Management*). He is also co-author of *Commitment in the Workplace:Theory, Research and Application*. His current research interests include the cross-cultural generalizability of the three-component model of commitment he developed with Natalie Allen, as well as the impact of organizational change on commitment.

LESLIE C. MOREY is Professor of Psychology at Texas A&M University. He received his Ph.D. in Clinical Psychology from the University of Florida, and has served on the faculty at Vanderbilt University, Harvard Medical School, the Yale University School of Medicine, and the University of Tulsa. He has published over 90 articles, books, and chapters on the assessment and diagnosis of mental disorders. He is the author of the Personality Assessment Inventory, Personality Assessment Screener, and the Interpretive Guide to the Personality Assessment Inventory, and has been an advocate of the construct validation approach in the development of taxonomy in mental disorder as well as in the measurement of elements in such taxonomies.

KEVIN R. MURPHY is a professor of Psychology at Colorado State University. He has served as President of the Society for Industrial and Organizational Psychology and is the Editor of *Journal of Applied Psychology*. He is the author of over ninety articles and book chapters, and author or editor of eight books, in the areas of performance appraisal, psychological testing, statistical power analysis, honesty in the workplace, and gender and work. Dr. Murphy has served as Chair of the Department of Defense Advisory Committee for Military Personnel Testing and has served on the National Academy of Sciences Committees on Performance Appraisal and on Drug Use in the Workplace, and the National Research Council Roundtable on Work, Learning and Assessment.

SAMPO V. PAUNONEN is a professor in the Department of Psychology at the University of Western Ontario, where he received his Ph.D. His research interests include person perception, personality assessment, factor analysis, and personnel selection.

MITCHELL G. ROTHSTEIN received his Ph.D. in industrial and organizational psychology in 1983 from the University of Western Ontario. He worked in industry and consulting for six years and then joined the Richard Ivey School of Business where he is currently

Associate Professor of Organizational Behavior. His research interests have focused on the relationship between personality and job performance, and more recently, career issues in international business. He has published articles in the *Journal of Applied Psychology, Personnel Psychology, Journal of Educational Psychology*, and *the Journal of Organizational Behavior*. He has consulted with a variety of organizations concerning recruitment and selection practices, performance appraisal, competency profiling, and management team building.

J. PHILIPPE RUSHTON is Professor of Psychology at the University of Western Ontario in Canada. He holds two doctorates from the University of London (Ph.D. and D.Sc.), is a Fellow of the John Simon Guggenheim Foundation, the American Association for the Advancement of Science, and the American, British, and Canadian Psychological Associations. His primary research interest is the sociobiology of human altruism. He has published nearly two hundred articles and six books, the latest of which is *Race, Evolution, and Behavior* (1995). Professor Rushton is listed in *Who's Who in Science and Technology, Who's Who in International Authors,* and *Who's Who in Canada.*

GERARD H. SEIJTS has been Assistant Professor in the Faculty of Management at the University of Manitoba since 1997. He earned his Ph.D. at the University of Toronto. Gerard teaches undergraduate and MBA courses in human resources management, decision-making, managerial negotiations, organizational behavior, and staffing and development. His research activities, spanning several journal articles, book chapters, and conference papers, cover a wide range of topics including, training and development, goal-setting, social cognitive theory, staffing, performance appraisal, and organizational justice.

WAYNE F. VELICER, Co-Director of the Cancer Prevention Research Center and Professor of Psychology at the University of Rhode Island, received his Ph.D. in Psychology from Purdue University in 1972. He has published more than 120 papers, book chapters, and books on a variety of topics, including health promotion, factor analysis/component analysis, time series analysis, and measurement development. He was identified as one of the highest impact authors in Psychology in both 1992 and 1996. He is one of the developers of the Transtheoretical Model of Change and is a pioneer in the development of expert system methodology for health promotion. He has been a Visiting Professor at the University of Western Ontario (Canada), Macquirie University (Australia), University of Maastricht (The Netherlands), and University of New South Wales (Australia).

PHILIP A. VERNON obtained his PhD from UC Berkeley in 1981 and is currently a Professor of Psychology at the University of Western Ontario. Vernon's research primarily involves behavior genetic and biological approaches to the study of individual differences. He is principal investigator of the Western Ontario Twin Project - a longitudinal investigation of personality and intelligence among 6-month to 6-year-old twins - and co-investigator on a number of adult twin projects and studies of biological correlates of human intelligence and information-processing. Vernon has published numerous articles in the journals *Intelligence, Personality and Individual Differences* and elsewhere, and has edited three books. He was elected President Elect of the International Society for the Study of Individual Differences in 1999.

FOREWORD

Sampo V. Paunonen

It has been over 30 years since the publication by Douglas Jackson and Samuel Messick of *Problems in Human Assessment*. That book was a compilation of classic articles intended by the authors to serve as a reference for important conceptual and empirical problems in the area of psychological measurement existing at the time. It was reprinted in 1978, demonstrating that many of the articles it contained were indeed classics worthy of being read despite the advances in knowledge over the years. And now, in the year of Jackson's 70th birthday, it seems both timely and fitting to publish this volume, entitled *Problems and Solutions in Human Assessment:Honoring Douglas N. Jackson at Seventy*.

It is expected that this book will become an indispensable source of information for all those who are interested in the measurement of individual differences. Moreover, this book is intended as a tribute to Professor Jackson and his lifelong study of problems in psychological measurement. As the title of this book suggests, we the authors offer some solutions to those problems. The common thread that connects the various chapters contained herein is the fact that all of the proposed solutions have been inspired, in one way or another by Professor Jackson's focus on deductive, construct-driven strategies and his remarkable empirical and theoretical work in the area of human assessment.

The editors of this volume do not mean to imply, by its title, that all measurement issues have now been solved. On the contrary, some problems are recalcitrant and obstinately defy analysis. There have been some recent developments in our science, however, such as new item response models, multivariate analytic methods, Monte Carlo simulation techniques, and computerized testing procedures, some of which are discussed in the present chapters. These developments ultimately might provide the technology necessary to resolve some of the still outstanding issues in human assessment.

It is our hope as authors of these works that we can humbly provide solutions to some extant problems in human assessment and, at the same time, formally acknowledge our indebtedness to Douglas N. Jackson for his important contributions to our own advancement as scientists.

PREFACE

This book deals broadly with the assessment of individual differences, an area that has occupied a place of prominence in both the practice and science of psychology for the past century and before. But the impact has not been limited to psychology; innovations and controversies in the assessment of individual differences have generated shock waves affecting sociology, education, and a number of other behavioral sciences as well as the fields of management and organizational behavior. Accordingly, the assessment of individual differences is conspicuous in early through to advanced training in psychology (often under the guise of "measurement," "psychological testing," or "personality assessment"), and well-trained specialists in this area have no shortage of career opportunities.

In covering the assessment of individual differences, this book pays tribute to the interests and activities that Douglas N. Jackson has incorporated into his career as a psychologist. He has been (and still is) in the midst of central controversies in personality and multivariate statistics, has set the standards for the development of many measures of individual differences, and continues to be a leader in putting academic findings to practical use. He has also inspired generations of students with his mastery of complex concepts and as a personal example of the ability to balance several simultaneous areas of research. Consistent with the focus of Jackson's research, the theme of this book will be how the use of deductive, construct-driven strategies in the assessment of individual differences leads to benefits in terms of the applicability of the assessment instruments and the clarity of the conclusions that can be drawn from the research.

Jackson's own assessment instruments, including the *Personality Research Form*, the *Jackson Personality Inventory*, and the *Jackson Vocational Interest Survey*, are among the most highly-lauded measures of individual differences in use today. Collectively, the chapters of this book provide a valuable source of information on the scale development and validation strategies Jackson has championed in creating his assessment tools, the conceptual and philosophical underpinnings of his approach, specific quantitative techniques that are integral to his scale development strategies, and promising directions that future researchers in this area might explore. Consequently, we expect that this volume will appeal to academics and practitioners of various disciplines (e.g., psychology, sociology, management) who are involved in, or have an interest in, the development or validation of individual differences measures.

The book is divided into three main sections, one on fundamental conceptual and methodological issues in the assessment of individual differences, one on the construct-oriented assessment of individual differences within the domain of personality, and one on the construct-oriented assessment of individual differences in industrial/organizational psychology.

Quite naturally, the first section begins with a view of the "big picture" in the assessment of individual differences. In Chapter 1 Samuel Messick discusses the ultimate standard by which assessment instruments are gauged, namely, validity. Messick cogently explicates and justifies his position on the role of values in considerations of testing and test validation. One of Jackson's closest friends and colleagues, and a prolific and highly influential author in the area of individual differences assessment for more than 40 years, Messick also provides some insights into the process by which societal goals and values are incorporated into the concept of validity. We are honored to have the opportunity to include in this volume what may be Messick's final published work, he passed on shortly after completing his chapter.

One of the hallmarks of the assessment instruments developed by Jackson is their ability to suppress the confounding effects of socially desirable responding. The second chapter, by Helmes, begins by providing a brief history of the concept of social desirability, starting with the work of Edwards, Block, Jackson and Messick, and Marlow and Crowne. The elaboration of social desirability as a distinct construct, and the effect and methodological control of this construct as a contaminant of individual differences measures is delineated in terms of past, present, and future directions.

Common factor analysis and principal components analysis are arguably the two most prevalent quantitative techniques used in the identification and explication of constructs for the purposes of individual differences assessment. Thus, the third chapter, by Velicer, Eaton and Fava, covers a central issue in the use of these two techniques, that is, how one determines the "correct" number of constructs. Velicer et al. review the number of factors/components problem and its many proposed solutions, including Velicer's own inventive solution.

Chapter 4, by Jamshidian and Bentler, addresses an additional concern relevant to the use of factor analysis and covariance structure modeling for construct explication and identification. Specifically, factor analysis and covariance structure modeling, as they are often undertaken, result in inaccurate estimates of the standard errors of loadings, which, in turn, can lead to inaccurate decision-making regarding construct interpretation. Jamshidian and Bentler discuss this problem and derive new methods by which it can be attenuated.

Section II begins with a concrete illustration of how the deductive, construct-driven approach to test development, which has been championed by Jackson, can be applied in the assessment of individual differences. Specifically, in Chapter 5, Holden traces the development of an instrument used in the evaluation of the dysfunctional personality.

Paunonen, in Chapter 6, extends Jackson's ideas to cross-cultural issues in the assessment of personality and the investigation of personality structure. As Paunonen shows, the construct validation procedures championed by Jackson can provide more stringent evidence than previously available to scholars who are working to discover which personality traits are generalizable across cultures and which, if any, are culture-specific.

Chapter 7 by Morey outlines his work in adapting the principles advocated by Jackson in the development of the *Personality Assessment Inventory*. This multiscale instrument for the assessment of psychopathology embodies the sequential application of principles derived from theory with the incorporation of empirical data at several steps to refine the item pool before composing the final scales.

In Chapter 8, Rushton, a long time collaborator of Jackson, and co-organizer (with Jackson) of a conference on scientific excellence, provides a summary of research which has assessed individual differences with the goal of identifying personality constructs and necessary preconditions for the fostering of scientific excellence.

Chapter 9 by Vernon closes Section II with a discussion of recent advances and future directions in the study of personality and cognitive abilities including research on basic cognitive processing components of mental ability; univariate and multivariate behavioral genetic studies of intelligence and personality; and studies of a number of biological and physiological correlates of human intelligence and mental abilities. Vernon credits Jackson's assessment instruments such as the *Personality Research Form* and the *Multidimensional Aptitude Battery* as providing the basic tools necessary for much of this research.

Section III documents the influence that Jackson's work has had in spawning important advances in the area of I/O psychology. Rothstein and Goffin's Chapter 10 provides an analysis of how the use of deductive, construct-driven strategies in the assessment of individual differences has influenced a number of theoretical and methodological advances in industrial/organizational psychology. In particular, discussion focuses on the assessment of applicant personality traits in the employment interview, the use of personality measures for predicting job performance, the suppression of nuisance variance due to faking, and innovations in the use of meta-analysis to determine the validity of personality measures in personnel selection.

Chapter 11, by Goffin, Rothstein and Johnston, provides an empirical demonstration of the usefulness of Jackson's *Personality Research Form* in predicting job performance. Using a sample of managers from a large organization, results show that the *PRF* surpasses another popular test with respect to the prediction of performance and suitability for promotion. Aside from its empirical contributions, this chapter raises the broader issue of whether or not past I/O researchers' implicit assumption that all personality tests have comparable levels of predictive validity, is tenable.

Few issues in industrial/organizational psychology have generated as much controversy as the use of integrity/honesty tests in the identification of potentially counterproductive employees. A core problem in this area is the general confusion as to the constructs that should, and are, being assessed by these tests. Consistent with the Jacksonian emphasis on construct validation and explication, in Chapter 12 Murphy addresses this concern and a number of additional issues relevant to the intelligent application of integrity/honesty tests.

In addition to the advances in personality assessment associated with the Jacksonian approach to measurement, industrial/organizational psychology has also benefited in other areas. Using the example of organizational commitment, Allen and Meyer (Chapter 13) illustrate how Jackson's construct driven methodology for scale construction can be applied to measure important work-related attitudes.

In Chapter 14, Seijts and Latham focus on a prominent individual differences construct in work motivation, namely, goal commitment. They discuss and critique currently available measures of goal commitment and explore heretofore unrealized measurement opportunities for this construct from the Jacksonian perspective.

Finally, in Chapter 15 Jackson describes the major influences underlying his development as a researcher. Much of the collected wisdom that he has acquired in a preeminent career spanning more than 40 years (and counting) is offered in distilled form.

With the breadth of his interests, any volume of reasonable length will fail to do justice to some area of Jackson's research, nonetheless, we believe the chapters in this volume do address the focal areas of psychology that have been at the heart of this man's work. We hope that it provides a similar type of inspiration to further generations in the same way that Jackson has inspired the contributors to this volume.

Our Editors at Kluwer Academic; Robert Chametsky, Scott Delman, and Michael Williams, have been extremely supportive and accessible throughout this project. Mary Panarelli, the Editorial Assistant at Kluwer could not have been more helpful in her courteous, prompt, and thorough replies to our innumerable questions. Jennifer Spicer was responsible for the care and expertise devoted to the final formatting and indexing of this work – a huge task throughout which she has somehow remained cheerful.

Financial support from the Social Sciences and Humanities Research Council of Canada facilitated the completion of this volume. A special thanks goes to those who selflessly donated their time to reading through chapters of this book and providing authors with constructive feedback. We extend our appreciation to Michael Ashton, Robert Gardner, Gary Groth-Marnat, Douglas Jackson, Arthur Jensen, Harry Murray, Adelheid Nicol, Del Paulhus, Susan Pepper, Sam Paunonen, Corinne Reid, Rosie Rooney, and Christian Vandenberghe, as well as to those who preferred not be mentioned by name. We thank Howard Wainer and Kathy Howell of Educational Testing Service for their assistance in locating Samuel Messick's chapter after his death. Finally, to Bea, Celia and Karl Goffin, thanks for your understanding regarding all the weekends and late nights I spent working on this.

Richard D. Goffin
Edward Helmes

SECTION I: CONCEPTUAL AND METHODOLOGICAL INFLUENCES IN THE ASSESSMENT OF INDIVIDUAL DIFFERENCES

The chapters in this section illustrate some crucial issues relevant in the consideration of the construct validity of assessment tools. Psychological constructs and the measures that instantiate them are fundamental to the study of personality, considered broadly in all its aspects. To those who study personality as it is reflected in natural language, this means that one may consider the domain of intelligence to be subsumed in some way as a personality construct, even though this is rarely done in practice. Nevertheless, this broad conception of personality proves one way of encapsulating the range of Jackson's interests. His work in test development alone spans not just traditional areas of personality, but also vocational interests, and intelligence. In addition, a cornerstone of Jackson's teaching has been that one cannot have an adequate measure of a construct if one did not have already an adequate theory of the construct.

The introductory chapter is a continuation of the theme promoted by Samuel Messick during the last several years that construct validity can imply that the consequences of test use may be as important, if not more so, than other aspects of construct validity. As he has recognized here and in other places, many specialists in the field do not agree with his position. Perhaps sensitized by the internal discussions at Educational Testing Service that may have arisen in response to the public criticism of test use, Messick was consistent in his defense of test use. He also, however, places the responsibility for the use and misuse of tests in the hands of both test developers and users, adopting a wider view of professional responsibility than many psychologists agree with. This chapter represents one of his last papers on this topic. His death during the preparation of this book was a huge loss to the field of psychological assessment.

The history of social desirability as a confounding factor in the assessment of personality dates at least to the 1930s, but the relevant debates were most active during the early years of Jackson's career. Chapter 2 provides a brief history of the debates over desirability, and summarizes Jackson's procedures for controlling the influence of desirability in the construction of multiscale inventories. The confounding of desirability with content has generated much heat, but surprisingly little active research since the 1960s work of Crown and Marlowe (1960, 1964) on the need for approval.   The research program of Del Paulhus during his development of the Balanced Inventory of Desirability Responding (BIDR, Paulhus, 1997) has been a notable exception.   Such developments are most likely to result in improved understanding of desirability and the cognitive processes involved in responding to personality test items.   Increased understanding at a theoretical level then leads to improved assessment instruments.   This is the essence, of course, of the recommendations made by Jackson (1971).

Anyone who has examined a manual for one of Jackson's personality or vocational interest tests will have seen his reliance on multivariate analysis for both test development and validation.   An article by Jackson and the first author of Chapter 3, Wayne Velicer (Velicer & Jackson, 1990), led to a series of comments and rebuttals regarding the relative advantages and weaknesses of component analysis and factor analysis.   In this volume, Velicer and his colleagues explore in further detail another troublesome topic in factor or component analysis, that of the best method of determining the number of factors or components in an exploratory analysis.

While Jackson's work emphasized the practical side of multivariate analysis, he used statistical theory where appropriate. In Chapter 4, Mortaza Jamshidian, and Jackson's long-time colleague and former student, Peter Bentler, use their knowledge of multivariate statistics to explore a practical problem that can arise in some forms of multivariate data analysis that are commonly used in the interpretation of constructs.   Specifically, they develop an improved means of standard error estimation that is more accurate than most currently-used methods when a correlation matrix is analyzed rather than a covariance matrix.

REFERENCES

Crowne, D. P., & Marlowe, D. (1960). A new scale of social desirability independent of psychopathology. *Journal of Consulting Psychology*, **24**, 349-354.
Crowne, D. P., & Marlowe, D. A. (1964). *The approval motive.* New York: Wiley.
Jackson, D. N. (1971). The dynamics of structured personality tests: 1971. *Psychological Review*, **78**, 229-248.
Velicer, W. F., & Jackson, D. N. (1990). Component analysis versus common factor analysis: Some issues in selecting an appropriate procedure. *Multivariate Behavioral Research*, **25**, 1-28.

1 CONSEQUENCES OF TEST INTERPRETATION AND USE: THE FUSION OF VALIDITY AND VALUES IN PSYCHOLOGICAL ASSESSMENT[1]

Samuel Messick

This paper addresses the role of social values in educational and psychological measurement, with special attention to the consequences of testing as validity evidence, which is an inherently value-dependent enterprise. The primary measurement standards that must be met to legitimize a proposed test use are those of reliability, validity, and fairness, which are also value-laden concepts. Evidence of reliability signifies that something is being measured; the major concern is score consistency or stability. Evidence of validity circumscribes the nature of that something; the major concern is score meaning. Evidence of fairness indicates that score meaning does not differ consequentially across individuals, groups, or settings; the major concern is comparability.

The appropriate level of reliability depends on the meaning of the construct being measured because some constructs are conceived theoretically to be more consistent or stable than others. Hence, evidence of reliability consistent with the construct's meaning is simultaneously also evidence of construct validity. Within these limits, the measurement intent is to achieve sufficient score consistency or stability to warrant the use of the scores in decision making. Another way of putting it is that the uncertainty involved in determining score levels should be inconsequential for the proposed test use.

Validity is mainly concerned with the meaning and consequences of measurement. Accordingly, validation studies aim to accrue convergent evidence supportive of score meaning and its action implications as well as discriminant evidence discounting plausible rival interpretations. Validity is a unitary concept, which means that fundamentally there is only one kind of validity, namely, construct validity. However, several complementary forms of evidence need to be integrated in construct validation, evidence bearing on test content, score structure, substantive processes, generalizability, external relationships, and testing consequences.

In general, fairness implies impartiality, and the question arises as to how fairness is manifested in educational and psychological measurement. In particular, the impartiality entailed in test fairness is achieved through comparable construct validity across individuals, groups, and settings. That is, score levels should have the same meaning and consequences in different population groups and environmental contexts. This does not imply that fair test use yields equal group outcomes, however, because fair tests may validly document unequal outcomes resulting from, among other things, unequal opportunities to learn as well as differential experiences in learning and development.

The discussion thus far implies that both reliability and fairness are actually different sub-topics subsumed under the overarching concept of validity. Indeed, reliability is treated here in terms of the generalizability aspect of construct validity. In contrast, fairness is discussed as a topic in its own right in order to highlight the complexity of the value choices and consequences entailed in fairness judgments in relation to validity judgments.

Thus, by virtue of focusing on the role of values in educational and psychological measurement, this paper emphasizes the value-laden nature of validity and fairness as psychometric concepts. However, validity and fairness are not just psychometric principles. They are themselves social values that have meaning and force outside of measurement whenever judgments and decisions are made. We must keep in mind this broader meaning because it informs the public's mind as to what is valid and fair. Ultimately, our psychometric considerations need to be justified in this public arena.

THE VALUES OF VALIDITY AND FAIRNESS

Validity is an overall evaluative judgment of the degree to which empirical evidence and theoretical rationales support the adequacy and appropriateness of interpretations and actions based on test scores or other modes of assessment (Messick, 1989). Validity is not a property of the test or assessment as such, but rather of the meaning of the test scores. Hence, what is to be validated is not the test or observation device per se but rather the inferences derived from test scores or other indicators (Cronbach, 1971) – inferences about score meaning or interpretation and about the implications for action that the interpretation entails. Broadly speaking, then, validity is an inductive summary of both the existing evidence for and the potential consequences of test interpretation and use.

To validate an interpretive inference is to ascertain the degree to which multiple lines of evidence are consonant with the inference, while establishing that alternative inferences are less well supported. To validate an action inference requires not only evidence of score meaning but also justification of value implications and action outcomes, especially appraisals of the relevance and utility of the test scores for particular applied purposes and of the social consequences of using the test scores for applied decision making. Thus the key issues of test validity are the interpretability, relevance, and utility of scores, the import or value implications of scores as a basis for action, and the functional worth of scores in terms of social consequences of their use.

Although different sources and mixes of evidence are required to support particular score-based inferences, validity is a unitary concept in the sense that score meaning as embodied in construct validity underlies all score-based inferences. Hence, all validation is construct validation. Furthermore, because value implications as a basis for action are integral to score meaning, construct validation has to include an appraisal of these value implications in terms of the actual and potential consequences of test use.

This point was forcefully made by Cronbach (1988) in his treatment of validation as persuasive argument: " the argument must link concepts, evidence, social and personal consequences, and values" (p.4). A special concern is to guard against adverse consequences that are traceable to sources of invalidity such as construct under-representation or construct-irrelevant variance (Messick, 1989, 1995). Indeed, it is difficult even to isolate questions of the value implications of score interpretations from questions of the validity of those interpretations. Even the meanings of the words "valid" and "value" derive from the same Latin root, valere, meaning "to be strong." From this perspective, validity judgments are value judgments.

This fusion of validity and values in test interpretation and use is especially salient in connection with testing consequences. This is the case because consequences are evaluated in a validity arena where social values abound, namely, in terms of test fairness. As we have seen, test fairness is a validity issue because fairness implies comparable validity across individuals, groups, and settings (Willingham, 1998; Willingham & Cole, 1997). The key problem in test fairness is legitimizing the meaning of the term "comparable" in terms of value choices.

The remainder of this paper explores the role of values in test validity and fairness in more detail. First, six main aspects of the validation process are examined; many of which entail important value issues and value choices. Next, we consider some of the value issues that need to be addressed in establishing the fairness of the test development process as well as the fairness of test use. Finally, the controversy over consequences as validity evidence is confronted, as is the value-dependence of such evidence.

VALIDITY OF TEST INTERPRETATION AND USE

In essence, test validation is empirical evaluation of the meaning and consequences of measurement, taking into account extraneous factors in the applied setting that might erode or promote the validity of local score interpretation and use. Because score meaning is a construction that makes theoretical sense out of both the performance underlying the score and its pattern of relationships with other variables, the psychometric literature views the fundamental issue as construct validity.

Recurrent Questions of Validity

To evaluate the meaning and consequences of measurement is no small order, however, and requires attention to a number of persistent validity questions, such as:

- Are we looking at the right things in the right balance?
- Does the assessment adequately cover the content domain? Has anything important been left out?
- Does our way of looking, especially the choice of stimulus and response formats, facilitate the expression of competence or other processes, or are sources of invalidity or irrelevant variance introduced that bias the scores or judgments?
- Is the scoring system consistent with the structure of the domain about which inferences are to be drawn or predictions made?
- Are there plausible rival interpretations of score meaning or alternative implications for action and, if so, by what evidence and arguments are they discounted?
- Are the scores reliable and are their properties and relationships generalizable across the contents and contexts of use as well as across pertinent population groups?
- Are the value implications of score interpretations empirically grounded in terms of observed outcomes, especially if pejorative in tone, and are they commensurate with the score's trait implications?
- Do the scores have utility for the proposed purposes in the applied setting?
- Are the scores applied fairly for these purposes, that is, consistently and equitably across individuals and groups?
- Are the short- and long-term consequences of score interpretation and use supportive of the general testing aims and are there any adverse side-effects traceable to test invalidity?

The general thrust of such questions is to seek evidence and arguments to discount the two major threats to construct validity – namely, construct under-representation and construct-irrelevant variance – as well as to evaluate the action implications of score meaning.

CONSTRUCTING CONSTRUCT VALIDITY

Validity is now widely viewed as an integral or unified concept (APA, 1985). Therefore, establishing validity requires the collection and integration of multiple complementary forms of evidence to answer an interdependent set of questions such as those just considered. To make this explicit, it is illuminating to differentiate unified validity into several distinct aspects to underscore issues and nuances that might otherwise be downplayed or overlooked.

In particular, six distinguishable aspects of construct validity are highlighted: *content, substantive processes, score structure, generalizability, external relationships,* and *testing consequences.* In effect, these six aspects function as general validity criteria or standards for all educational and psychological measurement (Messick, 1989, 1995).

These six aspects of construct validity take the construct to be measured as a given. However, there is a critical prior step in test design, if not in test validation, that must be carefully negotiated because it is profoundly value-laden. This is the stage of construct choice for the particular testing purpose. Although this choice is greatly influenced by salient variables operative in the criterion domain, there is usually ample leeway for social values to intrude. Is it not at least in part a value decision when reading and mathematics are privileged over other abilities in high-school graduation examinations and in college admissions (Willingham & Cole, 1997) or when intelligence test scores are used in placing children in special education programs (Heller, Holtzman, & Messick, 1982)? Approaches to circumscribing the nature of the construct being measured are addressed by the six aspects of construct validity that we turn to next. Although these considerations may not determine construct choice, they can certainly modify the nature of that choice. Especially pertinent in this regard are the content, substantive, and structural aspects of construct validity.

The content aspect of construct validity (Lennon, 1956; Messick, 1989) includes evidence of content relevance and representativeness as well as of technical quality (e.g., appropriate reading level and unambiguous phrasing). Key issues here are specifying the boundaries of the content domain to be assessed and selecting tasks or stimulus questions that are representative so that all important parts of the domain are covered. The aim is to assemble a representative sample of tasks or items tapping knowledge, skills, or other attributes relevant to the purpose of the testing. Expert professional judgment is usually relied upon to document content relevance and representativeness.

The substantive aspect of construct validity refers to the psychological processes (of thought, motive, or feeling) underlying both task or item performance and the correlations across items. There are two important points: One is the need for tests that assess domain processes in addition to traditional coverage of domain content; the other is the need to move beyond traditional professional judgment of content to accrue empirical evidence that the assumed cognitive, conative, or affective processes are actually at work. Thus, the substantive aspect adds to the content aspect of construct validity the need for empirical evidence of response consistencies or performance regularities reflective of domain processes (Embretson, 1983; Loevinger, 1957; Messick, 1989), In one form or another, the substantive aspect calls for models of the cognitive processes required by the assessment tasks.

The structural aspect appraises the degree to which the score scales are consistent with the structure of the domain being measured. The internal structure of the assessment should reflect the internal structure of the construct domain. Scoring models should be rationally consistent with what is known about structural relations inherent in behavioral manifestations of the construct in question (Loevinger, 1957; Peak, 1953). The theory of the construct domain should guide not only the creation of assessment tasks but also the development of scoring criteria and rubrics.

The generalizability aspect examines the extent to which scores and interpretations are consistent across assessment tasks, populations, and settings (Cook & Campbell, 1979; Feldt & Brennan, 1989; Shulman, 1970). An assessment should provide representative coverage of the content and processes of the construct domain being tested, so that the score interpretation not be limited to the particular sample of assessed tasks but be generalizable to the construct domain more broadly. Evidence of such generalizability depends on the degree of correlation of the assessed tasks with other tasks representing the construct or aspects of the construct. This issue of generalizability of score inferences across tasks and contexts goes to the very heart of score meaning. Indeed, setting the boundaries of score meaning is precisely what generalizability evidence is meant to address.

In one sense, the generalizability aspect of construct validity intersects with reliability in that it refers to the consistency of performance across the tasks, occasions, and raters of a particular assessment (Feldt & Brennan, 1989). But in a second sense, generalizability refers to transfer or the consistency of performance across tasks or items that are representative of the broader construct domain. Transfer refers to the range of tasks that performance on the assessed tasks facilitates the learning of or, more generally, is predictive of (Ferguson, 1956). Phrased more broadly to make clear that personality as well as ability tests are encompassed, transfer refers to the range of behaviors that the assessed behaviors facilitate the learning or acquisition of or are predictive of.

The issue of generalizability is especially relevant to performance assessments, which are typically limited to a small number of tasks because each performance task requires an extensive amount of time. There is a conflict in performance assessment between time-intensive depth of examination on any one task and the number of tasks needed for representative domain coverage. This conflict must be carefully negotiated in designing and interpreting performance assessments (Wiggins, 1993).

The external aspect of construct validity refers to the extent to which performance on a test is related to other test and nontest behaviors, the correlations to be either high or low as predicted by the theory of the construct being assessed. Thus, the meaning of the scores can be substantiated externally by appraising the degree to which empirical relationships with other measures, or the lack thereof, are consistent with that meaning.   That is, the constructs represented in the assessment should rationally account for the external pattern of correlations.

It is especially important to examine the external relationships between the test scores and criterion measures of the desired behaviors the test is intended to predict when using the scores for selection, placement, licensure, certification of competence, program evaluation, or other accountability purposes in applied settings.   Once again, the construct theory points to the relevance of potential relationships between the test scores and criterion measures, and empirical evidence of such links attests to the utility of the scores for the applied purpose.

The consequential aspect of construct validity includes evidence and rationales for evaluating the intended and unintended consequences of score interpretation and use in both the short and long term. Ideally, there should be no adverse consequences associated with bias in scoring and interpretation, with unfairness in test use, or with negative effects on teaching and learning.

Testmakers are mainly concerned with minimizing negative impact on individuals and groups due to any source of test invalidity such as construct underrepresentation or construct-irrelevant variance (Messick, 1989). That is, validity is compromised when the assessment is missing something relevant to the focal construct that, if present, would have permitted the affected examinees to display their competence. Similarly, scores may be invalidly low because the measurement contains something irrelevant that interferes with the affected examinees' demonstration of competence. In contrast, adverse consequences associated with valid measures of an individual's current status – such as validly low scores resulting from poor teaching or limited opportunity to learn – are not the testmakers' responsibility but the test users'. Adverse consequences resulting from valid assessment are problems not of measurement but of social or educational policy.

VALIDATION AS EVIDENCE-BASED ARGUMENT

From the discussion thus far, it should be clear that test validity cannot rely solely on any one of these complementary forms of evidence in isolation from the others. Neither does validity require any one form, or a high level of every form, if there is good overall evidence supporting score meaning. What is required is a compelling argument that the available evidence justifies the test interpretation and use, even though some pertinent evidence may be lacking.

The six aspects of construct validity apply to all educational and psychological measurement, including performance assessments or other alternative assessment modes. Taken together, they provide a way of addressing the multiple and interrelated validity questions that need to be answered in justifying score interpretation and use. In constructing the validity argument, one can set priorities about the forms of evidence needed to justify the inferences drawn from test scores by focusing on the vulnerable points in the argument that require support (Kane, 1992; Shepard, 1993). The key point is that the six aspects of construct validity provide a means of checking that the rationale or argument linking the evidence to the inferences drawn touches the important bases. If not, an argument should be provided that explains why such omissions are defensible (Messick, 1995).

FAIR ASSESSMENT AND EQUITABLE TREATMENT

There remains an important, overarching issue in the validity of test use, namely, test fairness. A central question in test validity asks whether any adverse consequences derive from sources of test invalidity such as construct underrepresentation or construct-irrelevant variance, which bears directly on the appropriateness and acceptability of outcomes. A central question in test fairness asks whether the consequences of test use are appropriate and acceptable, which relates directly to the validity of the inferences drawn from the test scores. Thus, the concept of fairness in assessment is impossible to divorce from the concept of validity because the two share a mutuality of meaning and import.

Fairness, like validity, is not just a psychometric issue. It is a social value, and there are alternative points of views about its essential features. In essence, fairness implies impartiality, with an absence of prejudice or favoritism. In regard to test use, this impartiality derives from comparable construct validity. A fair test is one that yields comparably valid scores from person to person, group to group, and setting to setting (Willingham, 1998). So, for instance, if an assessment yields scores that consistently underestimate ability levels for members of a particular group, then the test would be considered unfair to that group. Or if an assessment is interpreted to measure a single construct across groups, but in actuality measures different constructs in different groups, it would also be unfair.

ALTERNATIVE VIEWS OF FAIRNESS: PROCESS OR OUTCOME

Although there are alternative views as to what constitutes test fairness, most of them relate back in one way or another to the central idea of comparable validity. For instance, the 1998 draft revision of the *Standards for Educational and Psychological Testing* cites four alternative views of fairness commonly found in the technical and popular literature. Two of these views characterize test fairness, respectively, as the absence of bias and as equitable treatment of all examinees in the testing process.

Bias arises when deficiencies in the test itself result in different meanings for scores earned by different subgroups. An example is item content that differentially reflects the cultural or geographical background of different examinees or groups. Fairness as equitable treatment of all examinees in the testing process requires that examinees have a comparable opportunity to demonstrate their competence or, more generally, their standing on the construct being measured. Fair treatment includes such factors as comparable testing conditions and equal access to test familiarization and practice materials. There is general agreement that tests should be free from bias and that all examinees should be treated equitably in the testing process. These first two views refer to test fairness in ways that stop just short of requiring comparable validity across individuals, groups, and contexts, but they are quite compatible with the notion of comparable validity.

The other two views characterize test fairness, respectively, as equal opportunity to learn and as equality of testing outcomes. Opportunity to learn is an important issue to take into account when evaluating the comparability of score meaning across groups and is especially problematic when the scores are used to make high-stakes decisions about individuals. However, it is important to note that comparable score meaning does not necessarily imply the same or identical score meaning, as will be seen shortly in connection with efforts to accommodate tests to the needs of examinees with disabilities or those with limited English proficiency.

From one perspective, the notion that test fairness requires equality of testing outcomes is given some credence on the grounds that equality of outcomes should be the ultimate indicator of genuine equality of learning opportunities as well as of genuine equity of treatment. However, given current educational and social realities, the idea that test fairness requires overall passing rates to be comparable across groups is not generally accepted in the professional literature.

Indeed, the second two views refer not so much to fairness in testing as they do to equity of social and educational experience (Gordon, 1998). It is important not to confound test fairness with educational or social equity because the two need to be pursued in their own right and in different ways. Unequal outcomes and opportunities do not in themselves signify test unfairness because tests may validly document unequal individual or group outcomes that are reflective in part of unequal opportunity to learn.

It is also important to distinguish between equality (the state of being the same) and equity (treatment that is just under the circumstances) and to recognize that not all inequalities are inequities. Indeed, in education as in medicine, the watchword should not be equal treatment but, rather, treatment that is appropriate to the characteristic and sufficient to the need (Gordon, 1998). From this perspective, it was important that the Standards phrased one of the alternate views of test fairness just considered as equitable, not equal, treatment of all examinees in the testing process, thereby allowing room for accommodations to the different needs of examinees with handicaps or allowing use of tests translated into an examinee's best language (Willingham et al., 1988).

THE VALUES OF ACCOMMODATIONS IN TESTING

The issue of equity and the attendant desire to accommodate the testing process to the different needs of examinees with disabilities or those with limited English proficiency is a prime example of the role of social values in educational and psychological measurement. The pursuit of equitable testing accommodations goes to the very heart of comparable construct validity and test fairness.

In this regard, it is important to distinguish two kinds of comparability (Willingham et al., 1988). One kind, called score comparability, means that the properties of scores (such as reliabilities, internal relationships among items, and external relationships with other variables) are comparable across groups and settings. Score comparability is important in justifying uniform score interpretation and use for different groups and in different circumstances. The other kind, called task comparability, means that the test tasks elicit comparable cognitive processes across different groups and different settings.

Within task comparability, two types of cognitive processes may be distinguished: those that are relevant to the construct measured and those that are ancillary to the construct but nonetheless involved in task performance (Wiley, 1991). Comparability of construct-relevant processes is needed to sustain common score meaning across groups and contexts. Again, these processes need not be identical from person to person or from time to time for the same person, as long as it can be maintained that they represent alternative or substitutable construct-relevant processes, such as when different strategies are employed in a test of reasoning or problem solving.

Ancillary processes, in contrast, may in many cases be deliberately modified for some individuals or groups without jeopardizing score meaning. Such modifications, when they are possible, provide a fair and legitimate basis for accommodating tests to the needs of examinees with disabilities or those with limited English proficiency (Willingham et al., 1988). For example, a fair accommodation might be to read a mathematics test aloud to an examinee with visual impairment because reading is ancillary to the construct being measured. In this regard, the availability of multimedia stimulus and response modes on the computer promises generalized accommodation in computer-based testing to the various needs of examinees with disabilities (Bennett, 1998).

Thus, comparable validity – and hence, test fairness – does not require identical task conditions but, rather, comparable construct-relevant processes with inconsequential construct-irrelevant or ancillary processes that may be different across individuals and groups. Such accommodations, of course, have to be justified with evidence that score meaning and properties have not been unduly eroded in the process.

FAIRNESS ISSUES THROUGHOUT THE TESTING PROCESS

Fairness, like validity, cannot be properly addressed as an afterthought once the test has been developed, administered, and used. Fairness issues, like those of validity, must be confronted throughout the interconnected phases of the testing process, from test design and development, through administration and scoring, to interpretation and use (Willingham, 1998). Indeed, one of the most critical fairness issues occurs at the design stage, namely, the choice of the constructs to measure for the particular testing purpose. For example, consider the possible test requirements for awarding high-school diplomas. Graduation rates for males and females, as well as for language minority students, would be quite different if the tests emphasized reading and writing as opposed to science and mathematics (Willingham & Cole, 1997). Any limited number of subjects covered by the test would likely yield differential graduation rates for different groups because they underrepresent the broad construct of school learning and because students have differential opportunities to learn. Some alternatives are to assess school learning more comprehensively, to use more than one assessment mode such as high-school grades as well as test scores, and to justify any limited choice of subjects in terms of the social values of the school and community.

Construct choice is a critical issue for both fairness and validity because that choice determines test content, appropriate test formats, and test specifications. Ultimately, construct choice influences not only test development but also administration, scoring, interpretation, and use. Furthermore, the particular test use, in the first place, is critical in determining construct choice. Thus, these several decisions are interconnected, but the fairness issues involved at each stage are different and require different approaches.

There are other fairness considerations at the stage of test design and development. For example, the format of the items or the content used to contextualize an item may be more familiar to some examinees and groups than to others and may thereby create a disadvantage for some. Such potential bias in test questions is usually addressed empirically by examining whether individuals who have the same level of ability, but are members of different groups, have the same probability of getting the items correct.

Fairness issues arise in the administration of tests because of non-standard testing conditions. Examples include the use of test forms of unequal difficulty and providing a less-than-optimal testing environment (in terms of lighting, space, and temperature) that may disadvantage some examinees more than others. Fairness is also an issue whenever scoring is not completely objective, because subjective scoring is routinely threatened by biases associated with construct-irrelevant characteristics of the performance, the examinee, and the setting.

Fairness issues in connection with test use abound. Some examples are using measures that are less valid than others available, relying unduly on a single score, and basing decisions on an underrepresented view of the relevant construct when such uses result in differential individual or group impact (Willingham, 1998). A widespread and important use of tests is for selection, as in college admissions or job entry. Considerable attention has been given in the past to fair selection models, which by their very nature put heavy emphasis on comparable predictive validity but at the expense of comparable construct validity. Because these models expose alternative views of fairness as well as the specter of conflicting social values in the pursuit of fairness from different perspectives, we examine them next in more detail.

In the late 1960s and early 1970s, measurement specialists attempted to define fair selection in psychometric terms (Cleary, 1968; Cole, 1973; Linn, 1973; Thorndike, 1971). In one way or another, all of these fair selection models attempted to cope with the fact that any imperfect predictor fails to select members of a low scoring group in proportion to their criterion success rate. This is the case even when individuals having the same predictor score are equally likely to succeed regardless of group membership – that is, even when the predictor yields a common regression line for the different groups, which is Cleary's (1968) formulation of an unbiased predictor. Because fair test use implies that selection decisions will be equally appropriate in some sense regardless of an individual's group membership and because different selection systems yield different proportions of selected individuals in population groups displaying different test performance levels, questions of test fairness arise in earnest in selection settings. The problem for each of the fair selection models is to specify the meaning of the phrase in some sense.

Cleary's (1968) sense of fairness, as was just seen, is that individuals with the same predictor score should be equally likely to succeed regardless of group membership. From another viewpoint, Cole's (1973) conditional probability model of fair selection holds that applicants who can achieve a satisfactory criterion level should have an equal probability of being selected regardless of group membership. Several other models of fair selection were formulated and contrasted (e.g., Darlington, 1971; Einhorn & Bass, 1971; Linn, 1973, 1976; Thorndike, 1971), each of which assumed, either explicitly or tacitly, an unbiased criterion measure that is uniformly and fairly applied across groups. This unbiased criterion then serves as the standard for evaluating potential bias in the predictor measures.

Some of these models proved to be mutually incompatible and even contradictory (Petersen & Novick, 1976). It soon became apparent that each model accords a different importance or social value to the various quadrants of selected versus rejected and successful versus unsuccessful individuals in the different population groups (Dunnette & Borman, 1979). For example, one could emphasize equality in the rates of false negatives across groups, that is, equality in the rate of rejecting individuals who would have succeeded if selected. Moreover, the values accorded could be a function not only of desired criterion performance but also of desired individual and group attributes (Novick & Ellis, 1977). As a consequence, each model not only constitutes a different definition of fairness but also implies a particular ethical position (Hunter & Schmidt, 1976). Each view is ostensibly fair under certain conditions, so that arguments over the fairness of test use turn out in many instances to be disagreements as to what the conditions are or ought to be (Messick, 1989).

The core social problem in selection is the need to reduce subgroup differences in selection rate while minimizing any negative effects this might have on overall predictive validity. In an attempt to achieve such a trade-off, a National Research Council committee recommended the use of subgroup norming by means of within-group percentiles or some such device (Hartigan & Wigdor, 1989). The rationale is in tune with Cole's (1973) conditional probability model, but as an action proposal tantamount to the adjustment of subgroup scores it precipitated vigorous controversy (e.g., Gottfredson, 1994; Sackett & Wilk, 1994). In any event, the argument became moot when Congress expressly prohibited any form of score adjustment on the basis of race, color, religion, sex, or national origin (Civil Rights Act of 1991). In light of this Congressional prohibition, we must return to other views of fair selection.

With the recognition that fundamental value differences are at issue in fair selection, several utility models were developed that require specific value positions to be articulated (e.g., Cronbach, 1976; Gross & Su, 1975; Petersen & Novick, 1976; Sawyer, Cole, & Cole, 1976), thereby incorporating social values explicitly with measurement technology. However, the need to make values explicit does not determine or make easier the hard choices among them. At this point, it appears difficult if not impossible to be fair to individuals in terms of equity, to groups in terms of parity or the avoidance of adverse impact, to institutions in terms of efficiency, and to society in terms of costs and benefits all at the same time (Messick, 1989).

In principle, a workable balancing of the needs of each of the parties is likely to require successive approximations over time, with iterative modifications of selection procedures based on their consequences to date, so that the interests of none of the parties gets too far out of line. In practice, however, such balancing of needs and values almost always comes down to a political resolution. The challenge is that by recognizing the role of social values in educational and psychological measurement, we might be able to inform these political choices with evidence about effective policy alternatives and their consequences.

In any event, predictive validity, regardless of the selection model on which it is based, is not sufficient to signify test fairness. What needs to be comparable across groups and settings for fair test use is score meaning and the actions based thereon. That is, test fairness derives from comparable construct validity, which subsumes but goes beyond evidence of comparable predictive validity.

CONTROVERSIES OVER CONSEQUENCES

The elevation of construct validity to an overall validity framework for evaluating test interpretation and use has been highly controversial, especially with respect to the role of testing consequences as validity evidence contributing to score meaning. Critics argue vigorously that testing consequences should not be included as an integral part of validity. This is partly due to their misapprehension that the emphasis on adverse consequences traceable to sources of invalidity primarily reflects a concern with test misuse. For example, Wiley (1991) maintains that "the understanding of these use errors is conceptually and socially important, but involves social and moral analyses beyond the scope of test validation...and would needlessly complicate the conception and definition of test validity" (p.89). Popham (1997) believes that one of the motives for including consequences as validity evidence "was surely to draw our attention to the unsound uses of test results" (p. 12).

On the contrary, the motivation was to draw attention to unanticipated side effects of legitimate test use, especially if unanticipated adverse effects are traceable to sources of invalidity such as construct underrepresentation and construct-irrelevant variance. Of course, procedural errors and unsound interpretations would invalidate a particular local test use, and such misuse should not contribute to the validation process. By restricting their understanding of the consequential basis of construct validity to the effects of test misuse, these critics find it easy to argue that the validity of score inferences is separable from and orthogonal to the consequences of test misuse (Mehrens, 1997; Popham, 1997; Tenopyr, 1996). The argument is easy because it is basically true but immaterial. However, it is not possible to separate score meaning from the consequences of legitimate test interpretation and use. The unanticipated consequences of legitimate score interpretation and use bear not only on the justification of the use but also on the soundness of score meaning and, hence, are an integral part of the validation process (Messick, 1998).

Other critics (e.g., Brandon, 1996) contend that the consequential basis of construct validity is either circular or redundant, or both. They agree that adverse consequences signal invalidity only if traceable to sources of invalidity such as construct underrepresentation or construct-irrelevant variance. However, they argue that these sources of invalidity are identified and taken into account using the methods associated with Messick's (1995) other five validity aspects bearing on content, substantive processes, score structure, generalizability, and external relationships. Therefore, for these critics, consequences are unnecessary for examining validity.

However, even after diligently applying the methods of the other five validity aspects, every test still underrepresented its construct to some degree and contains sources of irrelevant variance, if for no other reason than it is a test and not a criterion performance (Loevinger, 1957). Test makers usually maintain that this remaining invalidity is inconsequential until confronted with evidence to the contrary. This is precisely why unanticipated consequences constitute an important form of validity evidence. Unanticipated consequences signal that we may have been incomplete or off-target in test development and, hence, in test interpretation and test use (Messick, 1998).

Testing consequences are inherently value-laden because their import is contingent on the value system brought to bear in evaluating them. Hence, the consequential basis of validity is value-dependent, a complexity that leads critics to reject it and to turn to the evidential basis in the hope that it is value-independent (Markus, 1998). However, value-neutral as well as theory-neutral facts are problematic in the postmodern world, so the evidential basis of validity can hardly be considered independent of values (Messick, 1989). But neither is the consequential basis independent of evidence.

This interplay of facts and values is one reason that the validation process needs to be rhetorical as well as scientific. In the process of validation, one needs to craft a persuasive argument linking constructs, evidence, and values (Cronbach, 1988), which is the rhetorical part of the enterprise. The scientific part relies on convergent and discriminant evidence involving multiple measures and multiple methods. In any event, the operation of social values in test design, development, interpretation, and use cannot be avoided but must be carefully negotiated in testing practice in the cause of both validity and fairness.

Indeed, there are signs that the measurement field is moving beyond the question of whether or not testing consequences should be part of validity (Yen, 1998). Instead, questions are being asked about how such consequences might be examined and who is responsible for collecting the evidence about consequences (Linn, 1998).

OVERVIEW

In sum, test use depends for its legitimacy on adherence to established principles of reliability, validity, and fairness. These principles are organized within an overarching conception of construct validity. The form and level of desired reliability depend on the meaning of the construct being measured while test fairness depends on comparable construct validity across groups and settings (Messick, 1989; Willingham, 1998). Conceptions of test fairness entailing only selected aspects of construct validity, such as the fair selection models based on comparable predictive validity, are not sufficient in themselves to justify fair test use. What is needed are comparable score meaning across groups and settings as well as comparable test uses based on the action implications of the construct meaning. That is, the purpose of the testing and the construct measured should mutually support or justify each other, in the sense that the testing purpose implies constructs to be measured and the construct choice implies testing purposes.

Pursuing test fairness as comparable construct validity requires a heavy burden of convergent and discriminant evidence bearing on test content, score structure, substantive processes, generalizability, external relationships, and testing consequences (Messick, 1995). From a practical standpoint, it would of course be more convenient and expedient to be able to base test fairness on only a selected aspect of construct validity such as comparable prediction across groups and settings. Apart from the insufficiency of the argument, however, there is also the danger that if evidence of comparable prediction were not forthcoming, the prize of fairness would be lost (possibly for the wrong reasons). In contrast, the pursuit of comparable construct validity is more flexible. With multiple complementary forms of evidence to be addressed, one does not have to rely on any one of them, nor is any one of them required. That is, just as no single form of evidence – whether content-based, criterion-related, or consequential – is sufficient to justify test interpretation and use, neither is any particular form of evidence necessary. What is necessary is a compelling rationale justifying score meaning and its action implications from the mosaic of available evidence, even though some pertinent evidence had to be forgone.

Fairness issues arise in each stage of the testing process from design and development, through administration and scoring, to interpretation and use. Thus, in the name of fairness, value judgments need to be made throughout the testing process, as they do in the name of validity throughout the validation process, especially in regard to testing consequences. The pervasive role of social values in educational and psychological measurement is not intrusive but rather integral to the assessment process because, in the last analysis, fairness judgments and validity judgments are value judgments.

NOTES

[1]Reprinted by permission of Educational Testing Service, the copyright holder.

REFERENCES

American Psychological Association, American Educational Research Association, & National Council on Measurement in Education.   (1985). *Standards for educational and psychological testing.* Washington, DC: American Psychological Association.

Bennett, R. E. (1998). Computer-based testing for examinees with disabilities: On the road to generalized accommodation (pp. 181-191). In S. Messick (Ed.), *Assessment in higher education.* Mahwah, NJ: Erlbaum.

Brandon, P. R. (1996, June). Fatal flaw in consequential validity theory. AERA-D Division D: Measurement and Research Methodology. Available on-line at: http://lists.asu.edu/cgi-bin/wa?A2=ind9606&L=aera-d&F=&S=&P=5219.

Civil Rights Act of 1991. (November 21, 1991). Publ. L. No. 102-166, 105 Stat. 1071.

Cleary, T. A. (1968). Test bias: Prediction of grades of Negro and White students in integrated colleges. *Journal of Educational Measurement,* 5, 115-124.

Cole, N. S. (1973). Bias in selection. *Journal of Educational Measurement,* 10, 237-255.

Cook, T.D., & Campbell, D. T. (1979). *Quasi-experimentation: Design and analysis issues for field settings.* Chicago: Rand McNally.

Cronbach, L. J. (1971). Test validation. In R. L. Thorndike (Ed.), *Educational measurement* (2nd ed., pp. 443-507). Washington, DC: American Council on Education.

Cronbach, L. J. (1976). Equity in selection: Where psychometrics and political philosophy meet. *Journal of Educational Measurement,* 13, 31-41.

Cronbach, L. J. (1988). Five perspectives on validation argument (pp. 3-17). In H. Wainer & H. Braun (Eds.), *Test validity.* Hillsdale, NJ: Lawrence Erlbaum Associates.

Darlington, R. B. (1971). Another look at "cultural fairness." *Journal of Educational Measurement,* 8, 71-82.

Dunnette, M. D., & Borman, W. C. (1979). Personnel selection and classification systems. *Annual Review of Psychology,* 30, 477-525.

Einhorn, H. J., & Bass, A. R. (1971). Methodological considerations relevant to discrimination in employment testing. *Psychological Bulletin,* 75, 261-269.

Embretson (Whitely), S. (1983). Construct validity: Construct representation versus nomothetic span. *Psychological Bulletin,* 93, 179-197.

Feldt, L. S., & Brennan, R. L. (1989). Reliability. In R. L. Linn (Ed.), *Educational Measurement* (3rd ed., pp. 105-146). New York: Macmillan.

Ferguson, G. A. (1956). On transfer and the abilities of man. *Canadian Journal of Psychology,* 10, 121-131.

Gottfredson, L.S. (1994). The science and politics of race-norming. *American Psychologist,* 49, 955-963.

Gordon, E. (1998). Human diversity and equitable assessment (203-211). In S. Messick (Ed.), *Assessment in higher education.* Mahwah, NJ: Erlbaum.

Gross A.L., & Su, W. (1975). Defining a "fair" and "unbiased" selection model: A question of utilities. *Journal of Applied Psychology,* 60, 345-351.

Hartigan, J. A., & Wigdor, A. K. (Eds.) (1989). *Fairness in employment testing: Validity generalization, minority issues, and the General Aptitude Test Battery.* Washington, DC: National Academy Press.

Heller, K. A., Holtzman, W. H., & Messick, S. (Eds.) (1982). *Placing children in special education: A strategy for equity.* Washington, DC: National Academy Press.

Hunter, J. E., & Schmidt, F. I. (1976). Critical analysis of the statistical and ethical implications of various definitions of test bias. *Psychological Bulletin*, **83**, 1053-1071.

Kane, M. T. (1992). An argument-based approach to validity. *Psychological Bulletin, 112*, 527-535.

Lennon, R. T. (1956). Assumptions underlying the use of content validity. *Educational and Psychological Measurement, 16*, 294-304.

Linn, R. L. (1973). Fair test use in selection. *Review of Educational Research, 43*, 139-161.

Linn, R. L. (1976). In search of fair selection procedures. *Journal of Educational Measurement, 13*, 53-58.

Linn, R. L. (1998). Partitioning responsibility for the evaluation of the consequences of assessment programs. *Educational Measurement: Issues and Practice, 17*(2), 28-30.

Loevinger, J. (1957). Objective tests as instruments of psychological theory. *Psychological Reports, 3*, 635-694 (Monograph Supplement, 9).

Markus, K. (1998). Science, measurement, and validity: Is completion of Samuel Messick's synthesis possible? *Social Indicators Research*, in press.

Mehrens, W. A. (1997). The consequences of consequential validity. *Educational Measurement: Issues and Practice, 16*(2), 16-18.

Messick, S. (1989). Validity. In R. L. Linn (Ed.), *Educational measurement* (3rd ed., pp. 13-103). New York: Macmillan.

Messick, S. (1995). Validity of psychological assessment: Validation of inferences from persons' responses and performances as scientific inquiry into score meaning. *American Psychologist, 50*, 741-749.

Messick, S. (1998). Test validity: A matter of consequence. *Social Indicators Research, in press*.

Novick, M. R., & Ellis, D. D. (1977). Equal opportunity in educational and employment selection. *American Psychologist, 72*, 306-320.

Peak, H. (1953). Problems of observation. In L. Festinger & D. Katz (Eds.), *Research methods in the behavioral sciences* (pp.243-299). Hinsdale, IL: Dryden.

Petersen, N. S., & Novick, M. R. (1976). An evaluation of some models for culture-fair selection. *Journal of Educational Measurement, 13*, 3-29.

Popham, W. J. (1997). Consequential validity: Right concern-wrong concept. *Educational Measurement: Issues and Practice, 16*(2), 9-13.

Sackett, P. R. & Wilk, S. L. (1994). Within-group norming and other forms of score adjustment in preemployment testing. *American Psychologist, 49*, 929-954.

Sawyer, R. L., Cole, N. S., & Cole, J. W. L. (1976). Utilities and the issue of fairness in a decision theoretic model for selection. *Journal of Educational Measurement, 13*, 59-76.

Shepard, L. A. (1993). Evaluating test validity. *Review of Research in Education, 19*, 405-450.

Shulman, L. S. (1970). Reconstruction of educational research. *Review of Educational Research, 40*, 371-396.

Tenopyr, M. L. (1996, April). Construct-consequences confusion. Paper presented at the annual meeting of the Society for Industrial and Organizational Psychology, San Diego.

Thorndike, R. L. (1971). Concepts of culture fairness. *Journal of Educational Measurement, 8*, 63-70.

Wiggins, G. (1993). Assessment: Authenticity, context, and validity. *Phi Delta Kappan, 75*, 200-214.

Wiley, D. E. (1991). Test validity and invalidity reconsidered. In R. E. Snow & D. E. Wiley (Eds.), *Improving inquiry in the social sciences: A volume in honor of Lee J. Cronbach* (pp. 75-107). Hillsdale, NJ: Erlbaum.

Willingham, W. W. (1998). A systemic view of test validity (213-242). In S. Messick (Ed.), *Assessment in higher education*. Mahwah, NJ: Erlbaum.

Willingham, W.W., & Cole, N. S. (1997). *Gender bias and fair assessment*. Hillsdale, NJ: Erlbaum.

Willingham, W. W., Ragosta, M., Bennett, R. E., Braun, H., Rock, D.A., & Powers, D. E. (1988). *Testing handicapped people*. Boston: Allyn & Bacon.

Yen, W. M. (1998). Investigating the consequential aspects of validity: Who is responsible and what should they do? *Educational Measurement: Issues and Practice, 17*(2), 5.

2 THE ROLE OF SOCIAL DESIRABILITY IN THE ASSESSMENT OF PERSONALITY CONSTRUCTS

Edward Helmes

Social desirability has had a checkered history in personality assessment. Its role has ranged from one of several "response styles" (Jackson & Messick, 1958) to being the focus of entire symposia, books (Berg, 1967), and heated debates in the literature. It has a comparatively short history as a personality characteristic, first coming to prominence in the 1950s in the work of Allen L. Edwards (1953, 1957). Since then, its popularity in the literature has waxed and waned, although social desirability retains an unusual position within personality assessment. This uncertainty as to its status as a legitimate attribute worthy of study is in part because of its history but also because of its inherent nature as a construct. To some, it is a source of irrelevant error on a test that should be minimized if not eliminated. To others, it is a meaningful construct in its own right (Crowne, 1979). Of course, these two positions are not mutually exclusive, which leads to the conceptual difficulties over the nature of social desirability. This chapter will not attempt to unravel all of the links of social desirability. I will concentrate here upon its role in the development of personality instruments. Of necessity, this will lead to some discussion of its nature as a construct. To do that, only some of the relevant history needs to be understood. This discussion will not incorporate the perspective that views social desirability as synonymous with "faking good" (Furnham, 1986), but will be more in keeping with Jackson's narrower definition that corresponds closely with the working definitions of Edwards. These definitions are elaborated upon later in the chapter, but at this point it is worth noting that both are pragmatic working definitions. Neither Jackson nor Edwards provided full definitions of social desirability, but instead relied upon the consensual meaning of the term in the English language and the operational definition of the concept in the scales that were developed to measure social desirability.

This brief history will be summarized in this chapter, along with an outline of the measures that have been used to measure social desirability. At that point, I will spend some time on an analysis of social desirability as a personality construct. It is only then that a discussion of its role in personality assessment can be undertaken in any meaningful way. The nature of social desirability as a construct is, of course, inextricably entwined with scales that purport to measure it. As constructs are inevitably embodied in their measurement processes, this will form the core of the discussion of the role of social desirability in test construction.

A BRIEF HISTORY OF SOCIAL DESIRABILITY

Much of the debate over social desirability has occurred in the context of the larger debate over what have been called response styles. Jackson, along with Messick and other colleagues, has played a major role in this debate. Response styles were defined as characteristics of an individual that are consistent across time and situations in terms of a systematic pattern of responding to personality and attitude items on the basis of something other than the semantic content of the items (Jackson & Messick, 1958). An example of a response style is to use only the middle three points on every seven- and nine-point rating scale that is encountered. If such a style is only temporary and limited to that particular occasion, then it is termed a "response set". An example is if a respondent feels under pressure to respond quickly and so endorses every item on the personality test that is being completed on that day as 'true'. This incident of 'yea-saying' would be termed a response set as this pattern is not consistent over time. Not all writers in the area have been consistent in their use of these terms, which has not improved the quality of the debate. Paulhus (1991) provides a good review of the topic of response bias in questionnaires and scales. Messick (1991) reviews the arguments over the role of social desirability and acquiescence from the 1960s and refutes the arguments made at that time by Block (1965) and Rorer (1965) that were so influential at the time.

Individual differences in this tendency to respond to social desirability would be conceptualized as a response style, a characteristic of people that is consistent over time and situations. When the situation involves completing a set of self-descriptive personality items, differences in the properties of the items in terms of their perceived social desirability interact with the stylistic tendencies of the people. When the manifest semantic content of the items is itself either highly desirable or highly undesirable, the social desirability of these items is easily confounded with the overt content. The interpretation of the responses to these items then becomes ambiguous. Two examples of such a confounded interpretation come from the Minnesota Multiphasic Personality Inventory; Hathaway & McKinley, 1976), which has been at the focus of much of the controversy over social desirability. The content of MMPI item 8 relates to having a "full and interesting life". The interpretation of a "True" response to this item in terms of its content reflects satisfaction and contentment. However, its Social Desirability Scale Value (SDSV; Messick & Jackson, 1961) is 8.28 on a 9-point scale. A stylistic interpretation is that many people would endorse this item simply because it reflects a "good thing", regardless of how interesting or boring their own life actually was. Similarly, MMPI item 158 expresses a fear of losing one's mind. A positive endorsement of this item could reflect either an honestly expressed existing fear, or reflect the SDSV of 1.77, which would be interpreted as the denial of undesirable content, true or not. This attribute of social desirability as a property of both the test items and of the individuals who respond to those items has been one of the underlying causes of the continuing debates over the utility of social desirability as an explanatory construct.

Thus the challenge that arises during the process of test or scale construction is to determine whether one can improve the accuracy of the conclusions that one wishes to draw from the scale by minimizing the influence of social desirability or if one can improve the predictive power of the instrument by not doing so. I hope that some indication of the manner in which to proceed is one outcome of reading this chapter.

Concerns about the influence of social desirability in questionnaires dates back to the early 1930's and were reflected in the interest over such issues revealed in the validity scales of the MMPI. While there is clearly a strong continuity of concern over the issue, in many ways the modern literature on social desirability can be regarded as beginning in the mid-1950s. In 1953, Edwards published a brief article on social desirability and its relationship to the frequency of item endorsement (Edwards, 1953). Four years later, his book *The Social Desirability Variable in Personality Assessment and Research* (Edwards, 1957) appeared and research on the construct of social desirability mushroomed. The next 10 years saw extensive debate over the importance of social desirability in personality assessment in general and the MMPI in particular. The mid-1960s saw both the denigration of the importance of social desirability and response styles in two major reviews (Block, 1965; Rorer, 1965) and its elevation to official status as a personality attribute in its own right as the need for approval (Crowne & Marlowe, 1964).

Later years led to refinements of the various arguments over social desirability, with old debates reappearing in the late 1980s and early 1990s in the context of discussions of construct validity (Hogan & Nicholson, 1988; Edwards, 1990; Walsh, 1990; Nicholson & Hogan, 1990) and over the interpretation of scores that confound social desirability and content (Edwards, 1990, 1991, Block, 1990). In many ways, Messick (1991) provides the last word in this debate, arguing for the continued plausibility of the stylistic interpretation of responses to personality test items.

While the debate over social desirability was active in the field of personality assessment, refinements of the concept of social desirability in another branch of psychology led to its separation into two separate concepts. These developments followed an entirely different perspective on the nature of the construct of social desirability. This tradition followed Crowne and Marlowe (1964) in interpreting social desirability as a meaningful construct in its own right, and explored its ramifications through a variety of experimental and observational studies (Crowne, 1979, Chapter 6). Sackeim and Gur (1978) used the concept of self-deception to explain the lack of apparent awareness of inconsistencies between self-reports and physiological evidence of emotional reactions across a variety of contexts. The suggestion that conscious awareness did not always result in accurate self-reports fit with clinical experience to support the concept of self-deception. This work was congruent with previous suggestions by Meehl & Hathaway (1946) in their article on the development of the L and K scales of the MMPI. These writers then distinguished self-deception, an unconscious process, from its conscious counterpart, other-deception (Sackeim & Gur, 1979). Both traits appear to have strong relevance to the concept of social desirability in some manner. Indeed, Paulhus developed these ideas into a measurement instrument, the Balanced Inventory of Desirable Responding (BIDR; Paulhus, 1984). These developments will be discussed in more detail in the following section. Note that Jackson and Messick (1958; Damarin & Messick, 1965) had previously made similar distinctions. Jackson (1984) subsequently developed a measure of *Denial* that is distinct from his measures of social desirability. This distinction bears a close resemblance to the concepts later labeled by Paulhus and Reid (1991) as enhancement and denial.

DEFINITIONS OF SOCIAL DESIRABILITY

One of the major elements that has helped to perpetuate the debate over social desirability is the absence of a formal definition of the construct that is widely accepted and used. Certainly it was apparent from the first that the people asked to provide social desirability ratings of personality adjectives and items had absolutely no difficulty in providing these ratings, which were highly consistent and stable over time. Edwards (1957) defined socially desirable responding as "the tendency of subjects to attribute to themselves in self-description, personality statements with socially desirable scale values and to reject those with socially undesirable scale values" (p. vi). This definition focuses on the social desirability scale values for personality statements as providing the meaning for the construct. In the instructions to raters, no real definition of the construct is provided. The raters are to evaluate the degree to which items are socially desirable or socially undesirable when used to describe other people. (This description is paraphrased from instructions used in Edwards, 1970, p. 89). Thus the meanings of *socially desirable* and *socially undesirable* as used by Edwards are essentially those inherent in everyday English.

The later stages of the debate became more complex as definitions of "response styles" as distinct from "response sets" developed (Rorer, 1965). Jackson and

Messick (1961; 1962) elaborated and refined the role of social desirability and acquiescence by proposing that these two constructs defined a circumplex structure for the MMPI. Demonstrating such a structure required separating scales into true- and false-keyed subscales, and their arguments did not convince everyone (Block, 1972; Samelson, 1972; Bentler, Jackson & Messick, 1971). Much of this debate concerned the role of acquiescence, whether taken as the simple tendency to endorse items regardless of content, or in a more refined manner with agreement acquiescence distinguished from acceptance acquiescence. Agreement acquiescence was taken to be the tendency to agree with personality statements. Acceptance acquiescence was defined as "the tendency to consider characteristics as descriptive" (Jackson & Messick, 1965). Distinguishing one from the other required the construction of reversed items that retained the denotative meaning and connotative implications of the original, with only the direction of scoring reversed. Doing this successfully is not as easy as it first seems, and the different efforts at reversing items appear to have led to varying degrees of success. Further studies (Ross & Mirowsky, 1984) and reviews (Paulhus, 1991) pertaining to the effects of acquiescence in personality assessment have appeared in recent times. The debate over the role of acquiescence has largely faded, however, whereas interest in social desirability continues.

The interpretation of the role of social desirability as a meaningful construct largely came about through the work of Crowne and Marlowe (1964) on the "need for approval". This work came more from the traditions of experimental social psychology than from those of personality assessment, and viewed social desirability under the 'need for approval' label as an attribute of the person, as well as one inherent in self-report items. The scale that resulted from their research program, the Marlowe-Crowne Social Desirability Scale, is probably the most widely used measure of social desirability (Crowne & Marlowe, 1960). As a construct, the need for approval is fairly complex, as it includes aspects of both defensiveness and weak self-esteem. Marlowe and Crowne (1964) reported a variety of behavioral correlates, including reduced risk-taking and a tolerance of boring tasks. One important aspect of the development of the Marlowe-Crowne scale was the deliberate choice of item content that was not associated with poor adjustment or psychopathology (Marlowe & Crowne, 1960). The issue of adjustment and social desirability is discussed at more length later, but the essence of the Marlowe-Crowne scale is the combination of items that reflect culturally affirmative characteristics, but which are probably not true of the person, together with items that are characteristic of most people, but are also undesirable. An example of an item reflecting a positive attribution is: "I never hesitate to go out of my way to help someone in trouble". An example of the type of item reflecting a denial of negative content is: "I like to gossip at times". This model for the scale also confounds the two types of items with the direction of scoring. The positive attribution items are all keyed in one direction, while all the items involving a denial of negative content are keyed in the other direction. Despite this complication, the consequences of which are discussed below, the Marlowe-

Crowne scale formed the basis for the development of the construct of need for approval.

The two types of item content in the Marlowe-Crowne scale led to further analyses of the scale. Millham (1974) suggested that the internal structure of the Marlowe-Crowne scale was such that the two initial components of attribution and denial would separate. Additionally, the methodological confound of the direction of keying with the type of content did prove to lead to contradictory reports, in which some studies reported a single factor and others reported two factors, as might be expected for confounded variables (Ramanaiah, Schill, & Leung, 1977; Evans, 1979). When the content was revised to balance the direction of keying, then the interpretation of the scale as reflecting a unitary need for approval could be justified (Ramanaiah and Martin, 1980). At the same time, the dual elements of attribution and denial were partially supported in experimental studies of cheating (see Millham & Jacobson, 1978, 1980 for a summary of these studies). Factor analyses of the 33 Marlowe-Crowne items (Crino, Svoboda, Rubenfeld, & White, 1983; Reynolds, 1982) found that the first principal component accounts for less than 16% of the variance. This modest amount of variance accounted for suggests that additional components would be interpretable. Crino et al. only interpreted the first component. Reynolds (1982) interpreted one component, although the eigenvalue for a second component was 1.63, which again suggests that at least one other component could be interpreted. There does not appear to have been a direct confirmatory test of the number of distinct and replicable components or factors in the Marlowe-Crowne scale. Fischer and Fick (1993) report modest fit for confirmatory factor analyses of the original Ramanaiah et al. (1977) attribution and denial scales and substantially improved fit for scales with reduced numbers of items.

Given the relatively few studies on the topic, the internal structure of the Marlowe-Crowne is not at all clear. The fact that the two components used to form the scale are confounded with the direction of keying does not make the interpretation of its internal structure any easier, as whether the item refers to a positive or negative attribute also appears to be important in determining how to interpret the interaction of the direction of keying with the positive or negative valence of the items (Paulhus & Reid, 1991). It appears that the positive or negative phrasing of symptoms as they are expressed in typical personality scale items is highly relevant to how they are interpreted by respondents (Mook, Kleijn, & van der Ploeg, 1991). Despite its wide use and longevity, with these unanswered questions about the scale, and possible changes over time in the characteristics of the items (Ballard, Crino, & Rubenfeld, 1988), the Marlowe-Crowne scale may no longer be the first choice for many applications. The Social Desirability Inventory of Jacobson and his colleagues may provide the most sophisticated evaluation of attribution and denial (Jacobson, Kellogg, Maricauce, & Slavin, 1977; Jacobson, Brown, & Ariza, 1983), although it does not seem to have been widely used. In addition, other influences have acted to elaborate the nature of facets of social desirability even more.

These additional refinements support the distinction between two elements of the concept of approval. The separation of approval into the domains of impression management, or other-deception, and of self-deception arose experimentally in work by Millham and Kellogg (1980). Their work was derived from Hartshorne and May's (1928) *Studies in Deceit* in children and the studies that developed the MMPI Lie scale (Meehl & Hathaway, 1946). The distinction was embodied in the Self-Deception and Other-Deception Questionnaires of Sackeim and Gur (1979). There is a substantial body of evidence from factor analysis to support such a separation (Paulhus, 1984). The self-deception factor is associated with more subtle measures of defensiveness such as Byrne's (1961) scale and the MMPI K scale (Meehl & Hathaway, 1946). The other-deception factor is associated with more obvious measures of adopting overly positive self-presentation styles, such as the MMPI *Lie* scale and the Wiggins (1959) scale. Jackson's work in this area also supported this distinction, but he and Kusyszyn used the terms *desirability* and *defensiveness* (Kusyszyn & Jackson, 1968). Paulhus (1984) reported replicating this distinction among the social desirability scales that he used. Interestingly, the Marlowe-Crowne scale also loaded on both factors in his work as well. In addition, the analysis of subscales of the Marlowe-Crowne scale with subscales of the Edwards and Jackson social desirability scales gave two factors, with the scales from the Marlowe-Crowne loading a factor separate from the subscales from the other two instruments (Holden & Fekken, 1989). Taken together, this collection of results suggests that the Marlowe-Crowne scale should not be interpreted as a unidimensional scale.

In order to eliminate the confound of the direction of keying of items with the item content that is inherent in the Marlowe-Crowne scale, Paulhus (1984) devised the Balanced Inventory of Desirability Responding (BIDR). The BIDR assesses the two components of self-deception and other-deception or impression management (Paulhus, 1986) without the confound with the direction of keying that is present in the Marlowe-Crowne scale.

The role of social desirability in personality assessment remains fluid at this point. Many people continue to regard it as a confound that muddies the interpretation of scores on tests. When social desirability is taken as a property of items and scales, this school of thought would argue that it should be controlled in some way. Other researchers feel that social desirability is a meaningful construct related to emotional stability, as argued by Block (1965) over thirty years ago. When, however, social desirability is taken as an individual difference variable, the issues become more complicated (McCrae & Costa, 1983). Consequently, the issues involving social desirability remain current and complex. One issue of practical concern is the choice of a measure of social desirability. Several methods of assessing social desirability have been developed, but researchers and practitioners must make decisions about theoretical issues in addition to the pragmatic one of selecting a scale. These theoretical issues concerning the measures of social desirability are taken up next.

THE CONSTRUCT OF SOCIAL DESIRABILITY

The previous section raised the major issues to be considered in selecting a social desirability scale. These are the domain of content, the theoretical approach, and the measurement model.

Item Content

The domain of content in part reflects the chronological era in which issues related to social desirability were debated. The original social desirability measures were taken from the MMPI (Edwards, 1957; Wiggins, 1959). The Edwards scales tended to confound the undesirable content associated with psychopathology with ratings of social desirability, while the Wiggins scale appeared to reflect aspects of content that changed when people were asked to respond in a desirable manner. Given the nature of the content of tests of psychopathology, scales derived from such measures are often less appropriate for use with normal populations than are other scales because the content is both uncommon in normal populations and also likely be undesirable because of the psychopathology. The newer social desirability scale of Edwards (1963) makes use of more general content. The social desirability measure that was derived for use in Jackson's (1989) Basic Personality Inventory (Helmes, 1996) shares the problem of confounding with psychopathology in that it makes use of the items from each scale that have the most extreme social desirability scale values (Reddon, Holden, & Jackson, 1983). Thus it too could not be recommended for use with a general population.

The work of Marlowe and Crowne and much of the literature on self-deception are based upon non-clinical samples, often university students. The measurement of social desirability in such populations requires scales that do not reflect substantial psychopathology, which is relatively uncommon in such groups. Jackson's first published test, the Personality Research Form (Jackson, 1967), was intended for use with the general adult population and incorporated an appropriate social desirability scale that reflected content consistent with non-pathological characteristics. Of Jackson's multiscale personality inventories, only the Personality Research Form has a scale explicitly titled "Desirability". Jackson's definition of social desirability for this scale follows the practice of Edwards closely in using the common usage meaning. The manual (Jackson, 1984) defines a high scorer in this way: "Describes self in terms judged as desirable; consciously or unconsciously, accurately or inaccurately, presents favorable picture of self in responses to personality statements" (p. 7). This definition avoids both the problem of distinguishing conscious from unconscious activities and that of the accuracy of self-awareness.   As discussed below, the distinction of social desirability from other constructs relies both upon theoretical considerations and upon the empirical item selection procedures (Jackson, 1970).

Measurement Models

Theoretical considerations become important at several levels in an analysis of the construct of social desirability. One is at the broad level of the definition of what social desirability is and is not. The next level is then to consider if the definition requires refinement into subscales or facets. The empirical literature to date generally supports the distinction of the two facets of self-deception and other-deception, or of defensiveness and impression management. It is at this point that the measurement model becomes important. If one considers social desirability to be a unitary construct, as is implied by the definitions based upon the semantic content of *desirability*, then summing item responses to give a single scale score is a reasonable measurement model. If one conceptualizes social desirability as comprising two components, then two non-overlapping sets of items must be summed to give two separate scores, one for each component. If the two components are logically distinct, then there is no rationale for combining the two scores into one summary score. This independence should also be empirically demonstrable by scores that do not correlate highly with one another. A more sophisticated demonstration of the distinctiveness of two components would combine empirical results that are predicted by a previous theoretical analysis. Such an analysis incorporates the concept of discriminant validity to describe how the construct of social desirability differs from a related but theoretically distinct construct. This refinement can be illustrated by a consideration of scales from some of Jackson's inventories.

The model of social desirability in much of Jackson's work is a unidimensional one, as reflected by the use of conventional internal consistency reliability measures.   The model follows that of Edwards' initial definition of social desirability. The definition follows closely on to the common semantic meaning: worth having, pleasing, excellent, or advisable. Table 1 provides examples of items from the item pool for the PRF Desirability scale. They illustrate the mixture of implausibly positive attributes and reflections of common aspects of poor personal adjustment that are found on most social desirability scales. The balance of positively and negatively keyed items is one characteristic that is not found on most other desirability scales, and the examples show that such items need not be negations (although certainly many of the negatively-keyed items are indeed negations).

Table 1. Examples of Items from Jackson's Social Desirability Scale Item Pool[1]

---

1. My daily life includes many activities I dislike.
2. I get along with people at parties quite well.
3. I have never been really happy.
4. I am one of the lucky people who could talk with my parents about my problems.

The items in Table 1 do not reflect notable psychopathology, and thus avoid the confounding of undesirability with psychopathology that is seen in an item such as "Someone is trying to poison me". In both industrialized and agrarian societies, the majority often shuns individuals with serious psychological disturbances. Items that reflect maladjustment are almost invariably rated as socially undesirable since Edwards first began to obtain social desirability scale values. This association between undesirability and psychopathology may be inherent in the constructs (Morey, 1997), making the empirical distinction between the theoretically distinct constructs of social undesirability and psychopathology very difficult.

The examples used to illustrate the distinction of the trait definition of social desirability from those of other traits are the related concepts of Value Orthodoxy in the Jackson Personality Inventory (JPI; Jackson, 1976) and of Denial in the Basic Personality Inventory (BPI; Jackson, 1989). These scales were selected because of their conceptual similarity to the attribution and denial components of the Marlowe-Crowne scale. Despite the conceptual similarity, Jackson defined these scales in such a way as to be distinct from social desirability, and then maximized the distinctions through the process of item selection.

In order to see the distinctions drawn by the construct-based approach among related concepts in practice, it will help to examine these examples in more detail. The original definition of a high score on *Value Orthodoxy* for the Jackson Personality Inventory (1976) was: "Values traditional customs and beliefs; his values may be seen as "old fashioned," takes a rather conservative view regarding contemporary standards of behavior; opposed to change in social customs" (p. 11). Value Orthodoxy thus reflects belief in conventional standards of behavior. A scale such as this could easily attract positive responses from those who wished to attribute to themselves the conventional and desirable moral and social values and behaviors. To the extent that the respondents do not actually possess these values and exhibit these behaviors, such a scale could reflect the attribution component of socially desirable responding. The JPI-R (Jackson, 1994) changed the scale name to *Traditional Values*, which "assesses the degree to which individuals incorporate 'old' values, as opposed to more modern views regarding topics such as patriotism and relations between the sexes. It is a scale in which significant differences would be expected between young and older adults. In general, a high scorer would be expected to be more conservative, and a low scorer more liberal in his or her views on major cultural themes" (p. 23). The definition for both these scales has a common core that is preserved in spite of the changes at the item level to the revised scale and which emphasizes the link to conservative social and political values. Of course, these definitions are provided with the understanding that the effects of social desirability have already been minimized through the item selection process used by Jackson. Thus the correlation of the JPI-R Traditional Values scale with the PRF Desirability scale is only .29 (Jackson, 1994, p. 61).

The Denial scale has closer theoretical links to social desirability than do the Value Orthodoxy and Traditional Values scales. A high scorer on the Denial scale is described as "lacks insight into feelings and causes of own behavior. Avoids unpleasant, exciting, or violent topics. Relatively unresponsive emotionally" (Jackson, 1989, p. 6). This clearly corresponds to the characteristics of denial as used by other authors in discussing social desirability. Denial can be seen as a facet of a broad definition of social desirability, but one that is distinct from other facets. As such, the scale can be interpreted as "a measure of response bias appropriate for interpreting test-taking behavior rather than criterion behavior" (Jackson, 1989, p. 61). Similar item selection strategies to those for the JPI were used in the construction of the BPI. The influence of desirability on the BPI Denial scale has been minimized through the use of the Item Efficiency Index (Neill & Jackson, 1976), despite the degree of pathology inherent in the item content. The Denial scale loaded together with the MMPI *Lie* scale on a factor defined by measures of socially deviant attitudes (Jackson & Hoffman, 1987) and correlated highly (.58) with the MMPI *Lie* scale (Jackson, 1989, p. 66). At the same time, its correlations with other domains of psychopathology were less than .3, reflecting minimal associations with other dimensions of pathology.

Thus it can be seen that relatively fine distinctions can be made using the construct approach to the measurement of social desirability. In practice, however, this has rarely been done and the consequence has been substantial confusion and unproductive debate regarding the respective scales. Nevertheless, in order to conduct research on social desirability or to assess the construct in clinical practice, one must select from among the array of published measures.

Analysis of Existing Social Desirability Scales

The previous section indicates that the use of a construct approach to test construction can lead to scales that reflect relatively fine distinctions at a theoretical level. Most existing measures of social desirability were not constructed using such methods. Therefore, what recommendations can be made about the existing scales?

Ostensibly, the Marlowe-Crowne scale measures a single construct. By using the Marlowe-Crowne scale, one also would implicitly adopt the underlying model and its use of the concepts of attribution and denial. However, as was pointed out earlier, there is substantial evidence that in practice the Marlowe-Crowne scale reflects a combination of content and method variance associated with the confounding of social desirability with the direction of keying of the items that reflect attribution and denial. Despite its very wide use in practice for evaluating social desirability, the Marlowe-Crowne scale is not recommended here because of this.

The other major option in this choice is whether to use a unidimensional scale, such as that of Edwards or that from the PRF, or to use a measure that incorporates either the distinction between self- and other-deception or that between attribution and denial. Among the unidimensional scales, the use of the original Edwards SD scale carries the connotations of the psychopathology content, something avoided by using the revised 1963 Edwards scale. Similarly, the Desirability scale from the Personality Research Form shares the unidimensional, vernacular model used by Edwards and the content does not reflect psychological problems. The choices for scales for measuring attribution and denial are more limited, and the best option might be to use the revised scale of Jacobson and his colleagues (Jacobson et al., 1977, Jacobson et al., 1983). Similarly, the revised versions of the BIDR are both more sophisticated from the standpoint of item selection and are more widely used than the original Self-Deception and Other-Deception Questionnaires of Sackeim and Gur (1979) and would likely be preferred for most purposes.

Clearly there are multiple issues to be considered before addressing the role of social desirability in test construction. Jackson has been the major proponent of the importance of controlling irrelevant sources of variance, such as social desirability, during test construction. Therefore, it may be instructive to explore further some of the above points by examining his arguments and procedures for the control of social desirability, along with a brief review of how this was done in his multiscale inventories.

CONTROLLING SOCIAL DESIRABILITY

Serious concern over the confounding nature of social desirability leads to efforts to minimize its influence at the early stages of test development. West and Finch (1997) note that a disproportionate influence of socially desirable item content is a threat to the content validity of a scale. As one of the most influential advocates for the control of irrelevant sources of variance in psychological test scores, Jackson developed a variety of methods for evaluating the relative influence of social desirability at the item level. The primary means by which Jackson controlled for the influence of social desirability in his instruments has been through the *Differential Reliability Index* or DRI. The first published use of the

DRI was in the development of the *Personality Research Form* (Jackson, 1967). It was also outlined in two forms by Neill and Jackson (1970), one for use with point-biserial correlations and one for use with factor or component loadings. The first formula for the DRI is:

[1] $$\text{DRI} = [r_{is}^2 - r_{iD}^2]^{1/2}.$$

Here r_{is} is the correlation of the item with its own scale and r_{iD} is the correlation of the item with a measure of social desirability. The formula for using factor or component loadings is very similar:

[2] $$\text{DRI} = [b_{il}^2 - b_{iD}^2]^{1/2}.$$

In this case, b_{il} is the loading of an item on the factor or component that corresponds to the construct that the item is intended to measure. Generally this would be a rotated loading. In the same way, r_{iD} is the loading on the factor that corresponds to the social desirability dimension. Once again, in most circumstances this would be a rotated loading.

During the revision of the *Jackson Personality Inventory*, Jackson revised the DRI in order to adjust for the variance of the item. His revised DRI that was used in the *JPI-R* (Jackson, 1994) is:

[3] $$\text{DRI} = [r_{is}^2 - r_{iD}^2 + p(1-p)]^{1/2}.$$

Here of course, $p(1-p)$ represents the variance for the item in question, assuming that the item uses a true-false or agree/disagree format.

Jackson typically used the DRI as one criterion in the iterative process of item selection. Jackson's methods are outlined in a widely-cited book chapter Jackson (1970), while a review the following year (1971) outline the theoretical rationale in more detail., Various test manuals provide examples in greater detail (Jackson, 1967, 1976, 1989,1994). These descriptions clearly imply that in use, items that are retained on his tests have values of the DRI that are in excess of 0, and are preferably much higher than this. The higher the value of the DRI for an item, the higher the content saturation is for that item. Content saturation is the extent to which an item reflects the trait in question. Items with a negative DRI would be eliminated from further consideration early in the process of item analysis. Jackson's later scales, such as the BPI, used the Item Efficiency Index (Neill & Jackson, 1976), in which desirability might be one scale of several others under simultaneous consideration. In the case of the BPI, all the other scales were undesirable, so desirability was implicitly a factor in the development of the BPI scales.

There has been little use of the DRI outside of Jackson's own research. In part this may be due to its primary application in the development of multiscale inventories, which are comparatively uncommon. It may also be due to the comparative lack of quantitative sophistication and awareness of the role of social desirability among those who develop unidimensional personality tests, particularly those with a medical or other background that does not include test construction as part of the curriculum. Morey (1991) used the same principle in the construction of the *Personality Assessment Inventory*, but did not make explicit use of the DRI. Instead, Morey simple eliminated items which correlated more highly with a short form of the Marlowe-Crowne social desirability scale (Reynolds, 1982) than with their own, keyed scale. This procedure is both logically and computationally simpler than the use of the DRI, if less elegant from a mathematical perspective.

Alternative methods have been proposed and used that control for social desirability after the items have been selected for the scale. As such, they control for the confounding influence of social desirability in some way, but do not minimize its influence in the same fashion, as do Jackson's methods.

One of the most well-known approaches is the use of a forced-choice item format, in which the respondent must choose one of two items that have been matched in terms of social desirability. Rothstein and Goffin (this volume, Chapter 10) review the use of the forced choice method in industrial and organizational applications. Many of the issues that they discuss are equally relevant to personality assessment in other domains. The first wide application of this method was in the Edwards Personal Preference Inventory (Edwards, 1959). Of course, this necessarily means that the items have been scaled for social desirability, and that there is a single, common perspective on the social desirability of the items. This common view of social desirability may not always in fact be the case (Messick, 1960). Jackson, Wroblewski, and Ashton (1999) tailored the matching of items on desirability to the specific characteristics of the situation in which the test was being used. This approach did appear to improve the predictive validity of the measure. The forced-choice format also leads to ipsative scales, in which the sum of the scale scores for different individuals is a constant. Such scales are not useful for comparing different individuals because the same numerical score for two different people does not reflect the same absolute strength of the trait in question. Only differences between traits within the same person can be interpreted meaningfully. Ipsative scales are thus of less use in comparing individuals than are conventional scales in many applications.

Other methods operate primarily to alter the interpretation of scores after the instrument has been administered. In the simplest case, scores on a scale sensitive to social desirability are used to decide that some responses should be modified (as in the MMPI *K* scale), or that the person's test results should be discarded (e.g., Nederhof, 1985, Rothstein & Goffin, this volume, Chapter 10). Other approaches to the control of social desirability are overt efforts to induce responses that are less socially desirable, and presumably, are therefore more "honest". Examples range from simple instructions to respond honestly (see Lautenschlager, 1994), to instructions that include statements to the effect that the test has scales to detect such types of responding and so efforts to appear more desirable will be detected (e.g., Eysenck, Eysenck, & Shaw, 1974), to manipulations designed to convince that respondent that efforts to deceive will invariably be detected, the "bogus pipeline" (Jones & Sigall, 1971). While of varying degrees of utility, such methods are of limited applicability in the construction of tests, except for those that involve the instructions given to those who complete the items during the early stages of test development. Little is actually known about the efficacy and effectiveness of such approaches in practice. Varying sets of instructions may be used to evaluate the properties of items during modern sequential approaches to test construction.

Another approach to controlling the influence of social desirability is to remove the influence statistically, either through the use of a mathematical adjustment, multiple regression, or through analysis of covariance (Morf & Jackson, 1972). These approaches use a formal mathematical or statistical manipulation of the raw scores. A simple example is the subtraction of some proportion of the K scale score from certain other MMPI clinical scale scores. Yet another statistical approach is through Paulhus' factor deletion method (Paulhus, 1981). The use of this method assumes the independence of desirability from the content of other scales, while other statistical approaches, such as regression, impose a form of independence. If the contribution of social desirability would add to the predictability of a criterion, then the overall validity may suffer if social desirability is removed statistically. Once again, such methods are of more utility in the interpretation of test scores that did not have social desirability considered during development. Tests developed using strategies to minimize the influence of desirability are less likely to need additional efforts at score adjustment in the process of interpreting scale scores.

The question of whether the predictability of a criterion is reduced if social desirability is removed statistically illustrates an issue that has arisen repeatedly in the debates over social desirability. The issue is whether social desirability is open to interpretation as a meaningful source of valid variance (McCrae & Costa, 1983), as having interpretations consistent with it being a construct with meaningful individual differences, or not. The former is consistent with the interpretation of Marlowe-Crowne scale scores as reflecting *Need for Approval*, while the negative position interprets variance associated with social desirability as error variance. This chapter is not the forum for attempting to unravel such an issue. In many ways, however, the most useful perspective on social desirability is comparatively agnostic on the issue. That perspective is to view social desirability as a confounding variable. As such, its control will lead to more precise measurement of the construct of interest. Whether variance associated with social desirability is due to a response style or to a meaningful construct, the net result is the same. The variance that is associated with social desirability is almost always different at a conceptual level from that of the variable(s) in question. Social desirability is a separate and distinct construct under both interpretations, and to confuse and conflate social desirability with another construct does not aid either the interpretation of that construct or the advancement of knowledge. Therefore, the control of social desirability during the stage of test construction has both theoretical and empirical advantages, but also has costs in terms of the large number of items that are discarded in the process. A benefit is that those who later interpret the test scores can do so more efficiently and with a lower risk of inappropriate interpretations.

FUTURE DEVELOPMENTS

It appears obvious from the perspective of discriminant validity that a construct such as social desirability that is conceptually distinct from the construct of interest to a test developer should be kept empirically distinct as well. While this may be difficult to do in the case of inherently undesirable content such as psychopathology, it would appear that efforts to do so result in instruments that are shorter (Basic Personality Inventory) or more discriminating (Personality Assessment Inventory, (Morey, 1991, Chapter 7, this volume) than tests such as the Minnesota Multiphasic Personality Inventory that did not involve a deliberate effort to control the confounding influence of social desirability during test development. If a construct-based approach is used during the development of a new scale or test, then the preliminary conceptual analysis will quickly indicate the nature of the relationship of the construct in question to social desirability. In most cases, I expect that the relationship would indicate a degree of association, but a confirmation that the construct in question was not the same as social desirability. In such a case, it would then follow that a reasonable criterion in selecting items would be that items be associated more strongly with the construct of interest than with a measure of social desirability. This is the essence of Jackson's Differential Reliability Index (discussed in more detail earlier) and the principle behind the control of irrelevant sources of variance that he espoused in his 1970 description of his construct-based method of test construction. To the extent that developers of psychological tests make use of these principles in the future there should be increasing evidence of discriminant validity and improved precision of measurement for such instruments.

Future developments may also lead to increased interest in social desirability as a construct in its own right. One of the most basic issues to be resolved concerns the nature of social desirability as a construct. It is fairly clear that the Marlowe-Crowne scale is not measuring a precise unidimensional construct. Scales such as those used by Edwards and Jackson are interpreted as if they were measuring a single construct, but when various measures of social desirability are factor analyzed, such scales generally fall with one or other of two latent dimensions. Such factor analyses generally support the existence of two dimensions or facets of social desirability, self-deception and impression management (Paulhus, 1991). Paulhus (in press) has argued for a distinction within self-deception of facets of enhancement and denial.   The theoretical aspects of social desirability thus continue to develop in contrast to the view by some that these issues were resolved many years ago.

If there are indeed two dimensions of social desirability, then much of the debate over social desirability needs to be reinterpreted. The question of what scale of social desirability was used in a particular study becomes much more important, as it is clear that social desirability scales are not all measuring the same thing.

Those facets of social desirability then need further exploration as constructs in their own right.   Is self-deception related to the construct of repressive style? Where does impression management blend into lying and into malingering?   How is malingering distinct from these stylistic constructs?   It is quite possible that such questions can only be answered with new measures of social desirability.   In that case, the development of appropriate measures will provide both notable practical difficulties and stimulating theoretical challenges.

NOTES

1. Items from Form BB of the Personality Research Form reproduced with the permission of Research Psychologists Press.

REFERENCES

Bentler, P. M., Jackson, D. N., & Messick, S. (1971). Identification of content and style: A two dimensional interpretation of acquiescence. *Psychological Bulletin, 76*, 186-204.

Berg, I. A. (Ed.). (1967). *Response set in personality assessment.* Chicago: Aldine.

Ballard, R., Crino, M. D., & Rubenfeld, S. (1988). Social desirability response bias and the Marlowe-Crowne social desirability scale. *Psychological Reports, 63*, 227-237.

Block, J. (1965). *The challenge of response sets: Unconfounding meaning, acquiescence, and social desirability in the MMPI.* New York: Appleton-Century-Crofts.

Block, J. (1972). The shifting definition of acquiescence. *Psychological Bulletin, 78*, 10-12.

Block, J. (1990). More remarks on social desirability. *American Psychologist, 45*, 1076-1077.

Byrne, D. (1961). The repression-sensitization scale: Rationale, reliability, and validity. *Journal of Personality, 29*, 334-349.

Crino, M. D., Svoboda, M., Rubenfeld, S., & White, M. C. (1983). Data on the Marlowe-Crowne and Edwards social desirability scales. *Psychological Reports, 53*, 963-968.

Crowne, D. P. (1979). *The experimental study of personality.* Hillsdale, NJ: Lawrence Erlbaum Associates.

Crowne, D. P., & Marlowe, D. (1960). A new scale of social desirability independent of psychopathology. *Journal of Consulting Psychology, 24*, 349-354.

Crowne, D. P., & Marlowe, D. A. (1964). *The approval motive.* New York: Wiley.

Damarin, F. & Messick, S. (1965). *Response styles as personality variables: A theoretical integration.* (Educational Testing Service RB 65-10). Princeton, NJ: Educational Testing Service.

Edwards, A. L. (1953). The relationship between the judged desirability of a trait and the probability that the trait will be endorsed. *Journal of Applied Psychology, 37*, 90-93.

Edwards, A. L. (1957). *The social desirability variable in personality assessment and research.* New York: Dryden.

Edwards, A. L. (1959). *Manual for the Edwards Personal Preference Schedule* (Rev. Ed.). New York: Psychological Corporation.

Edwards, A. L. (1963). A factor analysis of experimental social desirability and response set scales. *Journal of Applied Psychology*, **47**, 308-316.

Edwards, A. L. (1970). *The measurement of personality traits by scales and inventories*. New York: Holt-Rinehart-Winston.

Edwards, A. L. (1990). Construct validity and social desirability. *American Psychologist*, **45**, 287-289.

Edwards, A. L. (1991). Social desirability and ego resiliency. *American Psychologist*, **46**, 250-251.

Evans, R. G. (1979). The relationship of the MarloweCrowne scale and its components to defensive preferences. *Journal of Personality Assessment*, **43**, 406-410.

Eysenck, S. B. G., Eysenck, H. J., & Shaw, L. (1974). The modification of personality and lie scale scores by special 'honesty' instructions. *British Journal of Social and Clinical Psychology*, **13**, 41-50.

Fischer, D. G., & Fick, C. (1993). Measuring social desirabilityShort forms of the Marlowe-Crowne social desirability scale. *Educational and Psychological Measurement*, **53**, 417-424.

Furnham, A. (1986). Response bias, social desirability and dissimulation. *Personality and Individual Differences*, **7**, 385-400.

Gur, R. C., & Sackeim, H. A. (1979). Self-deception: A concept in search of a phenomenon. *Journal of Personality and Social Psychology*, **37**, 147-169.

Hartshorne, H. & May, M. A. (1928). *Studies in the nature of character. Vol. 1. Studies in deceit*. New York: Macmillan.

Hathaway, S. R., & McKinley, J. C. (1976). *Minnesota Multiphasic Personality Inventory manual*. (2nd ed.). New York: Psychological Corporation.

Helmes, E. (1996). Performance of validity indices for the Basic Personality Inventoryunder random responding. Department of Psychology Research Bulletin No. 737. University of Western Ontario, London, Canada.

Hogan, R., & Nicholson, R. A. (1988). The meaning of personalitytest scores. *American Psychologist*, **43**, 621-626.

Holden, R. R., & Fekken, G. C. (1989). Three common social desirabilityscales: Friends, acquaintances, or strangers? *Journal of Research in Personality*, **23**, 180-191.

Jackson, D. N. (1967). *Personality Research Form manual*. Goshen, NY: Research Psychologists Press.

Jackson, D. N. (1970). A sequential system for personality scale development. In C. D. Spielberger (Ed.), *Current topics in clinical and community psychology Volume 2* (pp. 61-96). New York: Academic Press.

Jackson, D. N. (1971). The dynamics of structured personality tests: 1971. *Psychological Bulletin*, **78**, 229-248.

Jackson, D. N. (1976). *Jackson Personality manual*. Goshen, NY: Research Psychologists Press.

Jackson, D. N. (1984). *Personality Research Form manual*. (3rd ed.). Port Huron, MI: Research Psychologists Press.

Jackson, D. N. (1989). *Basic Personality Inventory manual*. Port Huron, MI: Sigma Assessment Systems.

Jackson, D. N. (1994). *Jackson Personality Inventory - Revised manual*. Port Huron, MI & London, Ontario: Sigma Assessment Systems.

Jackson, D. N. & Hoffman, H. (1987). Common dimensions of psychopathology from the MMPI and the Basic Personality Inventory. *Journal of Clinical Psychology*, **43**, 661-669.

Jackson, D. N., & Messick, S. (1958). Content and style in personality assessment. *Psychological Bulletin*, **55**, 243-252.

Jackson, D. N., & Messick, S. (1961). Acquiescence and desirabilityas response determinants on the MMPI. *Educational and Psychological Measurement*, **21**, 771-790.

Jackson, D. N. & Messick, S. (1962). Response styles on the MMPIComparison of clinical and normal samples. *Journal of Abnormal and Social Psychology*, **65**, 285-299.

Jackson, D. N. & Messick, S. (1965). Acquiescence: The nonvanishing variance component. *American Psychologist*, **20**, 498.

Jackson, D. N., Wroblewski, V. R., Ashton, M. C. (1999). *The impact of faking on employment test validity: Does forced-choice offer a solution?* Manuscript submitted for publication.

Jacobson, L. I., Kellogg, R. W., Maricauce, A., & Slavin, R. S. (1977). A multidimensional social desirabilityinventory. *Bulletin of the Psychonomic Society*, **9**, 109-110.

Jacobson, L. J., Brown, R. F., & Ariza, M. J. (1983). A revised multidimensional social desirability inventory. *Bulletin of the Psychonomic Society*, **21**, 391-392.

Jones, E. E. & Sigall, H. (1971). The bogus pipelineA new paradigm for measuring affect and attitude. *Psychological Bulletin*, **76**, 349-364.

Kusyzyn, I., & Jackson, D. N. (1968). A multi-method factor analytic appraisal of endorsement and judgment methods in personalityassessment. *Educational and Psychological Measurement*, **28**, 1047-1061.

Lautenschlager, G. S. (1994). Accuracy and faking of background data. In G. S. Stokes, M. D. Mumford, & W. A. Owens (Eds.). *The biodata handbook: Theory, research and applications*. Palo Alto, CA: Consulting Psychologists Press.

McCrae, R. R., & Costa, P. T. (1983). Social desirabilityscales: More substance than style. *Journal of Consulting and Clinical Psychology*, **31**, 882-888.

Meehl, P. E., & Hathaway, S R. (1946). The K factor as a suppressor variable in the Minnesota Multiphasic Personality Inventory. *Journal of Applied Psychology*, **30**, 525-526.

Messick, S. (1960). Dimensions of social desirability. *Journal of Consulting Psychology*, **24**, 279-287.

Messick, S. (1991). Psychology and methodology of response stylesIn P. E. Snow & D. E. Wiley (Eds.) *Improving inquiry in social science: A volume in honor of Lee L. Cronbach*. Hillsdale, NJ: Lawrence Erlbaum Associates.

Messick, S. & Jackson, D. N. (1961). Desirability scale values and dispersions for MMPI items. *Psychological Reports*, **8**, 409-414.

Millham, J. (1974). Two components of need for approvalscore and relationship to cheating following success and failure. *Journal of Research in Personality*, **8**, 378-392.

Millham, J., & Jacobson, L. I. (1978). The need for approvalIn H. London & J. E. Exner (Eds.), *Dimensions of personality*. (pp. 365-390). New York: Wiley.

Millham, J., & Kellogg, R. W. (1980). Need for social approval: Management or self-deception. *Journal of Research in Personality*, **14**, 445-457.

Mook, J., Kleijn, W. C., & van der Ploeg, H. (1991). Symptom-positively and –negatively worded items in two popular self-report inventories of anxiety and depression. *Psychological Reports*, **69**, 551-560.

Morey, L. C. (1991). *Personality Assessment Inventoryprofessional manual*. Odessa, FL: Psychological Assessment Resources.

Morey, L. C. (1997). Personality diagnosis and personality disorders. In R. HoganJ. Johnson & S. Briggs (Eds.). *Handbook of personality psychology* (pp. 919-946). San Diego: Academic Press.

Morf, M. E. & Jackson, D. N. (1972). An analysis of two response styles: True responding and item endorsement. *Educational and Psychological Measurement*, **32**, 329-353.

Nederhof, A. J. (1985). Methods of coping with social desirabilitybias: A review. *European Journal of Social Psychology*, **15**, 263-280.

Neill, J. A., & Jackson, D. N. (1970). An evaluation of item selection strategies in personality scale construction. *Educational and Psychological Measurement*, **30**, 647-661.

Neill, J. A. & Jackson, D. N. (1976). Minimum redundancy item analysis. *Educational and Psychological Measurement*, **36**, 123-134.

Nicholson, R .A., & Hogan, R. (1990). The construct validityof social desirability. *American Psychologist*, **45**, 290-292.

Paulhus, D. L. (1981). Control of social desirability in personality inventories: Principal-factor deletion. *Journal of Research in Personality*, **15**, 383-388.

Paulhus, D. L. (1984). Two-component models of socially desirable responding. *Journal of Personality and Social Psychology*, **46**, 598-609.

Paulhus, D. L. (1986). Self-deception and impression management in test responses. In A. Angleitner & J. S. Wiggins (Eds.), *Personality assessment via questionnaire: Current issues in theory and measurement*. (pp. 143-165). Berlin: Springer-Verlag.

Paulhus, D. L. (1991). Measurement and control of response bias. In J. P. Robinson, P. R. Shaver, & L. S. Wrightsman (Eds.), *Measures of personality and social psychological attitudes. Vol.1*. (pp. 17-59). San Diego: Academic Press.

Paulhus, D. L (in press). Socially desirable responding: The evolution of a construct. In H. Braun, D. Wiley, & D. N. Jackson (Eds.). *Under construction: The role of constructs in psychological and educational measurement*. Mahwah, NJ: Lawrence Erlbaum Associates.

Paulhus, D. L., & Reid, D. B. (1991). Enhancement and denialin socially desirable responding. *Journal of Personality and Social Psychology*, **60**, 307-317.

Ramanaiah, N. V., & Martin, H. J. (1980). On the two-dimensional nature of the Marlowe-Crowne Social Desirability Scale. *Journal of Personality Assessment*, **44**, 507-514.

Ramanaiah, N. V., Schill, T., & Leung, L. S. (1977). A test of the hypothesis about the two-dimensional nature of the Marlowe-CrowneSocial Desirability Scale. *Journal of Research in Personality*, **11**, 251-259.

Reddon, J. R., Holden, R. R., & Jackson, D. N. (1983). Desirability and frequency of endorsement scale values and endorsement proportions for items of the Basic Personality Inventory*Psychological Reports*, **52**, 619-633.

Reynolds, W. M. (1982). Development of reliable and valid short forms of the MarloweCrowne Social Desirability Scale. Journal of Clinical Psychology, **38**, 119-125.

Rorer, L. G. (1965). The great response-style myth. *Psychological Bulletin*, **63**, 129-156.

Ross, C. E., & Mirowsky, J. (1984). Socially-desirable response and acquiescencein a cross-cultural survey of mental health. *Journal of Health and Social Behavior*, **25**, 189-197.

Sackeim, H. A., & Gur, R. C. (1978). Self-deception, self-confrontation, and consciousness. In G. E. Schwartz & D. Shapiro (Eds.), *Consciousness and self-regulation: Advances in research and theory. Vol. 2.* (pp. 139-197). New York: Plenum.

Sackeim, H. A., & Gur, R. C. (1979). Self-deception, other-deception, and self-reported psychopathology. *Journal of Consulting and Clinical Psychology, 47*, 213-215.

Samelson, F. (1972). Response style: A psychologist's fallacy. *Psychological Bulletin, 78*, 13-16.

Walsh, J. A. (1990). Comment on social desirability. *American Psychologist*, **45**, 289-290.

West, S. G. & Finch, J. F. (1997). Personality measurement: Reliability and validity issues. In R. Hogan, J. Johnson, & S. Briggs (Eds.). *Handbook of personality psychology* (pp. 143-164). San Diego: Academic Press.

Wiggins, J. S. (1959). Interrelationships among MMPI measures of dissimulation under standard and social desirabilityinstructions. *Journal of Consulting Psychology, 23*, 419-427.

3 CONSTRUCT EXPLICATION THROUGH FACTOR OR COMPONENT ANALYSIS: A REVIEW AND EVALUATION OF ALTERNATIVE PROCEDURES FOR DETERMINING THE NUMBER OF FACTORS OR COMPONENTS

Wayne F. Velicer
Cheryl A. Eaton
Joseph L. Fava

The concept of a construct is central to many of the advances in the behavioral sciences during the second half of this century. Constructs serve to summarize, organize, and facilitate the interpretation of data. The concept of a construct also permits us to move directly from data analysis to theory development and testing. Factor analysis and component analysis are two very similar methods that facilitate the transition from dealing with a large number of observed variables to a smaller number of constructed or latent variables. Douglas Jackson employed factor or component analysis as an integral part of his sequential approach to the development of psychological measures (Jackson, 1970, 1971). It has become a standard part of measure development and is one of the most employed statistical procedures in the behavioral sciences.

A central purpose of both principal component analysis and factor analysis is to determine if a set of p observed variables can be represented more parsimoniously by a set of m derived variables ($m<p$). Application of these procedures involves a series of decisions. First, the researcher must design the study. This involves determining the number and nature of the observed variables and the nature and number of participants to sample. Recent studies (Guadagnoli & Velicer, 1988; MacCallum, Widaman, Zhang, & Hong, 1999; Velicer & Fava, 1987; 1998) have provided guidance in making what are typically the most important series of decisions. Second, the researcher must

select the method of analysis. This usually involves selecting either factor or component analysis and then selecting from among the different choices of factor or component methods. This is typically not as critical a decision since the different methods give very similar results for most data sets and for the well designed study in particular (Jackson & Chan, 1980; Velicer & Jackson, 1990a, 1990b). Third, the researcher must determine the number of factors or components to retain. This is typically a critical decision and will be discussed in detail below. Fourth, the researcher must determine the method of rotation to employ. This involves selecting between orthogonal or oblique rotation to simple structure and rotation to a theoretically specified target. A number of specific techniques exist within each category but little empirical guidance is available. Fifth, the researcher will have to generate scores on the new variables in order to either focus on feedback to the individual or to assess external validity. This is typically not a critical decision since alternative methods of calculating scores produce very similar results (Fava & Velicer, 1992a). The use of some multivariate methods like structural equation modeling avoids the need to generate scores explicitly.

This chapter will focus on one of the critical decisions in performing a factor or component analysis, determining the optimal number of components or factors to retain, i.e., determining the correct value of m. Recent simulation studies (Fava & Velicer, 1992b, 1996; Wood, Tataryn, & Gorsuch, 1996) have examined and empirically demonstrated the deleterious effects of over- and under-extraction of components and factors. Miss-specification of the correct number of components and factors lead to poor score pattern reproduction (Fava & Velicer, 1992b, 1996) and to poor factor loading pattern reproduction and interpretation (Wood, Tataryn, & Gorsuch, 1996). Fava and Velicer conducted simulation studies of the effects of over-extraction (1992b) and under-extraction (1996) for principal component analysis and maximum likelihood factor analysis under a wide variety of sample sizes, factor and component loadings, and variable to factor/component ratios. They concluded that under-extraction would be a serious problem in all situations that were studied and that over-extraction becomes more problematic as sample size and/or average loading size decreases. Wood et al. (1996) studied over- and under-extraction with principal axes factor analysis within a more limited set of conditions but found similar general results to Fava and Velicer (1992b, 1996). Both Fava and Velicer (1992b, 1996) and Wood et al. (1996) emphasize that researchers should employ the most accurate methods of determining the correct number of factors or components in order to minimize such problems.

Zwick and Velicer (1986) reviewed the most widely employed methods for determining the values of m and evaluated five procedures in a simulation study. Two procedures were recommended as highly accurate: Parallel Analysis (PA; Horn, 1965) and the Minimum Average Partial Correlation (MAP; Velicer, 1976a). One procedure was recommended as a useful adjunct, but not as a stand-alone procedure: Scree (Cattell, 1966). Two procedures were generally inaccurate and use was not recommended: the Chi-square test (Bartlett, 1950, 1951) and the widely used eigenvalue greater than one rule (Kaiser, 1960).

During the time since the Zwick and Velicer (1986) review, a great deal of additional work has been published on the problem. In particular, a large number of alternative implementations of the Parallel Analysis method have been proposed, additional empirical evaluations have appeared, and the logic of some of the procedures has been challenged. However, the Kaiser rule continues to be the most widely employed, largely because the most widely used statistical software packages continue to often include this method as the default option. The purpose of this chapter is to both review developments since the Zwick and Velicer (1986) review and to evaluate some of the alternative implementations of PA and MAP that have been proposed.

In this section, we will provide a brief review of some of the more widely recommended procedures for determining the number of factors or components to retain. We will evaluate each procedure on the basis of three criteria: Rationale, the justification for the procedure; Implementation, the ease of use; and Performance, the extent to which the procedure is likely to produce the correct answer. Table 1 provides a summary evaluation of nine procedures. The basis for these evaluations is described later in this section. Six procedures, two factor analysis procedures and four component analysis procedures, are briefly reviewed. We then provide a more detailed review of the three remaining procedures that will be the prime focus of this chapter: the Kaiser eigenvalue greater than one rule, Parallel Analysis and the Minimum Average Partial procedure. The Kaiser rule is included because of its popularity and the PA and MAP procedures are included because of their accuracy.

Table 1. A comparison of nine alternative methods on three evaluative criteria

Method	Rational	Implementation	Accuracy	Recommendation
Factor Analysis				
Known *A Priori*	Poor	Easy	Unknown	No
Maximum Likelihood	Poor	Moderate	Poor	No
Component Analysis				
Known *A Priori*	Poor	Easy	Unknown	No
Bartlett's Test	Poor	Moderate	Poor	No
Scree	Moderate	Easy	Mixed	Adjunct
Percent Variance	Poor	Easy	Poor	No
Kaiser Rule	Poor	Easy	Poor	No
Parallel Analysis	Moderate	Difficult	Very Good	Yes
MAP	Good	Difficult	Very Good	Yes

Factor Analysis and Component Analysis

Factor analysis and component analysis are two approaches, based on different conceptual models, which often produce very similar results. Velicer and Jackson (1990a) summarize some of the issues involved in the decision to select one of the two approaches. That paper and the associated comments (Bentler & Kano, 1990; Bookstein, 1990; Gorsuch, 1990; Loehlin, 1990; McArdle, 1990; Mulaik, 1990; Rozeboom, 1990; Schonemann, 1990; Steiger, 1990; Velicer & Jackson, 1990b; Widaman, 1990) provide a broad overview of the controversy surrounding the choice of approach.

The method for determining the number of factors or components is intimately tied to the choice of method of analysis. In this review, we will consider both factor analysis based methods and component analysis based methods, but the focus will be on principal component analysis. As we will see, there are more component analysis based methods available for this particular decision and they represent the methods of choice. However, for the researcher who prefers factor analysis, component analysis can be viewed as a preliminary step, with the value for the number of components providing a guide in specifying the number of factors. Alternatively, two of the best component analysis procedures, Parallel Analysis and MAP (see below) have been adapted for principal axes factor analysis and we will reference these versions in the discussion below. However, the vast majority of the work available on these two methods has occurred within the principal component analysis framework.

Procedures to be reviewed

In a review of textbooks, computer programs, and published research reports, nine methods were identified which have received adequate attention for inclusion in this review. Each of these methods is described in detail in the following sections. Two methods were based on the factor analysis model: the assumption that the correct value of m was known *A Priori* and the Chi-square test associated with maximum likelihood factor analysis. Seven methods were associated with component analysis: the known *A Priori* assumption and the Bartlett chi-square test that are analogous to the factor analysis methods, the Scree test, decisions based on the percent of variance accounted for, the eigenvalue greater than one rule, the Parallel Analysis procedure, and the MAP procedure. Of the component analysis procedures, three (a regression analysis approach to parallel analysis, a variation of the MAP procedure, and the percent variance rule) have been applied to principal axes factor analysis.

REVIEW OF FACTOR ANALYSIS PROCEDURES

Factor Analysis: Known *A Priori*

Occasionally it is recommended that the number of factors should be known *A Priori* as a precondition for performing the analysis. This is seldom supported by an explicit argument, but rather seems to provide a means of avoiding a discussion of the problem of determining the correct number of factors. In fairness, some authors would restrict the use of factor analysis to only confirmatory uses, but examples of applications where a rigid confirmatory approach is used are rare. This approach avoids the issue and cannot be viewed as a serious alternative. In some cases, the critical question of the study involves determining the correct value for the number of factors. In other cases, the researcher has an estimate that they believe is correct, but they wish to evaluate the accuracy of their hypothesis. The rationale for this procedure was judged to be *poor*, the ease of implementation is, of course, *easy* (since nothing is required), and the accuracy is *unknown* since it is not testable. *This procedure is not recommended.*

Factor Analysis: Maximum Likelihood Chi-square Test

A well-known statistical test associated with maximum likelihood factor analysis is the asymptotic Chi-square test. This method, when employed to determine the number of factors to retain, calculates the test statistic for each increase in the number of factors retained. When the test is not significant, the correct value of m is assumed to have been achieved. The test can be interpreted as testing whether the eigenvalues associated with the last p-m factors are all equal.

Five concerns exist with respect to this test. First, the test assumes a multivariate normal distribution. When the number of variables becomes even moderately large, this assumption is not likely to be appropriate. In addition, the statistic seems to be very sensitive to non-normality (Boomsma, 1983). Violations will result in over-extraction. Second, the test is a "badness-of-fit" test in that we are trying to find non-significance. In simple terms, this test is attempting to prove the null hypothesis, a goal of dubious logic that is more likely to be achieved by insuring that power (e. g. sample size) is smaller rather than larger. Third, the test may not be testing a hypothesis of interest to the researcher. The researcher is typically interested in "common factors," i.e., new composite variables that involve shared variance among two or more observed variables. Clearly, a variable could have an eigenvalue that is different from error but not involve common variance. The test, therefore, has a tendency to include factors defined by only one variable or defined primarily by one variable. Fourth, the number of factors retained will be at least partially a function of sample size (Bentler, 1980), a characteristic that a number of researchers view as a problem (Marsh, Balla, & McDonald, 1988). Fifth, even when all the conditions are met, the test has not been very accurate in evaluative studies (Tucker & Lewis, 1973; Hakstian, Rogers & Cattell,

1982; M. B. Richman, reported in Zwick & Velicer, 1986). Perhaps this performance is the result of the test being an asymptotic rather than an exact test.

In evaluating this test, we judged the rationale to be *poor* because it was not testing the hypothesis of interest to most researchers and because it represents an attempt to prove the null hypothesis. With respect to implementation, we judged the ease of implementation to be *moderate*. It is available in most statistical computer packages. On the other hand, it requires the selection of maximum likelihood estimation procedures when many researchers may prefer an alternative procedure and it requires some complex computer programming to implement. The accuracy was judged to be *poor* on the basis of available simulation studies and the fact that violation of the multivariate normality assumption and/or large sample sizes are likely to result in the retention of many more factors than is appropriate. *This procedure is not recommended.*

REVIEW OF COMPONENT ANALYSIS PROCEDURES

Component Analysis: Known *A Priori*

The identical issues and evaluation occur when this procedure is invoked for component analysis as with factor analysis. *This procedure is not recommended.*

Component Analysis: Bartlett's Chi-Square Test

A procedure for determining the number of components that parallels the maximum likelihood Chi-square test is Bartlett's (1950, 1951) test of significance of the residuals. The null hypothesis of the test is that, after the first m components are removed, the remaining eigenvalues are equal. Like the factor analysis test, this hypothesis is not identical to the concept of "common" components. In practice, one continues to remove components until the null hypothesis fails to be rejected, so this is also a "badness-of-fit" test. Gorsuch (1973) reports that Bartlett's significance test indicates the maximum, not necessarily the actual, number of components to extract and that it leads to the extraction of too many smaller, often trivial components. This is consistent with the criticisms of the test as not testing for "common" components and the goodness-of-fit approach. In a study comparing five different methods, Hubbard and Allen (1987) reported that Bartlett's test overestimated the number of components to retain. Zwick and Velicer (1982, 1986) found the accuracy of Bartlett's significance test decreased with smaller sample sizes, and was less accurate and more variable than the scree test. The test trended to underextract when sample sizes were small, particularly in the low saturation condition, and tended to overextract when sample sizes were large, particularly the high saturation condition (Zwick & Velicer, 1986).

The Bartlett test suffers from many of the same problems as the maximum likelihood chi-square test and was, therefore, evaluated similarly: *poor* on rationale, *moderate* on implementation difficulty, and *poor* on accuracy. *The use of this procedure is not recommended.*

Component Analysis: Scree Test

The scree test, another commonly used procedure for determining the number of components to retain, was proposed by Cattell (1966). With this method, one plots the eigenvalues and examines the plot to find where a break or a leveling of the slope of the plotted line occurs. At the point of the break, the number of components is indicated. The eigenvalues above the break indicate common components, while those below the break represent error variance. Problems arise with this method when there is not an obvious break or when there are several breaks, both of which lead to a more subjective judgment of the appropriate number of components.

Horn and Engstrom (1979) discuss the similarities between Cattell's scree test and Bartlett's significance test. Both methods are based upon the same rationale, with an examination of the contribution of the remaining components after *m* components have been extracted. Horn and Engstrom (1979) express a preference for the more explicit method of the significance test over the subjective method of the scree test, although they state the scree test is useful. Not all agree with this preference. Many studies have found this method to be reasonably effective in suggesting the correct number of components to retain (Cattell & Jaspers, 1967; Cattell & Vogelmann, 1977; Cliff, 1970; Linn, 1968; Tucker, Koopman, & Linn, 1969; Zwick & Velicer, 1982). Zwick and Velicer (1982) found the scree test to be the most accurate of four methods for determining the number of components, especially in situations with large sample sizes and with strong components. Hakstian, Rogers, and Cattell (1982) found the scree test to be less accurate with low communality data, which resulted in an over-identification of the number of factors. The scree test has also been found to be less accurate with smaller sample sizes (Cliff & Hamburger, 1967; Linn, 1968). In a later study, Zwick and Velicer (1986) found the scree test to be more variable and less accurate than several other methods when more complex patterns, i.e., those which included unique and complex items, were considered.

The use of a visual rationale rather than a computational or algebraic rationale should not result in automatic rejection of this method. The visual argument parallels the algebraic argument of the Bartlett test (see Horn & Engstrom, 1979), but has potential to avoid some of the over-extraction problems because the trivial factors will not be visually compelling. Therefore, the rationale was judged to be *moderate*. The implementation was judged to be *easy* since computer programs typically produce the eigenvalue. The results from studies evaluating the accuracy of the test have been mixed. *The Scree procedure is recommended as an adjunct to other procedures, but not as a stand-alone procedure.*

Component Analysis: Percent Variance

This rule involves the imposition of any arbitrary minimum amount of variance, say 70%, that the extracted components have to account for. The origin of this rule is from principal component analysis. In the usual procedure, all the variables are standardized to unit variance and the analysis is performed on the correlation matrix. The total variance for the p observed variables is equal to p. Each eigenvalue can be interpreted as representing the variance of a new component. The sum of the eigenvalues of the m retained components represents the total variance of the retained components. The ratio of the sum of the eigenvalues for the retained components to the total variance is the percent of the variance accounted for by the components. The cutoff for the "acceptable" amount seems to be arbitrary and differs from authority to authority. This rule has also been applied to principal axes factor analysis. The principal axes method utilizes the reduced correlation matrix where the diagonal has been reduced by the subtraction of the unique variance estimates so the total variance no longer equals p. For this reason, the percent of variance accounted for will be less with component analysis than for the corresponding principal axes solutions. Sometimes the acceptable value for principal axes is erroneously applied to component analysis resulting in severe over-extraction.

A counter example will serve to illustrate problems associated with this rule. Assume you have 20 variables and 4 components, each of which is measured by 5 variables with high loadings. The 4 components account for 75% of the variance, which exceeds the 70% cut off that you are using. This represents an ideal situation with an easily interpretable and replicable pattern. Assume that you then augment the variable set with an additional 20 variables which represent pure error variance. A 4 component solution now accounts for 37.5% of the variance and the inclusion of a large number of unique components representing only error would have to be included to achieve the minimum cutoff that you are employing. The inaccuracy of any cutoff could be easily demonstrated in a simulation study by manipulating the size of the loadings, the correlation between the factors or components, and the number of unique variables included. The percent of variance rule was judged to be *poor* in rationale, *easy* to implement, and *poor* in accuracy. *Use of this rule is not recommended.*

Component Analysis: Kaiser Test

The most commonly used method for determining the number of components to retain in a principal component analysis is the eigenvalue greater than one rule proposed by Kaiser (1960). With this method, all components with an eigenvalue greater than unity are retained.

The rationale of the eigenvalue greater than one rule has been challenged in recent years. Guttman (1954) originally presented the rule to determine the lower bound of the number of common factors of a correlation matrix in the population. He did not suggest its use as a basis for determining the number of factors, so we view the occasional reference to it as the Kaiser-Guttman Rule as incorrect. Gorsuch (1983) criticized the applied use of the criterion for determining the number of factors rather than determining the lower bound for the number of factors. Schonemann (1990) questioned the accuracy of this rule as providing the lower bound.

A second rationale for the use of the eigenvalue greater than one rule has been the intuitively appealing argument that one would only want to retain factors which account for more variance (greater than 1.0) than the original variable. A third rationale for the use of this rule has been the statement by Kaiser (1960) that the eigenvalue must be greater than 1.0 for the reliability to be positive. However, Cliff (1988) demonstrated that this statement is incorrect: the reliability of components cannot be determined from the size of the eigenvalues. According to Cliff (1988), Kaiser's statement was based upon the incorrect application of the Kuder-Richardson 20 (K-R 20) formula for the reliability of a composite. In actuality, the reliability of a component is determined by the reliability of the measures. As a result, the rationale for this procedure was judged as *poor*.

The eigenvalue greater than one rule is *easy* to implement. No specialized technical or statistical knowledge is required to use the method. The eigenvalue greater than one rule is the default method for all major statistical software packages. This ease of implementation has contributed to the wide use of this method, even after numerous studies have demonstrated the poor performance of the method as compared to many other available methods.

Although the eigenvalue greater than one rule criterion is a very popular method, it has been shown to lead to over-extraction of the number of components (Cattell & Jaspers, 1967: Hubbard & Allen, 1987; Lee & Comrey, 1979; Linn, 1968; Revelle & Rocklin, 1979; Yeomans & Golder, 1982; Zwick & Velicer, 1982, 1986). Typically, in situations with low commonalities, the number of components retained by this rule is related to the number of variables (*p*) in ratios ranging from p/3 to p/5 rather than the actual structure of the data (Zwick & Velicer, 1982). Gorsuch (1983) suggests this method is appropriate as an approximate estimation of the number of factors in cases with less than 40 variables, a large N, and an expected number of factors between 1/3 and 1/5 of the number of variables. This method was judged to be *poor* in accuracy. *The use of this procedure is not recommended.*

Component Analysis: Parallel Analysis

Horn (1965) introduced the parallel analysis method for determining the number of factors as an alternative to the Kaiser rule. A set of random data correlation matrices, with the same number of variables and participants as the observed data, is generated. The average of the eigenvalues across the set of random data matrices is calculated. The eigenvalues of the observed data are then compared to the averaged eigenvalues of the random data. Components are retained as long as the eigenvalue of the observed data exceeds the eigenvalue of the random data. Figure 1 illustrates the PA procedure for a set of simulated data.

One problematic area is the determination of how many random data correlation matrices should be included. Although Horn (1965) used one random data correlation matrix in his introduction of parallel analysis, he proposed that the averaged eigenvalues should give the appropriate curve when the number of matrices is "reasonably large". Crawford and Koopman (1973) found no

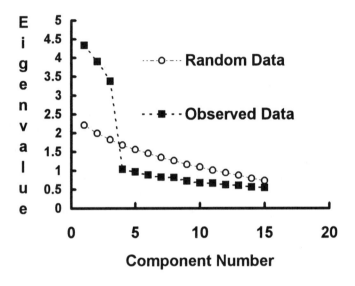

Figure 1. An illustration of the Parallel Analysis Procedure (Random Generation, 100 Matrices; M = 3, P = 24, N = 75, CS = .60).

significant difference in the accuracy of parallel analysis with eigenvalues from one random correlation matrix as compared to the averaged eigenvalues across 100 random correlation matrices. Longman, Cota, Holden, and Fekken (1991) found that accuracy was greater with 40 than 3 replications, but concluded that the difference in accuracy was not significant. As a result, they recommend parallel analysis based upon a few replications.

Due to the computational difficulty encountered when implementing this method, much recent work has been focused on developing alternatives to avoid the necessity of generating multiple correlation matrices. One alternative is the development of regression equations for predicting the random eigenvalues. Montanelli and Humphreys (1976) introduced the first regression equation for use in determining the number of factors to retain in principal axes factor analysis. The equation predicts the common (base 10) logarithms of the latent roots of random correlation matrices, with squared multiple correlations (SMC) on the diagonal. The regression equation is:

[1] $\text{Log } \lambda_i = a_i + b_{Ni} \log (N - 1) + b_{pi} \log \{(p\ (p\text{-}1)/2)\text{-}(I\text{-}1)\ p\}$

where a is the intercept; b_{Ni} and b_{pi} are regression coefficients; N is the number of observations; p is the number of variables; and I is the ordinal position of the eigenvalue. This equation estimates about half of the eigenvalues.

Allen and Hubbard (1986) developed the first regression equation for use with principal component analysis. Their study varied the number of variables from 5 to 50 in steps of 5. The number of participants included 30, 60, 90, 120, 240, 500, and 1000. All N and p combinations which satisfied the restriction that $N > 3p/2$ were examined. For cases with a sample size less than 240, 50 replications were employed. For those cases with a sample size of 240 or more, 30 replications were used. They presented the following equation for predicting the natural logarithms of latent roots of random data correlation matrices with unities on the diagonals:

[2] $\text{Ln } \lambda_i = a_i + b_i \ln (N\text{-}1) + c_i \ln \{(p\text{-}I\text{-}1)(p\text{-}I+2)/2\} + d_i \ln (\lambda_{i\text{-}1})$

where a is the intercept; b, c, and d are the regression weights; N is the number of observations; p is the number of variables; I is the ordinal position from 1 to $(p\text{-}2)$; and λ_0 equals 1. This equation predicts all eigenvalues except the last two. It is appropriate for situations with up to 50 variables.

Longman, Holden, and Fekken (1991) report the observance of anomalies with the Allen and Hubbard (1986) equation. They describe situations in which the eigenvalues predicted from the Allen and Hubbard (1986) regression equation initially decrease as expected, then begin to increase. Longman, Cota, Holden, and Fekken (1989a) introduced a second regression equation for predicting eigenvalues from random data correlation matrices with principal component analysis. They suggest it is easier to calculate, and yields improved results as compared to the equation of Allen & Hubbard (1986). The values for the number of variables were 5, 10, 15, 20, 25, 35, and 50. The number of participants included 50, 75, 100, 125, 150, 175, 200, 300, 400, and 500. After considering several variations of regression equations, the following equation was recommended:

[3] $\text{Ln } (\lambda_i) = a_i \ln (N_i) + b_i \ln (p_i) + c_i \{\ln (N_i) \ln (p_i)\} + d_i$

where a, b, c, and d are the regression weights; N is the number of observations; p is the number of variables; and i is the ordinal position from 1 to $(p\text{-}2)$. If p is 35 or less, the equation predicts $p\text{-}2$ eigenvalues. If p is greater than 35, then it is recommended that only the first 33 eigenvalues be predicted.

A third regression equation for predicting the eigenvalues of random correlation matrices was proposed by Lautenschlager, Lance, and Flaherty (1989). The number of variables ranged from 5 to 50 in increments of 5. The number of participants included 50, 75, 100, 150, 200, 300, 400, 500, 750, and 1000. Those N and p combinations which met the $N > 3p/2$ restriction were examined. The addition of a p/N term to the Allen and Hubbard equation improved the accuracy of the prediction of the first, and therefore subsequent, eigenvalues. This equation is:

[4] $\text{Ln } \lambda_i = a_i + b_i \ln (N\text{-}1) + c_i \ln \{(p\text{-}I\text{-}1)(p\text{-}I\text{+}2)/2\} + d_i \ln (\lambda_{i\text{-}1}) + e_i \, p/N$

where a is the intercept; b, c, d, and e are regression weights; N is the number of observations; p is the number of variables; and I is the ordinal position from 1 to $(p\text{-}2)$. This equation predicts up to 48 eigenvalues.

A second alternative to generating the multiple random data correlation matrices required to conduct parallel analysis is linear interpolation of tabled eigenvalues developed by Lautenschlager (1989a). These tables were generated by averaging the eigenvalues across random correlation matrices for 13 values of p, ranging from 5 to 80, and 12 values of N, ranging from 50 to 2000. The number of generated matrices was 100 when $p > 10$ and 200 for $p <= 10$. One first locates the table of eigenvalues corresponding to the N and p of the observed data. If there is no table for the exact value of N and p, the user then selects the values from the N and p tables that are above and below the desired value. Linear interpolation is then conducted on these values to obtain the eigenvalues for the specific values of N and p.

The rationale of parallel analysis is based upon the eigenvalue greater than one rule. Horn (1965) proposed parallel analysis specifically to address the inability of the eigenvalue greater than one rule to reflect sampling error. By comparing the eigenvalues of the observed data to the eigenvalues of randomly generated data instead of a fixed value of 1.0, random error is taken into account. Although this strengthens the rationale of this method, the criticisms of the eigenvalue greater than one rule rationale weakens the rationale for parallel analysis. The rationale for parallel analysis was judged to be *moderate*.

Three approaches to parallel analysis have been proposed: random data generation, regression equations, and tabled eigenvalues. There are a variety of alternative implementations of these methods.

Several computer programs are available for performing the random data generation method. The Longman, Cota, Holden, and Fekken (1989b) mainframe FORTRAN program and the IBM compatible personal computer program provided by Lautenschlager (1989b) provide random data eigenvalues. The regression equations may be implemented using available FORTRAN and BASIC programs for mainframe and IBM compatible personal computers. The estimated eigenvalues for the Allen &

Hubbard (1986) equation can be computed using the BASIC program presented by Hays (1987) or the FORTRAN program used in this study (Holden, Longman, Cota, and Fekken, 1989). The latter program also provides estimated eigenvalues for the Longman, Cota, Holden, and Fekken (1989a) equation. These programs require some skills or knowledge of computers that may be beyond what many users possess, especially users who are accustomed to using statistical software packages.

The tabled eigenvalues method provided by Lautenschlager (1989a) is the most accessible of all parallel analysis methods. However, it is rather cumbersome to use. If one needs to interpolate across both N and p for a large number of variables, the process can become fairly extensive. At this time, no computer program is available which would calculate the eigenvalues by this method. The availability of such a program would greatly simplify the use of this method. Given this, and that the random data generation and regression equation programs are absent from standard statistical software packages and the use of these alternative methods of implementing parallel analysis requires some advanced computer skills, implementation was judged to be *difficult*.

The Zwick and Velicer (1986) study provided the best available evidence supporting the accuracy of the parallel analysis procedure. In that study, the random data generation method was very accurate across a wide variety of conditions. It was more accurate than the eigenvalue greater than one rule, Cattell's scree test, and Bartlett's significance test for the number of components. Other studies, such as Hubbard and Allen (1987), have also provided support for the accuracy of the procedure but have been much more limited in scope. The accuracy of the procedure was judged as *very good* but this evaluation does not necessarily apply to all available approaches to parallel analysis.

The performance of the regression equations has not been extensively evaluated. In presenting their alternate equations to the Allen and Hubbard (1986) equation, Longman, Cota, Holden, and Fekken (1989a) provide only limited evidence that the alternate regression equations are superior to the Allen and Hubbard (1986) equation. They compared their equation with the Allen and Hubbard equation on five combinations of N and p by calculating the correlation between the actual and predicted eigenvalue. For all five combinations, the Longman, Cota, Holden, and Fekken equation was more accurate than the Allen and Hubbard equation.

Lautenschlager (1989a) compared the tabled eigenvalue method to the regression equations proposed by Allen and Hubbard (1986) and Lautenschlager, Lance, and Flaherty (1989). He suggests the tabled eigenvalues method is generally more accurate than the Allen and Hubbard (1986) regression equation and the Lautenschlager, Lance, and Flaherty (1989) regression equation. For the three regression equation approaches and the tabled value approach, there has not been a study that evaluates the ability of the method to accurately determine m. Since this is the ultimate criterion for each of these methods, such studies are critical. An empirical study of the alternative approaches to parallel analysis will be reviewed later in this chapter.

Component Analysis: Minimum Average Partial (MAP) Procedure

The MAP method (Velicer, 1976) was developed for use with principal components analysis. Each component is partialed out of the correlation matrix and a partial correlation matrix is calculated. For each value of m, the average of the squared correlations of the off-diagonal partial correlation matrix is computed. The number of components to retain is indicated at the point where the average squared partial correlation reaches a minimum. Figure 2 illustrates the MAP procedure.

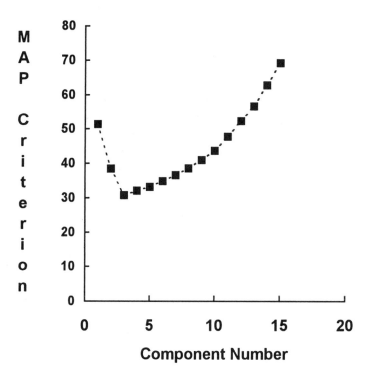

Figure 2. An Illustration of the MAP Procedure (Trace of the Squared Partial Correlation Matrix; M = 3, P = 24, N = 75, CS = .60).

The matrix of partial correlations is obtained by first computing the partial covariance matrix,

[5] $\mathbf{C} = \mathbf{R} - \mathbf{A}\,\mathbf{A}'$

where $\mathbf{C}$ is the partial covariance matrix, $\mathbf{R}$ is the correlation matrix, and $\mathbf{A}$ is the pattern matrix. The partial correlation matrix is then computed

[6] $\mathbf{R}^* = \mathbf{D}'\,\mathbf{C}\,\mathbf{D}$

where $\mathbf{R}^*$ is the matrix of partial correlations and $\mathbf{D}$ is the diagonal of the partial covariance matrix. The MAP procedure involves determining when the matrix of partial correlations most approximates an identify matrix, i.e., determining the value m for which

[7] $\mathbf{R}^* = \mathbf{I}$

The problem is to develop a summary statistic based on the $\mathbf{R}^*$ matrix to make this comparison. Velicer (1976) presented the following equation for calculating the MAP criterion.

[8] $\mathrm{MAP}_m = \Sigma \Sigma \, (r_{ij}^*)^2 / (p\,(p-1))$

where r_{ij}^* is the value in row i and column j of the matrix of partial correlations and p is the total number of observed variables.

An alternative way of defining this MAP criterion involves the trace, or sum, of the eigenvalues of the squared matrix of partial correlations as each of the m components are extracted. The number of variables is subtracted from the trace, and the remainder is then divided by the number of off-diagonal elements in the matrix, $(p\,(p-1))$. The resulting value equals the MAP criterion. This can be represented as,

[9] $\mathrm{MAP}_m = \Sigma \Sigma \, (r_{ij}^*)^2 / (p\,(p-1)) = (\mathrm{Trace}\;\mathbf{R}^{*2} - p) / (p\,(p-1))$

Velicer (1976) described the logic of the procedure as follows: as common variance is partialled out of the matrix for each successive value of m, the MAP_m criterion will continue to decrease. At the point where the common variance has been removed and only unique variance remains, the MAP_m criterion will begin to rise. Thus, the MAP criterion separates common and unique variance, and retains only components consisting of common variance. This rationale reflects the original rationale used by Spearman and is the criterion used for developing an optimum solution for factor analysis by Howe (1956; also see Morrison, 1976).

If one examines the general formula presented by Velicer (1976) for computing a partial correlation,

$$[10] \quad r_{ij \cdot y} = \frac{r_{ij} - (r_{iy} * r_{jy})}{((1 - r_{iy}^2) * (1 - r_{jy}^2))^{1/2}}$$

one sees that the partial correlation coefficient will decrease as long as the numerator decreases more than the denominator. When the denominator begins to decrease more than the numerator, the partial correlation coefficient will then begin to increase. The latter would occur when there is a high correlation of a component with one variable and low correlation with all the other variables, indicating the presence of unique rather than common component. The minimum average partial correlation procedure for determining the number of components to retain was judged to have a *good* rationale.

The current means of implementing the MAP procedure is the CAX (Component Analysis Extended) FORTRAN computer program (Velicer, Fava, Zwick, & Harrop, 1990) [1]. Reddon (1985) has published a short FORTRAN program. Evans (1992, personal communication) has provided a short SAS routine [1]. Hofer (1992, personal communication) has developed an executable FORTRAN program based on the CAX program that can run in a personal computer [1]. Gorsuch (1991) includes a principal axes factor analysis version in his UNIMULT program. None of the major statistical software packages include the MAP procedure analysis implementation. Since the programs that are available require skills beyond the execution of standard software packages, the MAP procedure was judged as *difficult* to implement.

The MAP method was found to be comparable to the scree test and more accurate (Zwick & Velicer, 1982) than the eigenvalue greater than one rule and Bartlett's significance test for the number of components. In a later study with more complex data, Zwick and Velicer (1986) demonstrated that the MAP criterion was more accurate than the Kaiser rule, Cattell's scree test, and Bartlett's significance test for the number of components. The accuracy of this method was judged to be *very good* and it will be a major focus of this study.

REVIEW OF EMPIRICAL STUDY

Two methods of determining the number of components, parallel analysis and the minimum average partial correlation, are clearly the methods of choice. A recent empirical evaluation study (Eaton, Velicer, & Fava, 1999) evaluated the performance of several variations of each of these methods. Six alternative methods of parallel analysis and three variations of the MAP procedure were selected for evaluation. As the most commonly used method, the eigenvalue greater than one rule was also included. The methods were evaluated across different factors known to affect the performance of these methods.

Decision Rules Evaluated

The following methods of parallel analysis were examined:
1. R5, the generation of 5 random correlation matrices and averaging of eigenvalues across the matrices.
2. R100, the generation of 100 random correlation matrices and averaging of eigenvalues across the matrices.
3. AH, the regression equation presented by Allen and Hubbard (1986).
4. LCHF, the regression equation proposed by Longman, Cota, Holden and Fekken (1989a).
5. LLF, the regression equation introduced by Lautenschlager, Lance, and Flaherty (1989).
6. TAB, interpolation from the tables of mean criterion eigenvalues provided by Lautenschlager (1989a).

Three versions of the MAP procedure were included. The previously studied MAP criterion is based upon the square of the trace of the correlation matrix. Occasionally, the decline and increase in the MAP values over the values of m is a gradual one, making the determination of the exact stopping point to be based on relatively minor differences. Other variations, which may display a sharper directional change from the removal of common to unique variance, were considered by examining two factors: the matrix summary statistics and the power of the matrix under consideration.

The trace of a matrix is one of three summary statistics (the trace, the determinant, and the largest root) which are used to summarize matrices in multivariate procedures. The largest root is the largest eigenvalue. The determinant is the product of the eigenvalues. For each value of m, the matrix of partial correlations will contain m zero eigenvalues, which will result in a value of zero for the determinant. Therefore, the determinant was excluded from consideration as a variation of the MAP criterion. The two remaining matrix summary statistics, the trace and the largest root, are both viable options.

The power of the matrix under consideration may also be varied. The current calculation of the MAP criterion is based on the squared matrix (Trace $\mathbf{R}^* = p$ which excludes the first power). The fourth power also contains potential as a possible alternative of calculating the criterion.

The following MAP variations were examined:
1. TR2, the previously studied version consisting of the trace of the matrix of squared partial correlations.
2. TR4, the trace of the matrix of partial correlations to the fourth power.
3. LR - the largest root of the matrix of partial correlations.

(Only one of the possible three versions of the largest root of the matrix of partial correlations was employed since the first, second, and fourth powers of the largest root mathematically produce the same result. Table 2 summarizes the choices.)

One additional method included in this study was the eigenvalue greater than one rule. As the most commonly employed method in applied use, this method served as a baseline to evaluate the alternative methods.

Table 2. Summary of Alternative Procedures for Implementing the MAP Procedure

| Power | Function of Partial Correlation Matrix | | |
	Trace	Determinant	Greatest Root
1	P	0	LR [Tested]
2	TR2 [Tested]	0	Same as LR
4	TR4 [Tested]	0	Same as LR

TR2 = Trace, partial correlation matrix, second power (Note: Current MAP procedure)
TR4 = Trace, partial correlation matrix, fourth power
LR = Largest root, partial correlation matrix

Design of the Study

The methods used here involve the generation of data sets in which the number of components (factors) is known. The accuracy of each method for determining the number of components is determined by evaluating how effectively the method estimates the correct number of components. Factors known to influence the accuracy of these methods include sample size (N), the number of variables (p), the ratio of the number of variables per component (p: m), and the component saturation (CS). Component saturation refers to the size of the loadings and can be interpreted as the correlation between an observed variable and the component. These factors were varied in an attempt to determine the performance of the methods under selected conditions. Values were selected for the levels of these factors according to two criteria: 1) those which best represent values which are found in applied research settings and 2) those which have been demonstrated to differentiate the accuracy of decision methods in other Monte Carlo studies.

1. The number of variables (p) was set at 24, 48, and 72. The value of 24 was selected to reflect a small data set, 48 a moderate data set, and 72 a larger data set.

2. Three levels of sample size (N) were selected to be included in this study: 75, 150, and 300. The value of 75 is considered to be a low sample size, while 150 has been recommended (Velicer, Peacock, & Jackson, 1982; Guadagnoli & Velicer, 1988) as a minimum to provide adequate results when the component saturation and the number of variables per component are sufficient. When the number of variables per component or the component saturation are at minimum ranges, the larger sample size of 300 is recommended (Guadagnoli & Velicer, 1988; Velicer & Fava, 1998).

3. The levels of the number of variables, p, and the number of components, m, were selected to ensure that the variables per component ratio was held constant at 4:1 and 8:1. The ratio of 4:1 is viewed as just over the minimum number of variables needed to define a component, and the ratio of 8:1 represents a moderately strong component. The p: m ratio has repeatedly (Guadagnoli & Velicer, 1988; Velicer & Fava, 1987, 1998; Yeomans & Golder, 1982; Zwick & Velicer, 1982, 1986) been found to influence the accuracy of the results, with more variables per component producing more stable values. For p = 24, m was set at 3 and 6; for p = 48, m was set at 6 and 12; and for p = 72, m was set at 9 and 18.

4. The magnitude of the component saturation, has repeatedly been found to be one of the factors having the greatest effect on accuracy within principal components analysis (Guadagnoli and Velicer, 1988; Hakstian, Rogers, and Cattell, 1982; Anderson, Acito, and Lee, 1982; Yeomans and Golder, 1982; Velicer and Fava, 1987,1998; Zwick and Velicer, 1982, 1986). The three levels of component saturation were .40, .60, and .80 that represent low, medium, and high component saturation, respectively.

Data Generation

The procedure previously employed by Guadagnoli and Velicer (1988,1991), Velicer, Peacock, and Jackson (1982), Velicer and Fava (1987), and Zwick and Velicer (1982, 1986) was utilized. The population correlation matrices were generated in the following manner: 1) the component pattern, **A**, based upon the combination of values for p, m, and CS was created, 2) the pattern matrix was multiplied by its transpose (**A'**) which resulted in a matrix $\mathbf{R}_1$ ($\mathbf{R}_1 = \mathbf{A}\,\mathbf{A}'$), and 3) values of 1.0 were substituted in the diagonal of the $\mathbf{R}_1$ matrix which added error and created a correlation matrix, $\mathbf{R} = \mathbf{R}_1 + \mathbf{D}^2$, of full rank. While this procedure follows the factor analysis model, an equivalent correlation matrix could be generated from a component analysis model. All data generated is from a multivariate normal distribution.

Population correlation matrices were generated for each of the 54 combinations of the 3 X 3 X 3 X 2 design. For each of the population correlation matrices, five sample correlation matrices were then generated employing a program by Montanelli (1975). This program is based on a method proposed by Odell and Feiveson (1966). Guadagnoli and Velicer (1991) evaluated how many samples are required for a study of this type and five was considered adequate.

A principal component analysis was performed on each of the resulting 270 correlation matrices. The number of components retained by each of the methods was then computed. The following section presents the procedures used to compute the number of components for each method.

Computation of M

The value for the number of components retained by the eigenvalue greater than one rule was calculated by counting the number of eigenvalues that were greater than 1.0.

The number of components retained by the three MAP variations was computed by adapting the CAX FORTRAN program (Velicer, Fava, Zwick, & Harrop, 1990). The program was expanded to include the calculation of the trace of the matrix of partial correlations to the fourth power and the largest root of the matrix of partial correlations.

For the six parallel analysis methods, the eigenvalues of the simulated data were compared to the eigenvalues produced by the random data correlation matrices, the three regression equations, and the interpolated table values provided by Lautenschlager (1989a).   Several computer programs were utilized to determine the number of components for these methods. For random data parallel analysis, the generation of the random correlation matrices and the averaging of the random data eigenvalues was performed using the PAM FORTRAN program presented by Longman, Cota, Holden, and Fekken (1989b). The implementation of the regression equations for estimating the eigenvalues of the equations presented by Allen and Hubbard and by Longman et al. were completed with the PAR FORTRAN program (Holden, Longman, Cota, & Fekken, 1989). This program was adapted to also estimate the eigenvalues for the equation proposed by Lautenschlager, Lance, and Flaherty (1989).

Results of the Study

The results are organized into two separate comparisons of the performance of the ten methods. The first comparison is based on all valid estimates provided by each method. Some of the procedures had a poorer performance than other procedures simply because they provided estimates for almost all cases while the comparison method only provided estimates for a limited number of well-defined cases.   The second comparison was restricted to only those cases where all ten procedures produced legitimate estimates and, therefore, all ten methods were evaluated on the same cases.

Measures of Method Performance

There were four criteria of method performance calculated for each of the ten methods evaluated in this study:

1. The number of cases where the procedure produced an acceptable estimate.
2. The mean of the deviation from correct.
3. The standard deviation of the deviation from correct.
4. The percent of cases where the estimate was exactly correct.

A critical criterion was the number of cases where the procedure produced an acceptable estimate, as the results of the other three statistics are dependent on this criterion.

The accuracy of the number of components given by each method was computed by subtracting the number of components indicated (m estimated) for the simulated data from the correct number of components (m) for each sample of that combination of N, p, p: m, and CS. A value of 0 indicated the method was correct for that case. The average of the deviation scores was then computed. Values of 0 indicate that the method was accurate on the average. Negative values indicate that the method overestimated on the average, while positive values indicate that the method underestimated the correct number of components on the average.

The standard deviation of the averaged deviation scores was also calculated as a measure of variability for each method. A high standard deviation indicates considerable variability in estimating m in the different conditions. If a method produced a large number of both overestimates and underestimates the mean of the deviation scores could be near zero, producing the illusion of accuracy but the standard deviation would detect the problem.

The percent of the total cases available where the estimate of the number of components was exactly correct was computed. This is a severe criterion that treats both small and large errors exactly the same.

First Comparison

Two sets of inappropriate estimates ($m = 0$ and $m = p - 2$) were observed and eliminated from consideration. While the retention of zero components is possible, e. g., if the correlation matrix represents a set of independent variables, no such examples were included in this study. It is more difficult to imagine a realistic example where p – 2 was the correct value of m and no such examples were included in this study. These values are better treated as indicators of method misperformance. For the regression equation methods, the value of $p - 2$ could occur when the observed eigenvalues remained greater than the estimated eigenvalues until $p - 2$ components were retained, the maximum possible value. There were 22 occurrences of this situation with the Allen and Hubbard (1986) equation and 12 occurrences with the Lautenschlager, Lance, and Flaherty (1989) equation.

For all the parallel analysis and MAP methods, zero was the minimum possible value that could be obtained. For the six parallel analysis methods, whenever the first randomly generated, estimated, or tabled eigenvalue is greater than the first eigenvalue of the observed data, the method indicates 0 components. The three minimum average partial correlation methods may also give 0 as a value for the number of components. The average correlation of the correlation matrix before any components are partialed out is used as the initial minimum value that is compared to the subsequent values of the partial correlation matrix. A value of 0 is given for m when the partialling out of components does not result in a reduced value for the correlation matrix.

The situations in which the value of 0 occurred were consistent across all methods. The situations occurred at the lower variables per component ratio (55 out of 57 at $p{:}m = 4{:}1$) and at lower component saturation (55 cases at CS = .40, 2 cases at CS = .60). Among the parallel analysis methods, solutions of $m = 0$ occurred twice for the Lautenschlager, Lance, and Flaherty equation (1989) and once for the random data generation with 5 replications, random data generation with 100 replications, and the tabled eigenvalues method. For the MAP methods, there were 38, 13, and 1 solutions of $m = 0$ for the trace of the squared matrix of partial correlations, the trace of the matrix of partial correlations to the fourth power, and the largest root of the matrix of partial correlations, respectively.

Once these inappropriate values were eliminated, the first measure of method performance was examined with the data collapsed across all levels of the four factors (N, p, $p{:}m$, and cs). Figure 3 summarizes the number of cases out of a possible 270, where each method produced a legitimate estimate.

The two random data generation parallel analysis methods, two of the MAP methods, and the eigenvalue greater than one rule produced an estimate on 95.2 to 100% of the matrices. The other methods produced an estimate in fewer cases, due to either the presence of inappropriate values or the limitations of the methods. The tabled eigenvalues method produced an estimate in 88.5% of the matrices. Tabled values were not available for $N = 75$ and $p = 72$. The three parallel analysis regression methods produced an estimate for 58.5 to 66.7% of the matrices. The application of the equation approach is limited to the range of values of N and p on which the equations were developed. Since 50 is the maximum number of variables for the three regression equations, the conditions of $p = 72$ and $N = 75$, 150, and 300 had to be omitted from the examination.

On the three other measures of method performance, all methods except the Kaiser rule performed well. The methods that exhibited the best performance, as indicated by lower average deviation score, lower variability, and a higher percent of correct estimates were also the methods with valid estimates for the greatest number of cases.

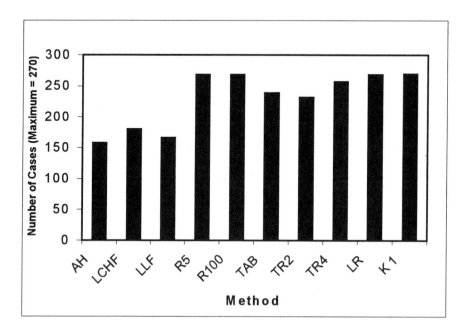

Figure 3. The number of cases (out of a possible 270) where each of the ten methods produced a legitimate estimate of M.

Second Comparison

The methods were next compared on only those cases where all ten methods produced an estimate. The number of cases for this comparison was 137, or 50.7%. The results of this second comparison will be described briefly.

On the three remaining measures of method performance, a consistent pattern of results was observed across the measures. The six parallel analysis methods and the MAP trace of the matrix of partial correlations to the fourth power were highly accurate. The Kaiser rule and the MAP largest root method were the least accurate.

The mean of the deviation from the correct value ranged from -.13 to .07 for the most accurate methods. Figure 4 illustrates this result.

For the percent of correct estimates, the eight most accurate methods produced accuracy rates close to 90%. Figure 5 illustrates the percent of cases where the methods produced exactly the correct estimate for m.

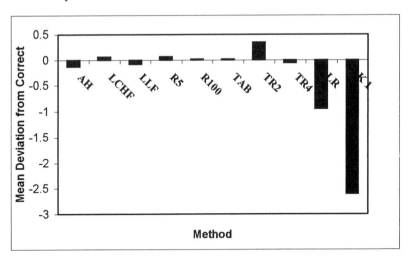

Figure 4. The mean deviation from the correct value of M for each of the ten methods.

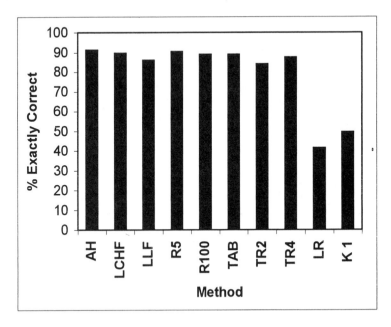

Figure 5. The percent of cases where each of the ten methods produced an exactly accurate estimate of M.

The same pattern of results was observed for the estimate of the deviation of the sample estimate from the population value for m. Figure 6 illustrates the results of this comparison. The first eight methods were all highly accurate. The Kaiser Rule and the MAP procedure based on the largest root were the most inaccurate with the Kaiser Rule overestimating the correct value by an average of 2.6 components. Among the MAP procedures, the trace to the fourth power was the best on this comparison.

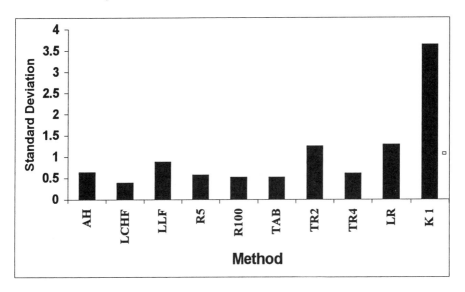

Figure 6. The standard deviation of the estimates produced by each of the ten methods.

SUMMARY AND ANALYSIS

In the first two sections of this chapter, we reviewed the most frequently recommended procedures for determining the number of factors or components to retain. In the third part of this chapter, we reviewed a recent empirical study that focused on different versions of three of these methods. Previously, we evaluated each procedure on the basis of three criteria: Rationale, the justification for the procedure; Implementation, the ease of use; and Performance, the extent to which the procedure is likely to produce the correct answer. We will now review the performance of the variations of the three methods with respect to both accuracy and the number of cases where the method produced an estimate. The next three sections discuss the eigenvalue greater than one rule, the six parallel analysis methods, and the three MAP versions.

Eigenvalue Greater Than One Rule

Performance. The eigenvalue greater than one rule was the least accurate and most variable of all methods. It consistently overestimated the number of components to retain. With the exception of the largest root MAP version, the eigenvalue greater than one rule also had the fewest percent of correct estimates.

Number of Cases. A strength of this method is the number of cases to which the method can be applied. Since this method relies only upon an examination of the eigenvalues, it can be performed on all cases.

Parallel Analysis Methods

Performance. Six variations of parallel analysis were examined. All of the versions produced very accurate estimates of the number of components to retain. Several problems with the regression equations were observed. The Allen & Hubbard (1986) equation and the Lautenschlager, Lance, & Flaherty (1989) equation gave the number of components as p-2 in some of the cases. It is problematic that these two regression equation methods do not give a viable solution in these conditions. A warning to the user that the observed eigenvalues never crossed the random eigenvalues would be helpful for interpreting the solution.

Linear interpolation from the tables of mean criterion eigenvalues provided by Lautenschlager (1989a) was also found to be an accurate method for determining the number of components. While it was comparable in accuracy to the regression equations, interpolation of the tabled values does not exhibit the problems of the regression equations.

The random data generation method was less accurate, more variable, and had the fewest percent of correct estimates of the parallel analysis methods when cases of $m = 0$ or $m = p - 2$ were excluded. After examining the six parallel analysis methods only for the cases where all methods apply, the performance of the random generation method was comparable or better than the other four methods. The use of 100 instead of 5 random correlation matrices only marginally improved the accuracy of the method.

Number of Cases. The variations of parallel analysis differed on the number of cases that were examined for each method. The random data generation method was applied with the total number of correlation matrices in this study, 270. After excluding those solutions of $m = 0$, this method gave estimates for 99.6% of the matrices.

The tabled eigenvalues method could be used on 240 of the 270 correlation matrices. The further reduction for the one case of an estimation of $m = 0$ resulted in this method being employed on 88.5% of the 270 matrices.

The regression equations were implemented on the fewest number of the correlation matrices. The three equations are limited to the values of N and p from which they were developed. The three equations were applied to 180 of the 270 matrices. After excluding the solutions of $m = 0$ and $m = p - 2$, the equations gave viable solutions for 58.5% to 66.7% of the correlation matrices. This limitation is a considerable factor in selecting a decision method. Since the three regression equations, and to a lesser extent, the tabled eigenvalue method could not be applied to all cases, it could be argued that the study was designed to the disadvantage of these methods. However, the fact that these procedures do not apply to many cases represents a real drawback to their use on a wide variety of problems. Since initial correlation matrices of 100, 200 or even 300 variables are fairly common, these procedures would be precluded from many regular applications.

MAP Rules

Performance. The performance of the three versions of the minimum average partial correlation method were examined and found to give estimates of m of varying accuracy. Overall, the largest root of the matrix of partial correlations produced was the least accurate of the MAP methods. The trace of the matrix of partial correlations to the fourth power generally performed better than the original method, the trace of the squared matrix of partial correlations. It was more accurate, less variable, and had a greater percent of correct estimates across conditions, although often the difference between the two methods was very slight.

Number of Cases. The three MAP methods were applied to all of the correlation matrices generated in this study. After excluding those cases with a value of $m = 0$, the three methods estimated the number of components for 85.9%, 95.2%, and 99.6% of the 270 matrices for the trace of the squared matrix of partial correlations, the trace of the partial correlation matrix to the fourth power, and the largest root of the partial correlation matrix, respectively.

Conclusions

On the basis of the review of the literature and results of this and previous empirical evaluation, we have reached the following conclusions.

1. Of the methods examined, the MAP methods have the strongest rationale.
2. The eigenvalue greater than one rule is the easiest decision method to implement.
3. The MAP methods, the random data generation parallel analysis method, and the eigenvalue greater than one rule were implemented on all 270 correlation matrices and, therefore, demonstrated the widest applicability.
4. The parallel analysis methods were the most accurate, followed closely by the MAP methods.

5. The eigenvalue greater than one rule was extremely inaccurate and was the most variable of all the methods. Continued use of this method is not recommended.
6. The largest root variation of the three MAP methods had the greatest averaged accuracy, but also the lowest percent of correct estimates.
7. The trace of the matrix of partial correlations to the fourth power performed better than the original MAP version (the trace of the squared matrix of partial correlations.)
8. When solutions of $m = 0$ or $m = p - 2$ were excluded, the three regression equations and the tabled eigenvalues performed better than the random data generation method of parallel analysis.
9. When compared on the same cases, the random data generation with 100 replications and the tabled eigenvalues method displayed the best overall performance of the parallel analysis methods.

General Guidelines.

On the basis of this review of the available methods and the results of the existing empirical assessments, we can provide researchers with some guidelines for determining the number of factors or components to retain. First, if the researcher prefers factor analysis to component analysis, it would still be advisable to perform a component analysis in the initial stages of the analysis and use one of the component methods to guide the choice of m since no satisfactory alternatives are available within factor analysis. Second, a combination of MAP and Parallel Analysis should be employed. Third, scree may be a useful adjunct. Fourth, the methods should be used as a guide but not the final solution. The interpretability of the final solution is critical. If MAP and PA procedures indicate the retention of a component but it is not well identified and interpretable, adding additional measures of that construct and a second administration is recommended. Velicer and Fava (1998) provide guidance about variable and subject sampling. Sixth, continued use of the Kaiser rule is not recommended and this method should be eliminated as the default option from statistical software packages.

NOTES

This research was partially supported by grants CA 50087, CA 63045, and CA 27821 from the National Cancer Institute. For further information, contact Wayne F. Velicer, Cancer Prevention Research Center, 2 Chafee Rd., University of Rhode Island, Kingston, RI 02881. E-mail address: VELICER@URI.EDU. Website: WWW.URI.EDU/RESEARCH/CPRC

[1] Available from the authors of this paper.

REFERENCES

Allen, S. J & Hubbard, R. (1986). Regression equations for the latent roots of random data correlation matrices with unities on the diagonal. *Multivariate Behavioral Research, 21*, 393-398.

Anderson, R. D., Acito, F. & Lee, H. (1982). A simulation study of three methods for determining the number of image components. *Multivariate Behavioral Research*, **17**, 493-502.

Bartlett, M. S. (1950). Tests of significance in factor analysis. *British Journal of Psychology, Statistical Section*, **3**, 77-85.

Bartlett, M. S. (1951). A further note on tests of significance in factor analysis *British Journal of Psychology, Statistical Section*, **4**, 1-2.

Bentler, P. M. (1980). Multivariate analysis with latent variables: Causal modeling. In M. R. Rosenzweig & L. W. Porter (eds.), *Annual Review of Psychology*, (pp. 419-454). Stanford, CA: Annual Reviews, Inc.

Bentler, P.M. & Kano, Y, (1990). On the equivalence of factors and components. *Multivariate Behavioral Research*, **51**, 67-74.

Bookstein, F. L. (1990). Least squares and latent variables. *Multivariate Behavioral Research*, **25**, 75-80.

Boomsma, A. (1983). *On the robustness of LISREL (maximum likelihood) estimates against small sample sizes and non-normality.* Unpublished doctoral dissertation, kijksuniversiteit Gronigen, the Netherlands.

Cattell, R. B. (1966). The scree test for the number of factors. *Multivariate Behavioral Research*, **1**, 245-276.

Cattell, R. B. & Jaspers, J. (1967). A general plasmode for factor analytic exercises and research. *Multivariate Behavioral Research Monographs*, **3**, 1-212.

Cattell, R. B. & Vogelmann, S. A. (1977). A comprehensive trial of the scree and Kaiser-Guttman criteria for determining the number of factors. *Multivariate Behavioral Research*, **12**, 289-325.

Cliff, N. (1970). The relation between sample and population characteristic vectors. *Psychometrika*, **35**, 163-178.

Cliff, N. (1988). The eigenvalue greater than one rule and the reliability of components. *Psychological Bulletin*, **103**, 276-279.

Cliff, N. & Hamburger, C. (1967). Study of sampling errors in factor analysis by means of artificial experiments. *Psychological Bulletin*, **68**, 430-445.

Crawford, C. B. & Koopman, P. (1973). A note on Horn's test for the number of factors in factor analysis. *Multivariate Behavioral Research*, **8**, 117-125.

Eaton, C. A., Velicer, W. F., & Fava, J. L. (1999). *Determining the Number of Components: An Evaluation of Parallel Analysis and the Minimum Average Partial Correlation Procedures.* Manuscript under review.

Fava, J. L., & Velicer, W.F. (1992a). An empirical comparison of factor, image, component, and scale scores. *Multivariate Behavioral Research*, **27**, 301-322.

Fava, J. L., & Velicer, W.F. (1992b). The effects of overextraction on factor and component analysis. *Multivariate Behavioral Research*, **27**, 387-415.

Fava, J. L., & Velicer, W.F. (1996). The effects of underextraction in factor and component analysis. *Educational and Psychological Measurement*, **56**, 907-929.

Gorsuch, R. L. (1973). Using Bartlett's significance test to determine the number of factors to extract. *Educational and Psychological Measurement*, **33**, 361-364.

Gorsuch, R. L. (1983). *Factor Analysis. (2nd ed.)* Hillsdale, N. J.: Lawrence Erlbaum.

Gorsuch, R. L. (1991). *UniMult Guide.* Altadena, CA: UniMult.

Guttman, L. (1990). Common factor analysis versus component analysisSome well and little known facts. *Multivariate Behavioral Research*, **25**, 33-39.

Guttman, L. (1954). Some necessary conditions for common factor analysis. *Psychometrika*, **19**, 149-162.

Guadagnoli, E. & Velicer, W. F. (1988). Relation of sample size to the stability of component patterns. *Psychological Bulletin*, **103**, 265-275.

Guadagnoli, E. & Velicer, W. (1991). A comparison of pattern matching indices. *Multivariate Behavioral Research*, **26**, 323-343.

Hakstian, A. R., Rogers, W. T., & Cattell, R. B. (1982). The behavior of number-of-factors rules with simulated data. *Multivariate Behavioral Research*, **17**, 193-219.

Hays, R. D. (1987). PARALLEL: A program for performing parallel analysis. *Applied Psychological Measurement*, **11**, 58.

Holden, R. R., Longman, R. S., Cota, A. A., & Fekken, G. C. (1989). PAR: Parallel analysis routine for random data eigenvalue estimation. *Applied Psychological Measurement*, **13**, 192.

Horn, J.L. (1965). A Rationale and test for the number of factors in factor analysis *Psychometrika*, **30**, 179-185.

Horn, J.L. & Engstrom, R. (1979). Cattell's scree test in relation to Bartlett's chi-square test and other observations on the number of factors problem. *Multivariate Behavioral Research*, **14**, 283-300.

Howe, H. G. (1955). *Some contributions to factor analysis.* Oak Ridge, TH: Oak Ridge National Laboratory.

Hubbard, R. & Allen, S. J. (1987). An empirical comparison of alternate methods for principal components extraction. *Journal of Business Research*, **15**, 173-190.

Jackson, D.N. (1970). A sequential system for personality scale development. In C.D. Spielberger (Ed.), *Current Topics in Clinical and Community Psychology*, (Vol. 2, pp. 61-96). New York: Academic Press.

Jackson, D. N. (1971). The dynamics of structured personality tests. *Psychological Review*, **78**, 229-248.

Jackson, D. N., & Chan, D. W. (1980). Maximum-likelihood estimation in common factor analysisA cautionary note. *Psychological Bulletin*, **88**, 502-508.

Kaiser, H. F. (1960). The application of electronic computers to factor analysis. *Educational and Psychological Measurement*, **20**, 141-151.

Lautenschlager, G. J. (1989a). A comparison of alternatives to conducting Monte Carlo analyses for determining parallel analysis criteria. *Multivariate Behavioral Research*, **24**, 365-395.

Lautenschlager, G. J. (1989b). PARANAL.TOK: A program for developing parallel analysis criteria. *Applied Psychological Measurement*, **13**, 176.

Lautenschlager, G. J., Lance, C. E., & Flaherty, V. L. (1989). Parallel analysis criteria: Revised equations for estimating the latent roots of random data correlation matrices. *Educational and Psychological Measurement*, **49**, 339-345.

Lee, H. B. & Comrey, A. L. (1979). Distortions in a commonly used factor analytic procedure. *Multivariate Behavioral Research*, **14**, 301-321.

Linn, R. L. (1968). A Monte Carlo approach to the number of factors problem. *Psychometrika*, **33**, 37-71.

Loehlin, J.C. (1990). Component analysis versus common factor analysis: A case of disputed authorship. *Multivariate Behavioral Research*, **25**, 29-31.

Longman, R. S., Cota, A. A., Holden, R. R., & Fekken, G. C. (1989a). A regressionequation for the parallel analysis criterion in principal components analysis: Mean and 95th percentile eigenvalues. *Multivariate Behavioral Research*, **24**, 59-69.

Longman, R. S., Cota, A. A., Holden, R. R., & Fekken, G. C. (1989b). PAM: A double precision FORTRAN routine for the parallel analysis method in principal components analysis. *Behavior Research Methods, Instruments, and Computers*, **21**, 477-480.

Longman, R. S., Cota, A. A., Holden, R. R., & Fekken, G. C. (1991). *Implementing parallel analysis for principal components analysis: A comparison of six methods*. Unpublished manuscript.

Longman, R. S., Holden, R. R., & Fekken, G. C. (1991). Anomalies in the Allen and Hubbard parallel analysis procedure. *Applied Psychological Measurement*, **15**, 95-97.

MacCallum, R. C., Widaman, K. F., Zhang, S., & Hong, S. (1999). Sample size in factor analysis. *Psychological Methods*, **4**, 84-99.

Marsh, H.W., Balla, J. R., & McDonald, R. P. (1988). Goodness of fit indices in confirmatory factor analysis: The effect of sample size. *Psychological Bulletin*, **103**, 391-410.

McArdle, J.J. (1990). Principles versus principals of structural factor analysis. *Multivariate Behavioral Research*, **25**, 81-87.

Montanelli, Jr., R. G. (1975). A computer program to generate sample correlation and covariance matrices. *Educational and Psychological Measurement*, **35**, 195-197.

Montanelli, Jr., R. G. & Humphreys, L. G. (1976). Latent roots of random data correlation matrices with squared multiple correlations on the diagonal: A Monte Carlo study. *Psychometrika*, **41**, 341-348.

Morrison, D. F. (1976). *Multivariate Statistical Methods.* (2nd ed.). New York: McGraw-Hill

Mulaik, S.A. (1990). Blurring the distinctions between component analysisand common factor analysis *Multivariate Behavioral Research*, **25**, 53-59.

Odell, P. L. & Feiveson, A. H. (1966). A numerical procedure to generate a sample covariance matrix. *Journal of the American Statistical Association*, **61**, 199-203.

Reddon, J. R. (1985). MAPF and MAPS: Subroutines for the number of principal components. *Applied Psychological Measurement*, **9**, 97.

Revelle, W. & Rocklin, T. (1979). Very simple structure: An alternative procedure for estimating the optimal number of interpretable factors. *Multivariate Behavioral Research*, **14**, 403-414.

Rozeboom, W.W. (1990). Whatever happened to broad perspective? *Multivariate Behavioral Research*, **25**, 61-65.

Schonemann, P. H. (1990). Facts, fictions, and common sense about factors and components. *Multivariate Behavioral Research*, **25**, 47-51.

Steiger, J.H. (1990). Some additional thoughts on components, factors, and factor indeterminacy. *Multivariate Behavioral Research*, **25**, 47-51.

Tucker, L. R., Koopman, R. F., & Linn, R. L. (1969). Evaluation of factor analytic research procedures by means of simulated correlation matrices. *Psychometrika*, **34**, 421-459.

Tucker, L. R., & Lewis, C. (1973). A reliability coefficient for maximum likelihoodfactor analysis. *Psychometrika*, **38**, 1-10.

Velicer, W. F. (1976). Determining the number of components from the matrix of partial correlations. *Psychometrika*, **31**, 321-327.

Velicer, W. F. & Fava, J. L. (1987). An evaluation of the effects of variable sampling on component, image, and factor analysis. *Multivariate Behavioral Research*, **22**, 193-209.

Velicer, W. F. & Fava, J. S. (1998). The effects of variable and subject sampling on factor pattern recovery. *Psychological Methods*, **3**, 231-251.

Velicer, W. F., Fava, J. L., Zwick, W. R., & Harrop, J. W. (1990). *CAX* (Computer program). Kingston, RI: University of Rhode Island.

Velicer, W. F., & Jackson, D. N. (1990a). Component analysis versus common factor analysis: Some issues in selecting an appropriate procedure. *Multivariate Behavioral Research*, **25**, 1-28.

Velicer, W. F., & Jackson, D. N. (1990b). Component analysis versus common factor analysissome further observations. *Multivariate Behavioral Research*, **25**, 97-114.

Velicer, W. F., Peacock, A. C., & Jackson, D. N. (1982). A comparison of component and factor patterns: A Monte Carlo approach. *Multivariate Behavioral Research*, **17**, 371-388.

Widaman, K. F. (1990). Bias in pattern loadings represented by common factor analysis and component analysis*Multivariate Behavioral Research*, **25**, 89-95.

Wood, J.M., Tataryn, D. J., & Gorsuch, R. L. (1996). Effects of Under- and overextraction on principal axis factor analysis with varimax rotation. *Psychological Methods*, **1**, 254-365.

Yeomans, K. A. & Golder, P. A. (1982). The Guttman-Kaiser criterion as a predictor of the number of common factors. *The Statistician*, **31**, 221-229.

Zwick, W. R. & Velicer W. F. (1982). Factors influencing four rules for determining the number of components to retain. *Multivariate Behavioral Research*, **17**, 253-269.

Zwick, W. R. & Velicer W. F. (1986). Comparison of five rules for determining the number of components to retain. *Psychological Bulletin*, **99**, 432-442.

4 IMPROVED STANDARD ERRORS OF STANDARDIZED PARAMETERS IN COVARIANCE STRUCTURE MODELS: IMPLICATIONS FOR CONSTRUCT EXPLICATION

Mortaza Jamshidian
Peter M. Bentler[1]

INTRODUCTION

Because measurement scales of observed variables in social and behavioral sciences are often arbitrary, and because the sample correlation matrix, unlike the sample covariance matrix, is scale independent, analyses of correlation structures based on sample correlation matrices are desirable, and often done (e.g., Velicer & Jackson, 1990; Goffin & Jackson, 1992). The problem is that most popular covariance structure software is built around the sampling theory designed to analyze covariance structures. This theory is based on the multivariate sampling distribution of a covariance matrix, which is not the same as that of a correlation matrix. A number of papers have addressed problems relevant to this issue in the contexts of exploratory factor analysis (EFA), and confirmatory factor analysis (CFA). These address problems of parameter estimation, tests of hypotheses, and standard error estimation. Our main focus here will be on the problem of standard error estimation. This is critical to accurate decision-making regarding the interpretation of constructs and the necessity of parameters such as factor loadings as indicators of such constructs. Since typical practice in factor analysis is to interpret a factor by its highly loading variables in a standardized solution, it is also important to verify that such loadings are statistically significantly different from zero. For example, if one uses confirmatory factor analysis in a sequential system for personality scale construction (e.g., Jackson, 1970), it would be essential to be able to determine whether or not the loading of a particular item on the trait factor that it is hypothesized to reflect is significantly different from zero. Furthermore, confirmatory factor analyses of the higher-order structure of personality scales (e.g., Jackson, Paunonen, Fraboni, & Goffin, 1996) could not be meaningfully interpreted in the absence of accurate estimates of the standard errors of the parameters. The previous examples are only two of a multitude of possible examples where the estimation of standard errors assumes a prominent role in the evaluation of construct validity. In this paper, we provide some new methods to achieve this purpose.

When fitting covariance structure models, several approaches may be taken. The typical one is to fit the sample covariance matrix to the model, and then standardize the parameter estimates. An overriding motivation for this standardization is the problem of construct interpretation. For example, when fitting a factor analysis model one can obtain maximum likelihood estimates (MLE) by fitting the sample covariance, and then standardize the factor loadings. The standardized factor loadings are then also maximum likelihood estimates of their population counterpart. In addition, they are more interpretable. Not only are they scale independent, but standardized regression coefficients (factor loadings) and correlations among factors are easier to interpret than their unstandardized counterparts. Without meaningful scales for variables and factors, it is impossible to know whether a loading of, say, 6.3 is large and validates the interpretation of a construct. In contrast, it is much easier to conclude that a standardized regression coefficient of .8 is large, because standardized coefficients are inherently meaningful to most behavioral scientists. Nonetheless, in spite of the importance of standardized solutions, it is not widely appreciated that even regression programs almost never provide standard errors for standardized coefficients. Most likely this is because standard errors of standardized parameters, in general, are not a simple rescaling of the standard errors of the original parameter estimates. They require special computation, as we shall see.

Another approach is to fit the sample correlation matrix to the model, treating it as a sample covariance matrix of standardized observed variables. The idea is that since the analyzed observed variables in this case are scale-free, the parameter estimates will be scale free as well. Among others, Cudeck (1989) spells out the possible shortcomings of this approach with regard to parameter estimates, tests of hypotheses, and standard errors in the context of restricted covariance structure modeling. In a recent paper Yuan and Bentler (in press) also reviewed the literature relevant to fitting a sample correlation matrix, and discussed the problem of standard error estimation under various exploratory factor analysis models.

A third approach is to directly use the theory of the asymptotic distribution of correlations and to fit a structure directly to these correlations (e.g., Shapiro & Browne, 1990). This approach was implemented and evaluated in a study by Leung and Chan (1997) and found to be very promising. There is no issue about standardizing variables in this approach, however, standardizing factors representing constructs is not necessarily easy. While it is straightforward in the factor model, where factor variances can be arbitrarily set to 1.0, more general latent variable models such as the Bentler-Weeks (1980) or LISREL (Jöreskog

& Sörbom, 1988) models contain latent dependent variables that cannot be standardized without a complex nonlinear constraint routine. Steiger (1995) has emphasized the value of this approach.

To expand on the second approach a bit more, we introduce the properties of *scale invariance*, and *scale equivariance* that are commonly used in statistical literature (e.g., Lehmann & Casella 1998)[2]. Let $\mathcal{X} = (x_1, \cdots, x_N)$ be a sample of size N from a p-variate random variable which is parameterized by $\boldsymbol{\theta}$. Let $x_i^* = T(x_i)$, where $T(\cdot)$ is an arbitrary transformation. Then usually the counterpart of $\boldsymbol{\theta}$, corresponding to x_i^*'s, is $\boldsymbol{\theta}^* = \mathbf{h}(\boldsymbol{\theta})$, for some function $\mathbf{h}$ (e.g., Lehmann & Casella 1998, Chapter 3). Let $\widehat{\boldsymbol{\theta}} = M(\mathcal{X})$, be an estimator of $\boldsymbol{\theta}$, and similarly let $\widehat{\boldsymbol{\theta}}^* = M(\mathcal{X}^*)$. If $\mathbf{h}(\boldsymbol{\theta}) = \boldsymbol{\theta}$ and $\widehat{\boldsymbol{\theta}}^* = \widehat{\boldsymbol{\theta}}$, then the estimator M is said to be scale invariant with respect to transformation T. On the other hand, when $\mathbf{h}(\boldsymbol{\theta}) \neq \boldsymbol{\theta}$ and the estimator M satisfies $\widehat{\boldsymbol{\theta}}^* = M(\mathcal{X}^*) = \mathbf{h}(M(\mathcal{X})) = \mathbf{h}(\boldsymbol{\theta}^*)$, then the estimator is said to be equivariant with respect to the transformation T. In our context T is the transformation that scales the observed variables to have variance 1, and $\mathbf{h}$ is the transformation that scales the relevant latent variables to have variance 1.

If $x_i = \Lambda\xi + \epsilon$, under the usual assumption that the factors ξ are uncorrelated with the errors ϵ, the covariance structure

$$\Sigma = \Lambda\Phi\Lambda^T + \Psi,$$

results. As is usual in CFA, elements of the parameters (Λ, Φ, Ψ) may be fixed to arbitrary values and Ψ is assumed to be diagonal. The diagonal elements of Φ give the variances of the factors, which need not be 1.0. We denote the corresponding vector of free parameters by $\boldsymbol{\theta}$. Let $\widehat{\boldsymbol{\theta}} = (\hat{\Lambda}, \hat{\Phi}, \hat{\Psi})$ denote the MLE of $\boldsymbol{\theta}$ when the sample covariance matrix is fit, and let $\tilde{\boldsymbol{\theta}} = (\tilde{\Lambda}, \tilde{\Phi}, \tilde{\Psi})$ be the estimates obtained from a maximum likelihood procedure, when the sample correlation matrix is fit. If θ_i, the i-th parameter, is invariant with respect to MLE, then $\tilde{\theta}_i = \widehat{\theta}_i$, and the standard errors for this parameter in both procedures will be the same. On the other hand, if θ_i is equivariant with respect to MLE, then a simple rescaling of both $\tilde{\theta}_i$ and $\widehat{\theta}_i$ will lead to the same standardized estimate, however, in this case the same rescaling of standard errors generally will not lead to correct standard errors of the standardized parameter estimates. Finally, in some cases, θ_i is neither invariant nor equivariant. In these cases fitting the correlation matrix will lead to both erroneous parameter estimates and standard errors. Cudeck (1989) has given examples of each case and a detailed discussion.

While there are standard examples of invariant and equivariant models and parameters with respect to maximum likelihood estimation, in general it is not easy to identify whether a model or parameter possesses these properties. An alternative, proposed e.g., by Jöreskog (1978), is to fit a model of the form

$$\Sigma = D_\sigma P D_\sigma,$$

where P has the factor analysis structure defined above, and D_σ is a diagonal matrix with free parameters to be estimated. This structure is equivariant. It is fitted to data and the nonlinear restrictions $\text{diag}(P) = I$ are imposed, making P the population correlation matrix. This will lead to both correct parameter and standard error estimates. However, imposing the nonlinear restrictions can be in general difficult and costly. Browne and DuToit (1992) and Jamshidian and Bentler (1993) give methods of imposing nonlinear constraints when fitting covariance structure models.

In view of the above discussion, to insure appropriate parameter estimates and standard errors, a good approach is to fit the sample covariance matrix, standardize the parameter estimates, and correctly compute the standard errors for the standardized parameters. Browne (1982) seems to be the only reference that gives standard error estimates for the standardized factor loadings and uniquenesses for the confirmatory factor model. He gave formulas for the special case where $\Phi = I$ is fixed. It is easy to show that his estimates are based on what is referred to as the delta method (see e.g., Cudeck & O'Dell, 1994, for a discussion). Another approach to estimating the standard error of standardized variables is to use the bootstrap (Efron, 1982). This approach is apparently used in AMOS (Arbuckle, 1997). However, a criticism of it is that its computational cost can be very high. Also, there are many varieties of bootstrap methods, and it is not guaranteed that a standard bootstrap will always work reliably (e.g., Yung & Bentler, 1996).

Our focus here will be on restricted covariance structure models, and in particular our examples and discussions will focus on the confirmatory factor analysis model. We will give a general description of the delta method and provide the necessary formulas for a general CFA model. We examine a second order correction to the delta method, and give the necessary formulae. Additionally we will propose two hybrid methods that use bootstrap and linear approximations of the standardized parameters. In each case we will examine the efficiency, as well as accuracy of each estimator using three structures, with three varying sample sizes.

METHODS

In this section we will describe four methods of estimating the variance of the estimates of standardized parameters in covariance structure analysis. We will describe the methods in a general framework and give details for their implementation for the CFA model. Their extension to more general covariance structures will be obvious for some of the methods, and for others will require extra derivation of derivative formulas.

The Delta Method and a Quadratic Correction

Let λ_{ij}, ϕ_{ij}, $\psi_{i,j}$ denote the (i,j)th element of each of the matrices Λ, Φ, and Ψ respectively. The standardized parameters in each case are given by

[1]
$$\lambda_{ij}^* = \frac{\lambda_{ij}\phi_{jj}^{1/2}}{\sigma_{ii}^{1/2}}$$

$$\phi_{ij}^* = \frac{\phi_{ij}}{\phi_{ii}^{1/2}\phi_{jj}^{1/2}}$$

$$\psi_{ii}^* = \frac{\psi_{ii}}{\sigma_{ii}}$$

where

$$\sigma_{ii} = \sum_{k=1}^{m}\sum_{l=1}^{m}\lambda_{ik}\lambda_{il}\phi_{kl} + \psi_{ii}$$

is the i-th diagonal element of Σ. Note that ψ_{ii}^* is not fully standardized in the sense that the unique variate has not been transformed to unit variance, as would occur in a Sewell Wright type of standardization (e.g., Chou & Bentler, 1993). In that case, the variance parameter ψ_{ii} would become transformed to a standardized regression coefficient, but in factor analysis this type of standardization is usually not interesting. Let $\widehat{\theta} = (\hat{\Lambda}, \hat{\Phi}, \hat{\Psi})$ be an estimate of $\theta = (\Lambda, \Phi, \Psi)$. Then an estimate of the standardized parameters can be obtained by plugging-in the $\widehat{\theta}$ estimates in the formulas given in [1]. We denote the standardized estimates by $\widehat{\theta}^* = (\hat{\Lambda}^*, \hat{\Phi}^*, \hat{\Psi}^*)$. The form of the standardized parameters in the more general LISREL covariance structure model (Jöreskog & Sörbom, 1988) is for example given by Chou and Bentler (1993) and Bollen (1989, page 350). The problem that we consider here is that of obtaining standard errors for $\widehat{\theta}^*$.

We describe the problem in a general setting. Let $\hat{\theta}$ be an element of $\widehat{\theta}$, and $\hat{\theta}^*$ be the corresponding standardized element in $\widehat{\theta}^*$. Then $\hat{\theta}^* = h(\theta)$, where h is the function that transforms $\hat{\theta}$ to its standardized form. Assume that $\text{var}(\widehat{\theta}) = \Omega$. Since h is generally a nonlinear function of $\widehat{\theta}$, $\text{var}[h(\widehat{\theta})]$ is not an obvious function of Ω. The delta method is a common methodology used to approximate variance of nonlinear functions of random variables. It uses the first order Taylor expansion of $h(\widehat{\theta})$ around the true population parameter θ. This can be written as

[2]
$$h(\widehat{\theta}) \approx h(\theta) + (\widehat{\theta} - \theta)^T \dot{h}(\theta),$$

where we are assuming that θ and $\widehat{\theta}$ are column vectors, and $\dot{h}(\theta)$ is the column vector of the gradient of h evaluated at $\boldsymbol{\theta}$. Now using the approximation [2] we get

[3] $$\text{var}[h(\widehat{\boldsymbol{\theta}})] \approx \dot{h}(\boldsymbol{\theta})^T \Omega \dot{h}(\boldsymbol{\theta}).$$

Of course in practice $\boldsymbol{\theta}$ and Ω are not known, so the delta-method estimate will be

$$\widehat{\text{var}}[h(\widehat{\boldsymbol{\theta}})] = \dot{h}(\widehat{\boldsymbol{\theta}})^T \widehat{\Omega} \dot{h}(\widehat{\boldsymbol{\theta}}),$$

where $\widehat{\boldsymbol{\theta}}$ and $\widehat{\Omega}$ are usually unbiased, or asymptotically unbiased estimates of $\boldsymbol{\theta}$ and Ω. For example in the case where maximum likelihood estimation is used, $\widehat{\boldsymbol{\theta}}$ are the MLEs and $\widehat{\Omega}$ may be based on the Fisher or the observed information matrix.

The main ingredient needed to obtain the delta method approximation of variance of the standardized estimates, assuming that $\widehat{\boldsymbol{\theta}}$ and $\widehat{\Omega}$ are known, is the derivatives $\dot{h}(\boldsymbol{\theta})$. The necessary derivatives for the factor model are given in the Appendix. As noted in the introduction, Browne (1982) gave formulas for the variances for the standardized estimates of the factor model when $\Phi = I$. His formulas on the outset look different from the delta method estimates, as given here. It can be shown, however, that they are equal to these in the special case considered by him.

While, as we will see, in many cases the delta method gives good estimates of the variance of $\widehat{\boldsymbol{\theta}}^*$, there are cases where the linear approximation [2] does not hold well. It is natural in these cases to consider a two-term Taylor expansion. This is given by

[4] $$h(\widehat{\boldsymbol{\theta}}) \approx h(\boldsymbol{\theta}) + (\widehat{\boldsymbol{\theta}} - \boldsymbol{\theta})^T \dot{h}(\boldsymbol{\theta}) + \tfrac{1}{2}(\widehat{\boldsymbol{\theta}} - \boldsymbol{\theta})^T \ddot{h}(\boldsymbol{\theta})(\widehat{\boldsymbol{\theta}} - \boldsymbol{\theta}),$$

where $\ddot{h}(\boldsymbol{\theta})$ is the Hessian (matrix of second order derivatives) of h evaluated at $\boldsymbol{\theta}$. For simplicity, let $l(\widehat{\boldsymbol{\theta}})$ and $q(\widehat{\boldsymbol{\theta}})$ be the linear and quadratic terms in [4]. Then using the approximation [4] we have

$$\text{var}[h(\widehat{\boldsymbol{\theta}})] \approx \text{var}[l(\widehat{\boldsymbol{\theta}})] + \frac{1}{4}\text{var}[q(\widehat{\boldsymbol{\theta}})] + \text{cov}[l(\widehat{\boldsymbol{\theta}}), q(\widehat{\boldsymbol{\theta}})].$$

The delta method estimate [3] can be used to estimate $\text{var}[l(\widehat{\boldsymbol{\theta}})]$. Without any distributional assumptions on $\widehat{\boldsymbol{\theta}}$, and assuming finite fourth moments, the second term in [4] can be computed, but it will involve fourth moments that are generally computationally intractable. However, if the normality assumption $\widehat{\boldsymbol{\theta}} \sim \mathcal{N}(\boldsymbol{\theta}, \Omega)$ is reasonable and is made, then using standard multivariate statistics results (e.g., Schott 1997, Chapter 9) we obtain

$$\text{var}[q(\widehat{\boldsymbol{\theta}})] = 2\text{trace}[(\ddot{h}(\boldsymbol{\theta})\Omega)^2],$$

and as we show in the Appendix

[5] $$\operatorname{cov}[l(\widehat{\theta}), q(\widehat{\theta})] = 0.$$

So the variance of the standardized estimates can be estimated by

$$\operatorname{v\hat{a}r}[h(\widehat{\theta})] = \dot{h}(\widehat{\theta})^T \widehat{\Omega} \dot{h}(\widehat{\theta}) + \frac{1}{2}\operatorname{trace}[(\ddot{h}(\theta)\widehat{\Omega})^2],$$

where again $\widehat{\theta}$ and $\widehat{\Omega}$ are estimates of θ and Ω.

As compared to the delta method, the additional complexity of the quadratic approximation method is that of computing $\ddot{h}$. In general, however, the first order derivatives of h can be used in a finite difference method to obtain the second order derivatives. This avoids the need for analytic computation of the second order derivatives. Specific methods based on Richardson extrapolation are given by Jamshidian and Jennrich (1997, in press) for which they report very good accuracies.

When $\widehat{\theta}$ is MLE, under some regularity conditions which generally hold, $\widehat{\theta} \sim \mathcal{N}(\theta, \Omega)$ asymptotically with $\Omega = \frac{1}{N}\mathcal{I}^{-1}(\theta)$, where N is the sample size, and $\mathcal{I}(\theta)$ is the Fisher information matrix evaluated at θ (e.g., Ferguson 1996, page 121). There are also asymptotic theorems that give the delta estimate [3] as the asymptotic variance of $h(\widehat{\theta})$ (e.g., Ferguson 1996, page 45). But Ferguson (1996, pages 45-50), using a simple example showed that if $\dot{h}(\widehat{\theta})$ is close to zero, then in order for the delta estimates to be accurate a very large sample is required. It is in these cases that the second order correction will be useful. When the normality assumption holds, using [4], it can be concluded that the delta method underestimates the variance. As we will see, this is consistent with observations from our examples.

The Bootstrap Method with Control Functions

Among the methods discussed here, and for the problem considered here, the bootstrap method is the simplest method to implement. A nonparametric bootstrap procedure is as follows:

Step 1. Draw a simple random sample (with replacement) of size N from the raw data $\mathcal{X} = (x_1, \cdots, x_N)$. Denote the resulting sample by $\widetilde{\mathcal{X}} = (\tilde{x}_1, \cdots, \tilde{x}_N)$.

Step 2. Obtain an estimate $\widehat{\theta} = (\widehat{\Lambda}, \widehat{\Phi}, \widehat{\Psi})$, based on $\widetilde{\mathcal{X}}$.

Step 3. Calculate the standardized estimates $\widehat{\theta}^* = (\widehat{\Lambda}^*, \widehat{\Phi}^*, \widehat{\Psi}^*)$ [using $\widehat{\theta}$ and equations in [1] in the case of CFA].

Step 4. Repeat Steps 1-3 b times to obtain b bootstrap samples estimates of $\widehat{\theta}^*$. Denote these by $\widehat{\theta}^{*(1)}, \cdots, \widehat{\theta}^{*(b)}$.

Step 5. For each parameter θ^* obtain an estimate of the variance using

$$\frac{1}{b-1} \sum_{i=1}^{b} \left(\hat{\theta}^{*(i)} - \bar{\hat{\theta}}^* \right),$$

where $\hat{\theta}^{*(i)}$ is an appropriate element of $\widehat{\boldsymbol{\theta}}^{*(i)}$ corresponding to θ^*, and $\bar{\hat{\theta}}^* = \sum_{i=1}^{b} \hat{\theta}^{*(i)}/b$.

While this method is simple to implement, to achieve reasonable efficiency it may require a large number of bootstrap samples b, and thus become computationally expensive. A general idea, using what are called control functions, has been put forth to modify the bootstrap in order to increase the efficiency of the estimates for a given bootstrap sample size b (e.g., Efron & Tibshirani, 1993). This is what we will discuss next.

Let $g(\widehat{\boldsymbol{\theta}})$ be a function that approximates $h(\widehat{\boldsymbol{\theta}})$. Then using the obvious equality $h(\widehat{\boldsymbol{\theta}}) = g(\widehat{\boldsymbol{\theta}}) + [h(\widehat{\boldsymbol{\theta}}) - g(\widehat{\boldsymbol{\theta}})]$ we can write

$$\text{var}[h(\widehat{\boldsymbol{\theta}})] = \text{var}[g(\widehat{\boldsymbol{\theta}})] + \text{var}[h(\widehat{\boldsymbol{\theta}}) - g(\widehat{\boldsymbol{\theta}})] + 2\text{cov}[g(\widehat{\boldsymbol{\theta}}), \{h(\widehat{\boldsymbol{\theta}}) - g(\widehat{\boldsymbol{\theta}})\}].$$

The function g is referred to as the *control function*. If g is chosen such that its variance can be computed exactly, then one can obtain an estimate of $\text{var}[h(\widehat{\boldsymbol{\theta}})]$ by the following steps:

Step 1. Compute $\text{var}[g(\widehat{\boldsymbol{\theta}})]$, analytically.

Step 2. Obtain b bootstrap sample estimates $\widehat{\boldsymbol{\theta}}^{(1)}, \cdots, \widehat{\boldsymbol{\theta}}^{(b)}$ of $\widehat{\boldsymbol{\theta}}$, by resampling as explained in the bootstrap method.

Step 3. Let $d(\widehat{\boldsymbol{\theta}}) = h(\widehat{\boldsymbol{\theta}}) - g(\widehat{\boldsymbol{\theta}})$. Estimate $\text{var}[h(\widehat{\boldsymbol{\theta}})]$ by

$$\hat{\text{var}}[h(\widehat{\boldsymbol{\theta}})] = \text{var}[g(\widehat{\boldsymbol{\theta}})] +$$

$$\frac{1}{b-1} \sum_{i=1}^{b} [d(\widehat{\boldsymbol{\theta}}^{(i)}) - \bar{d}]^2 + \frac{2}{b-1} \sum_{i=1}^{b} [d(\widehat{\boldsymbol{\theta}}^{(i)}) - \bar{d}][g(\widehat{\boldsymbol{\theta}}^{(i)}) - \bar{g}]$$

where $\bar{d} = \sum_{i=1}^{b} d(\widehat{\boldsymbol{\theta}}^{(i)})/b$, and $\bar{g}$ is defined similarly.

As Efron and Tibshirani (1993, Chapter 23) point out, if the function g is a good approximation to h, then $\text{var}[h(\widehat{\boldsymbol{\theta}}) - g(\widehat{\boldsymbol{\theta}})] < \text{var}[h(\widehat{\boldsymbol{\theta}})]$ and as a result the control function will produce an estimate with lower variance for the same number of bootstrap samples b.

We propose and examine two control functions for covariance structures. One, which we refer to as the delta control function uses

$$g(\widehat{\boldsymbol{\theta}}) = h(\boldsymbol{\theta}) - \dot{h}(\boldsymbol{\theta})^T(\widehat{\boldsymbol{\theta}} - \boldsymbol{\theta}).$$

Obviously, $\boldsymbol{\theta}$ is not known. But all that is needed is the $\text{var}[g(\widehat{\boldsymbol{\theta}})]$. This we will approximate by the delta method estimate [3].

The second method uses a linear regression approximation to h. First, use the bootstrap sample of Step 2 above, and calculate $h[\widehat{\boldsymbol{\theta}}^{(i)}]$, for $i = 1, \cdots, b$. Then fit the regression model

$$h[\widehat{\boldsymbol{\theta}}^{(i)}] = \alpha + \boldsymbol{\beta}^T \widehat{\boldsymbol{\theta}}^{(i)} + e_i, \quad i = 1, \cdots, b$$

by least squares to obtain the estimates $\hat{\alpha}$ and $\hat{\boldsymbol{\beta}}$. Then use

$$g(\widehat{\boldsymbol{\theta}}) = \hat{\alpha} + \hat{\boldsymbol{\beta}}^T \widehat{\boldsymbol{\theta}},$$

whose variance can be estimated by

$$\text{vâr}[g(\widehat{\boldsymbol{\theta}})] = \hat{\boldsymbol{\beta}}^T \hat{\Omega} \hat{\boldsymbol{\beta}}.$$

A restriction of this method is that the size of the bootstrap sample b has to be at least as large as the number of parameters. The delta method does not have such a restriction. An advantage of the regression control function to that of the delta control function, however, is that it does not require computation of any derivatives. This computation is replaced by a linear least squares estimation that can be performed easily.

In the next section we will apply the methods described here to a few factor analysis examples, and compare their accuracy and efficiency.

EXAMPLES AND COMPARISONS

We consider application of the methods described above to three CFA examples, and in each case use three sample sizes of 75, 150, 500. These were chosen to examine the behavior of each method on small, moderate, and relatively large sample sizes. For all the examples we have generated data from a multivariate normal distribution with mean 0 and covariance to be described for each case.

For our first example we generated data using the covariance matrix

$$\begin{pmatrix}
6.982 & & & & & \\
4.686 & 6.047 & & & & \\
4.335 & 3.307 & 5.037 & & & \\
-2.294 & -1.453 & -1.979 & 5.569 & & \\
-2.209 & -1.262 & -1.738 & 3.931 & 5.328 & \\
-1.671 & -1.401 & -1.564 & 3.915 & 3.601 & 4.977
\end{pmatrix}.$$

This is a sample covariance matrix based on a set of real data described by Bollen (1989, page 259). The first three variables in this matrix were measures of sympathy whereas the last three were measures of anger, thus, a two-factor model is embodied here. The model that we fitted to the data in each case was a two-factor model with the last three factor loadings in the first factor and the first three factor loadings in the second factor fixed to zero. Also the first factor loading of the first factor, and the fourth factor loading of the second factor were fixed at 1. The factor covariance matrix Φ and diagonal elements of Ψ were free parameters to be estimated. There are a total of 13 parameters in this model. This model is the same as that fit by Bollen (1989) to the covariance matrix given above.

Our second example uses the population quantities

$$\Lambda = \begin{pmatrix} 1.0000 & 0 & 0 \\ 1.0000 & 1.0000 & 0 \\ 1.0000 & 1.0000 & 1.0000 \\ 0.7714 & 0 & 0 \\ 0.8641 & 0 & 0 \\ 0.8088 & 0 & 0 \\ 0.8580 & 0.8498 & 0 \\ 0.7214 & 0.8975 & 0 \\ 0.9368 & 0.7261 & 0 \\ 1.0002 & 1.0513 & 1.4441 \\ 1.2260 & 0.9903 & 1.0530 \\ 0.8382 & 0.7476 & 1.1497 \end{pmatrix}, \quad \text{diag}(\Psi) = \begin{pmatrix} 0.8627 \\ 1.0605 \\ 1.0889 \\ 1.2610 \\ 1.1061 \\ 1.2562 \\ 0.9247 \\ 1.4369 \\ 0.5789 \\ 1.1349 \\ 0.8844 \\ 1.3419 \end{pmatrix}$$

The covariance from which the data were generated was computed from $\Lambda\Lambda' + \Psi$. For this example $\Phi = I$ was fixed, and all the zero elements shown in Λ were fixed to zero in estimation as well. The elements that are not 0 or 1 in Λ, as well as the diagonal elements of Ψ were generated from a uniform distribution in the interval (.5,1.5). This example has 36 free parameters, and was used to examine the performance of the methods on a problem with a moderately large number of parameters.

Finally the data for our third example were generated using the population parameters

$$\Lambda = \begin{pmatrix} .2 & 0 \\ 1 & 0 \\ 1 & 0 \\ 0 & 1 \\ 0 & 1 \\ 0 & 1 \end{pmatrix}, \quad \text{diag}(\Psi) = \begin{pmatrix} 1 \\ 1 \\ 1 \\ 1 \\ 1 \\ 1 \end{pmatrix}.$$

All the elements shown as zero were fixed in estimation. Also $\Phi = I$ was fixed. This model has 12 parameters to be estimated. A special feature of this model is the small factor loading .2 which makes the example different from the others, as we will see. This makes the model marginally identified. For this example, a large sample size is required to estimate the parameters well.

To estimate the variance of the standardized parameter estimates $\widehat{\theta}^*$ for these examples, we will compare application of the following methods: Ordinary bootstrap (B), bootstrap with delta control function (BD), bootstrap with regression control function (BR), the delta method (D), and the quadratically corrected delta method (Q). For all of these methods, but the ordinary bootstrap, an estimate of $\Omega = \text{cov}(\widehat{\theta})$ of the nonstandardized estimates is required. For these methods, the sources of error are twofold. One is from approximating the general nonlinear function $h(\theta)$, by another function. For example, in the D, BD, and BR, methods, a linear approximation of h is used, and in the Q method a quadratic approximation to h is used. The second source of error is from estimating the covariance Ω by $\widehat{\Omega}$. For example, when $\widehat{\theta}$ is MLE, then a popular estimate of $\widehat{\Omega}$ is based on the information matrix, as mentioned. We are mainly interested in studying the performance of these methods in dealing with the first source of error. We will study both bias and efficiency of each of the estimates B, BD, BR, D, and Q. There is a vast literature that discusses different methods of estimating Ω. To include the errors from this estimation makes our comparisons complicated.

To concentrate on the first source of errors which stems mainly from the nonlinearity of h, we eliminate the second source of error by using what we will call the population value of Ω. We obtain this value based on a bootstrap sample of size 2000. While what we obtain is really not equal to Ω, in general it should be very close to it. Additionally, we use the 2000 bootstrap samples to obtain, again, what we refer to as the true or the population value of the variance of the standardized estimates $\text{var}(\widehat{\theta}^*)$. We use this to estimate bias.

We have experimented with using the information matrix estimate of Ω. To keep things simple, we do not report our experience in detail. Briefly, however, the results in terms of reduction of bias and efficiency are very much in parallel to what we will see shortly, except that the amount of bias in general is larger, mainly due to errors that result from estimating Ω by the information matrix. Obviously as N gets larger, the information matrix estimate of Ω gets closer to Ω and, as expected, the difference between the methods using the population value Ω and the information matrix estimate become very small.

We begin by examining the accuracy of the estimates obtained by each method. We will look at the absolute relative bias (ARB) for each estimate. This, we define as

$$\text{Absolute Relative Bias} = \left| \frac{\text{True} - \text{Estimate}}{\text{True}} \right|.$$

Roughly speaking, if this value is as large as .3, the estimate agrees with the true value, after rounding, to one significant digit of accuracy – and obviously smaller values of ARB indicate more accuracy of the estimates. For practical purposes we use .3 as the boundary for "acceptable" ARBs.

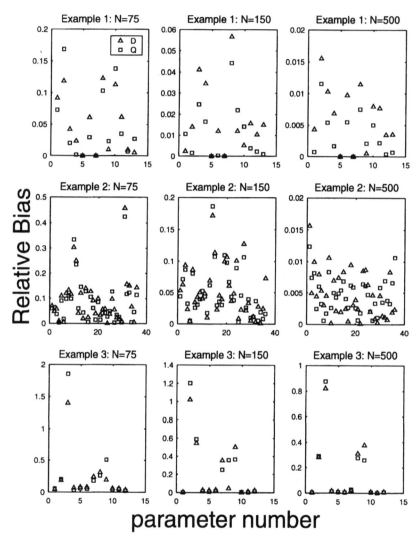

Figure 1. Absolute relative bias for the delta (D) method, and quadratic approximation (Q) method for Examples 1, 2, and 3 with sample sizes N=75, 150, and 500.

We start our comparison of absolute relative bias with the two least expensive methods, D and Q. Figure 1 shows the ARBs for these when applied to our examples. In this figure, and the subsequent figures, the horizontal axis indicates the parameter number. The free parameters are counted rowwise in Λ, Φ, and Ψ. The vertical axes, in all the figures, but Figure 3, are ARB values.

In Example 1, the ARBs are small for all three sample sizes. In particular, they are all below the acceptable value of .3. Also ARBs decrease as the sample size increases. In light of the asymptotic theory mentioned in Section 2, this is expected. The Q-method estimates have smaller ARBs, as compared to the D-method for most parameters in this example. The differences, however, in general are very small.

We also experimented with fitting a slightly different model to the data of Example 1. Instead of fixing two of the factor loadings to 1, we fixed two of the factor variances to 1. This results in the factor covariance ϕ_{21} to be scale invariant. When we applied the D and Q methods, the ARBs for both methods were 0 for this parameter. This is not a coincidence. When a parameter is invariant with respect to standardization, the standard error of its estimate should not change in the process of standardization. It can be shown that this is guaranteed for the methods that use D, or Q, either directly, or as control functions in bootstrap. Note that the ordinary bootstrap does not have this property.

For Example 2, as shown in Figure 1, the ARB again decreases for both D and Q methods as the sample size increases. Only for the case where $N = 75$ do two of the parameters have ARBs that exceed 0.3. While for most cases the Q estimate has a smaller ARB than the D estimate, the differences are again small. The maximum absolute difference for the D and Q ARBs for $N = 75$ and 150 is about .06, and for $N = 500$ is .008.

For Example 3, again we see the trend of reduced ARB as the sample size increases. For most cases the Q estimates have smaller ARBs than the D estimates. When $N = 75$, the D and Q variance estimates of $\hat{\lambda}_{31}^*$ and $\hat{\psi}_{33}^*$ are notably biased. For $N = 150$ this holds for $\hat{\lambda}_{21}^*$ and $\hat{\psi}_{22}^*$. For both of these cases, the population value of the unique variance was 1, but the estimated values were .3 and .03, respectively. To estimate these parameters more accurately, a larger sample is required. The estimates for the case of $N = 500$ were close to the population values. Again taking ARB = .3 as the acceptable cut-off point, for $N = 75$ and $N = 150$ all but four of the estimates in each case had ARBs larger than .3 for both the D and Q methods. When N is large, three of the D estimates were not acceptable, and only one of the Q estimates had an ARB larger than .3.

In Figure 2, we compare the absolute relative bias for B, BD, and BR. For each case 50 estimates were obtained based on bootstrap samples of size 250,

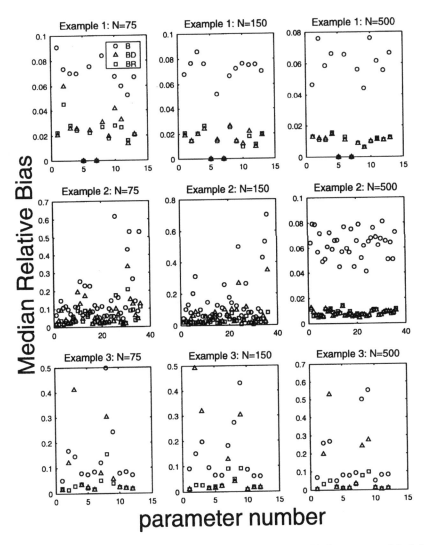

Figure 2. Absolute relative bias for the ordinary bootstrap (B), bootstrap with delta control function (BD), and bootstrap with regression control function (BR) for Examples 1, 2, and 3 with samples N=75, 150, and 500. The size of the bootstrap sample in each case is b=250.

and the median of the ARBs for the 50 estimates were plotted. Importantly, comparing Figure 1 to Figure 2, the relative biases for the BD and BR methods are in general lower than those for the D and Q methods. This is especially clear from the figures when $N = 75$, or 150. Another interesting observation is that for almost all the examples, the BD and BR methods have smaller ARBs than the ordinary bootstrap method, with this difference being notable, especially in Example 1. Comparing the BR and BD methods, in most cases BR has a smaller ARB than BD, and in a few cases the difference is notable. There are cases where BD shows less bias than BR, but the differences in these cases are relatively small and negligible. In all the examples the ARB values are smaller than the acceptable .3 value for the BR method. This also holds for BD in Examples 1 and 2. The BD method has the most bias in Example 3 for parameters for which the Delta method had the most bias in Figure 1. The reader is reminded that ARBs in Example 1 were set to zero for the fifth and seventh parameter, for the reason explained earlier.

We now compare the efficiencies of B, BD and BR, i.e., the relative variances of estimates. Figure 3 shows the $\log_{10}$-efficiencies of BD relative to B, and BR relative to B for all the examples considered. The efficiencies plotted were computed as follows: For each method bootstrap samples of size $b = 250$ were drawn to estimate the variances of the standardized parameter estimates. This process was repeated 50 times, each time drawing a different bootstrap sample. As a result 50 estimates of the variances based on each of the methods of B, BD, and BR were obtained. Then the ratio of variances of the 50 BD, and BR estimates to those of B were computed, and the $\log_{10}$ of these values were plotted. We plotted the $\log_{10}$-efficiencies, because the efficiencies themselves varied over a wide range. Nine plots are shown in Figure 1. These correspond to Examples 1, 2, and 3 and each case with data sets of size 75, 150, and 500.

Because the variances of the fifth and seventh elements of $\widehat{\theta}^*$ in Example 1 are zero, the $\log_{10}$ efficiencies for these parameters are set to 0 in the plot. The statements that we subsequently make ignore these two parameters. For Example 1, BD and BR are more efficient than the ordinary bootstrap with very significantly large efficiencies in some cases. The range of the efficiencies of BD and BR relative to the ordinary bootstrap method are 3 to 121 for BD, and 5 to 101 for BR. For $N = 75$, the BR method is more efficient than the BD method for all but one parameter, for which the efficiencies are very close. For $N = 150$ and 500, BD and BR are about equally efficient in this example.

For Example 2, when $N = 75$, three parameters are estimated more efficiently by the ordinary bootstrap method as compared to BD, and for $N = 150$ four of the estimates have this property. The BR method is more efficient than the ordinary bootstrap for all parameters in this example. In fact, the efficiency of BD relative to B is above 100 for a few parameters, and that for BR is above 1000 for a few parameters. In this example BR is generally more efficient than BD for sample sizes 75, and 150 . For $N = 500$, both BR and BD are more

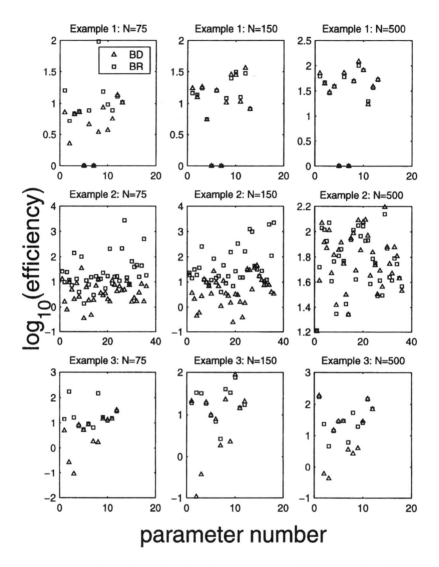

Figure 3. Log$_{10}$-efficiencies of the bootstrap-delta (BD) method, and the bootstrap-regression (BR) method relative to the ordinary bootstrap (B) for Examples 1, 2, and 3 with sample sizes N=75, 150, and 500. The size of the bootstrap sample in each case is b=250.

efficient than B, and in most cases the efficiencies of BD and BR are close.

As mentioned earlier, Example 3 is one where a large sample is required for the delta method estimates to be accurate. For $N = 500$, the BD estimates are less efficient than the B estimates for two of the parameters. The efficiency of BD, however, in general improves as N increases. The BR method is more efficient than the B method for all the parameters here, having efficiencies larger than 100 in a few of the cases. For this example the BR method is at least as efficient as the BD method, and in a few cases it is much more efficient.

A fair question is how large of a bootstrap sample is sufficient to obtain acceptable answers. A simulation study helps in answering this question. Since our main goal is to introduce methods, we have not done this here. However, we tried our examples with a bootstrap sample size of $b = 50$. The median absolute relative bias for each parameter estimate variance is given in Figure 4. The pattern of ARBs in Figures 2 and 4 are very similar. It is interesting to note that the BR estimates all have median ARBs that are less than .3. The bias for Example 2 estimates in both Figures 2 and 4 are very similar. Also when the sample sizes are large it seems that there is not much gain in going from a bootstrap sample of size 50 to 250. Finally, while these are not shown, the efficiencies for the BD and BR, as compared to B, when $b = 50$ are similar to those shown in Figure 3.

SUMMARY AND CONCLUSIONS

The delta method is an easy method to implement in order to obtain estimates of standard errors of standardized estimates in covariance structures. Surprisingly, this approach has not been implemented in popular covariance structure software. Our experience shows that the delta method estimates are acceptable, especially for problems with a large sample size. The method based on the quadratic approximation, proposed here, is an improvement over the delta method. Its effect is most significant when sample sizes are small, or $h(\boldsymbol{\theta})$ has large curvatures. Unfortunately, there is no easy measure to calibrate the gain in using the quadratic approximation method over the delta method. Several approaches that were tried proved unsuccessful.

The bootstrap method has been used to estimate variances of $\widehat{\boldsymbol{\theta}}^{*}$. Its critique, however, is the expensive computation it requires. The control function methods, introduced here, although slightly more complex to implement, seem to have significant gains both in terms of bias and efficiency, as compared to the ordinary bootstrap. Since they are considerably more efficient, one can comfortably use a smaller number of bootstrap samples. We have compared bias between two bootstrap sample sizes of 250 and 50. The results based on the bootstrap sample of size 50 are quite acceptable. A more detailed simulation study is desirable to determine acceptable bootstrap sample sizes. From the two

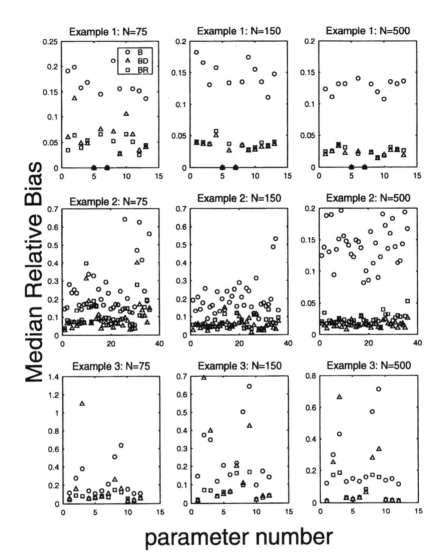

Figure 4. Absolute relative bias for the ordinary bootstrap (B), bootstrap with delta control function (BD), and bootstrap with regression control function (BR) for Examples 1, 2, and 3 with samples N=75, 150, and 500. The size of the bootstrap sample in each case is b=50.

control function methods, BR performed as well as or better than BD in almost all the cases. In some cases BR was significantly less biased than BD, and in those cases where BD had less bias than BR, the difference in bias was negligible. The only disadvantage of BR over BD is that the bootstrap sample size that it requires has to be at least as large as the number of parameters. There is no such restriction for the delta method. Of course, to implement the delta method, one is required to compute derivatives of h. This is not required by the BR method. This can be a major advantage of the BR method, especially for complex covariance structures. A final note is that the R-square value from the regression performed in the BR method may be used to calibrate the efficiency of this method relative to the ordinary bootstrap method. Determining the values of R-square that indicate improved efficiency deserves further study.

Further work also is needed to compare the methods proposed here to alternative approaches based on analysis of correlation rather than covariance structures, such as have been developed by Steiger (1995) and Leung and Chan (1997). Also, for convenience our development has been limited to ML estimation under normality though the approach clearly could be applied to any consistent estimator. Such additional work is not unimportant because, as our honoree has shown (Jackson & Chan, 1980), the ML approach may not always be the best choice to use in the factor analysis of empirical data.

The further development of improved estimates of standard errors of standardized parameters, such as those that were explicated in this chapter, has far reaching implications. Among other benefits, the construct validation of psychometric measures of a wide variety of human attributes from the domain of personality, industrial-organizational psychology, clinical psychology, and organizational behavior, may be advanced by this work.

APPENDIX

Derivatives of the Standardized Parameters of the Factor Model

The following first order derivatives are required for the delta method for the factor model.

$$\frac{\partial \lambda_{ij}^*}{\partial \lambda_{uv}} = \delta_{iu}\delta_{jv}\phi_{jj}^{1/2}\sigma_{ii}^{-1/2} - \frac{1}{2}\lambda_{ij}\phi_{jj}^{1/2}\frac{\partial \sigma_{ii}}{\partial \lambda_{uv}}$$

$$\frac{\partial \lambda_{ij}^*}{\partial \phi_{uv}} = \frac{1}{2}\sigma_{ii}^{-3/2}\phi_{jj}^{-1/2}\lambda_{ij}(\sigma_{ii}\delta_{ju}\delta_{jv} - \phi_{jj}\frac{\partial \sigma_{ii}}{\partial \phi_{uv}})$$

$$\frac{\partial \lambda_i^*}{\partial \psi_u} = -\frac{1}{2}\sigma_{ii}^{-3/2}\phi_{jj}^{1/2}\lambda_{ij}\frac{\partial \sigma_{ii}}{\partial \psi_u}$$

$$\frac{\partial \phi_{ij}^*}{\partial \phi_{uv}} = -\frac{1}{2}\phi_{ii}^{-3/2}\phi_{ij}\phi_{jj}^{-3/2}(\phi_{jj}\delta_{iu}\delta_{iv} - 2\phi_{ii}\phi_{jj}\phi_{ij}^{-1}\delta_{iu}\delta_{jv} + \phi_{ii}\delta_{ju}\delta_{jv})$$

$$\frac{\partial \psi_i^*}{\partial \lambda_{uv}} = -\frac{\psi_i}{\sigma_{ii}^2}\left(\frac{\partial \sigma_{ii}}{\partial \lambda_{uv}}\right)$$

$$\frac{\partial \psi_i^*}{\partial \phi_{uv}} = -\frac{\psi_i}{\sigma_{ii}^2}\left(\frac{\partial \sigma_{ii}}{\partial \phi_{uv}}\right)$$

$$\frac{\partial \psi_i^*}{\partial \psi_u} = \frac{\delta_{iv}(\sigma_{ii} - \psi_i)}{\sigma_{ii}^2}$$

where δ_{ij} is the Kronecker's Delta with values 1 when $i = j$ and 0 when $i \neq j$,

$$\frac{\partial \sigma_{ii}}{\partial \lambda_{uv}} = 2\delta_{iu}\sum_{k=1}^{m}\lambda_{ik}\phi_{kv}$$

$$\frac{\partial \sigma_{ii}}{\partial \phi_{uv}} = \lambda_{iu}\lambda_{iv}$$

$$\frac{\partial \sigma_{ii}}{\partial \psi_u} = \delta_{iu}$$

and all other derivatives are zero.

Derivation of Equation [5]

$$
\begin{aligned}
\mathrm{cov}(l(\widehat{\boldsymbol{\theta}}), q(\widehat{\boldsymbol{\theta}})) &= E\{l(\widehat{\boldsymbol{\theta}})[q(\widehat{\boldsymbol{\theta}}) - E\{q(\widehat{\boldsymbol{\theta}})\}]\} \\
&= E\{l(\widehat{\boldsymbol{\theta}})[q(\widehat{\boldsymbol{\theta}}) - \mathrm{trace}(\ddot{h}(\boldsymbol{\theta})\Omega)\}]\} \\
&= E\{l(\widehat{\boldsymbol{\theta}})q(\widehat{\boldsymbol{\theta}})\} \\
&= E\{(\widehat{\boldsymbol{\theta}} - \boldsymbol{\theta})^T \dot{h}(\boldsymbol{\theta})(\widehat{\boldsymbol{\theta}} - \boldsymbol{\theta})^T \ddot{h}(\boldsymbol{\theta})(\widehat{\boldsymbol{\theta}} - \boldsymbol{\theta})\} \\
&= \mathrm{trace}E\{(\widehat{\boldsymbol{\theta}} - \boldsymbol{\theta})(\widehat{\boldsymbol{\theta}} - \boldsymbol{\theta})^T \dot{h}(\boldsymbol{\theta})(\widehat{\boldsymbol{\theta}} - \boldsymbol{\theta})^T\}\ddot{h}(\boldsymbol{\theta}) \\
&= 0
\end{aligned}
$$

The last equality follows by a standard Theorem on functions involving the third moments of a multivariate normal distribution (e.g., Schott, 1997, pages 392-394).

Notes

1. Douglas Jackson was Bentler's dissertation chair on a problem in personality assessment at Stanford University 35 years ago, and ever since has provided inspiration and encouragement for work on improved quantitative methods in psychology.

Mortaza Jamshidian is an Assistant Professor, Department of Statistics, University of Central Florida, Orlando, Florida 32816-2370.

Peter M. Bentler is Professor, Departments of Psychology and Statistics, University of California, Los Angeles, 4627 Franz Hall, Los Angeles, CA 90024-1563.

2. These properties have been identified in psychometric literature (e.g., Cudeck, 1989; Krane & McDonald 1978; Swaminathan & Algina, 1978), however no uniform terminology has been used. Yuan and Bentler (in press) seem to be the first to use the statistical terminology.

REFERENCES

Arbuckle, J. L. (1997). *Amos users' guide version 3.6.* Chicago: Small-Waters.
Bentler, P. M., & Weeks, D. G. (1980). Linear structural equations with latent variables. *Psychometrika,* **45,** 289–308.
Bollen, K. A. (1989). *Structural equations with latent variables.* New York: Wiley.
Browne, M. W. (1982). Covariance structures. In D. M. Hawkins (Ed.) *Topics in applied multivariate analysis* (pp. 72-141). Cambridge: Cambridge University Press.
Browne, M. W., & du Toit, S. H. C. (1992). Automated fitting of nonstandard models. *Multivariate Behavioral Research,* **27,** 269–300.
Chou, C. P., & Bentler, P. M. (1993). Invariant standardized estimated parameter change for model modification in covariance structure analysis. *Multivariate Behavioral Research,* **28,** 97–110.
Cudeck, R. (1989). Analysis of correlation matrices using covariance structure models. *Psychological Bulletin,* **105,** 317–327.
Cudeck, R., & O'Dell, L. L. (1994). Applications of standard error estimates in unrestricted factor analysis: Significance tests for factor loadings and correlations. *Psychological Bulletin,* **115,** 475–487.
Efron, B. (1982). *The jackknife, the bootstrap and other resampling plans.* Philadelphia: SIAM.
Efron, B., & Tibshirani, R. J. (1993). *An introduction to the bootstrap.* New York: Chapman & Hall.
Ferguson, T. S. (1996). *A course in large sample theory.* New York: Chapman & Hall.
Goffin, R. D. & Jackson, D. N. (1992). Analysis of multitrait-multirater performance appraisal data: Composite direct product method versus confirmatory factor analysis. *Multivariate Behavioral Research,* **27,** 363–385.

94

Jackson, D. N. (1970). A sequential system for personality scale development. In C. D. Spielberger (Ed.), *Current topics in clinical and community psychology Volume 2.* (pp. 91-96). New York: Academic Press.

Jackson, D. N., & Chan, D. W. (1980). Maximum-likelihood estimation in common factor analysis: A cautionary note. *Psychological Bulletin,* **88**, 502–508.

Jackson, D. N., Paunonen, S. V., Fraboni, M. & Goffin, R. D. (1996). A five-factor versus six-factor model of personality structure. *Personality and Individual Differences,* **20**, 33-45.

Jamshidian, M., & Bentler, P. M. (1993). A modified Newton method for constrained estimation in covariance structure analysis. *Computational Statistics and Data Analysis,* **15**, 133–146.

Jamshidian, M., & Jennrich, R. I. (1997). Standard errors for EM estimation. In E. Wegman & S. Azen (Eds.), *Computing science and statistics,* **29**, 463-470.

Jamshidian, M., & Jennrich, R. I. (in press). Standard errors for EM estimation. *Journal of the Royal Statistical Society, Series B.*

Jöreskog, K. G., & Sörbom, D. (1988). *LISREL 7: A guide to the program and applications.* Chicago: SPSS.

Krane, W. R., & McDonald, R. P. (1978). Scale invariance and the factor analysis of correlation matrices. *British Journal of Mathematical and Statistical Psychology,* **31**, 218–228.

Lehmann, E. L., & Casella, G. (1998). *Theory of point estimation.* New York: Springer-Verlag.

Leung, Y. P., & Chan, W. (1997). Constrained generalized least squares and asymptotically distribution free estimation in correlation structure analysis. *American Statistical Association Proceedings of the Section on Government Statistics and Section on Social Statistics,* 422–427.

Schott, J. R. (1997). *Matrix analysis for statistics.* New York: Wiley.

Shapiro, A., & Browne, M. W. (1990). On the treatment of correlation structures as covariance structures. *Linear Algebra and Its Applications,* **127**, 567–587.

Steiger, J. H. (1995). *SEPATH in STATISTICA for windows.* Tulsa: StatSoft.

Swaminathan, H., & Algina, J. (1978). Scale freeness in factor analysis. *Psychometrika,* **43**, 581–583.

Velicer, W. F., & Jackson, D. N. (1990). Component analysis versus common factor analysis: Some issues in selecting an appropriate procedure. *Multivariate Behavioral Research,* **25**, 1–28.

Yuan, K. -H., & Bentler, P. M. (in press). On equivariance and invariance of standard errors in three exploratory factor models. *Psychometrika.*

Yung, Y. -F., & Bentler, P. M. (1996). Bootstrapping techniques in analysis of mean and covariance structures. In G. A. Marcoulides & R. E. Schumacker (Eds.), *Advanced structural equation modeling techniques* (pp. 195-226). Hillsdale, NJ: LEA.

SECTION II: CONSTRUCT-ORIENTED ASSESSMENT WITHIN THE DOMAIN OF PERSONALITY

Assessment of personality and psychopathology is difficult. Screening tests must be both brief and accurate, which is made more difficult by the need to screen for a wide range of possible psychological problems. This is, of course, the bandwidth-fidelity problem: assuming the number of items is held constant, one cannot assess a range of problems with the same degree of accuracy that one could assess a single disorder. There is no known solution to this dilemma, but that has not discouraged efforts to develop short screening tests. One common approach in the past has been to form short versions of longer tests. These efforts have commonly used the *Minnesota Multiphasic Personality Inventory* (*MMPI*). After a degree of popularity (Faschingbauer & Newmark, 1978), authoritative recommendations against this approach largely stifled additional research (Butcher & Hostetter, 1990).

A second common approach has been the development of specific short screening tests. Such tests are commonly based more upon clinical experience and perceived clinical demands than upon psychological theories. In this section, Ronald Holden outlines the development of a screening test that does have links to psychological theory, the *Holden Psychological Screening Inventory* (*HPSI*). The *HPSI* was developed using a test construction strategy that relied heavily upon the principles advocated by Douglas Jackson. The empirical results suggest the important advantages that may arise from the use of such an approach.

The assessment of personality and psychopathology by means of paper-and-pencil tests has largely been a concern of the English-speaking world. In cases where such tests have been used in other languages, the test in question has frequently been a translation from English. Such translations have not been without problems. In Chapter 6 Sampo Paunonen explores the conditions required for the successful application of constructs that are native to one culture and language to other cultures and languages. His chapter discusses the importance of theoretical analyses of the nature of the relevant constructs in the different cultures and the ways in which the application of a particular construct from one culture may be mismatched in another culture. He also notes the complexity of the empirical analyses necessary to demonstrate successfully that a construct can be appropriately assessed in two different cultures.

Leslie Morey is one of the few psychologists to take up the challenge of developing a multiscale inventory to challenge the dominance of the *MMPI* in the assessment of psychopathology. His development of the *Personality Assessment Inventory* (*PAI*) was founded upon considerations of the adequacy of psychological theory relating to the constructs to be assessed. He also adopted a complex sequential process of item analysis for the *PAI* that was based upon principles put forth by Jackson. The *PAI* represents a substantial advance in ease of use and clarity of interpretation. His work demonstrates that the methods advocated by Jackson are not exercises in complex multivariate statistics, but basic principles that can readily be applied to any domain in which sufficient theoretical knowledge exists to support construct-based methods.

Jackson's career has followed several productive tangents. One of these was an exploration of the nature of scientific productivity. Philippe Rushton describes how this interest led first to an international conference and then to an edited book on the topic. The explication of scientific productivity is close to the hearts of scientists in many fields, and Rushton's observations on the influences of research management practices upon scientific productivity will be of interest to many readers.

The final chapter in this section is by P. A. Vernon who deals with the relationship of personality to intelligence as assessed by two of the instruments developed by Jackson, the *Personality Research Form* (*PRF*) and the *Multidimensional Aptitude Battery* (*MAB*). The former has its roots in the theory of needs developed by Henry Murray (1938), while the latter is based upon the model of intelligence used by David Wechsler. There has been increasing interest in this area in recent years (Saklofske & Zeidner, 1995), and a notable amount of this research has involved the *PRF* and *MAB*. Here Vernon outlines the basic issues in studies of personality and intelligence and summarizes the studies in this field that have used the *MAB* and *PRF*.

REFERENCES

Butcher, J. N. & Hostetter, K. (1990). Abbreviating MMPI item administration: What can be learned from the MMPI for the MMPI-2? *Psychological Assessment*, **2**, 12-21.
Faschingbauer, T. S. & Newmark, C. S. (1978). *Short forms of the MMPI*. Lexington, MA: Lexington Books.
Saklofske, D. H. & Zeidner, M. (Eds.) (1995). *International Handbook of Personality and Intelligence*. New York: Plenum.

5 APPLICATION OF THE CONSTRUCT HEURISTIC TO THE SCREENING OF PSYCHOPATHOLOGY: THE HOLDEN PSYCHOLOGICAL SCREENING INVENTORY (HPSI)

Ronald R. Holden

This chapter describes the development and properties of the Holden Psychological Screening Inventory (HPSI; Holden, 1996), a brief multiphasic, self-report measure of psychopathology. HPSI scales reflect the higher-order dimensions associated with the orthogonal constructs of the Minnesota Multiphasic Personality Inventory (MMPI) that Douglas N. Jackson identified over 25 years ago. Further, construction of the HPSI employed the principles and procedures expounded by Jackson to foster the construct validity of an inventory's scales. Thus, in describing the development of the HPSI, this chapter provides a blueprint for the adaptation of construct-guided scale development, profoundly influenced by Jackson, to a specific test construction project.

HISTORY OF TESTING OF PSYCHOPATHOLOGY

The history of psychological testing may trace its roots back to Ancient China (Dubois, 1970; Jackson & Paunonen, 1980; Wiggins, 1973) where civil service examinations were putatively used in the selection and classification of civil servants. Although the verification of records pertaining to this history is subject to challenge (Bowman, 1989), it does seem logical that the formal assessment of individual differences in psychological functioning does indeed have a distant past. The birth of modern psychological testing is often associated with the anthropometric laboratory of Sir Francis Galton in the 1880s where emphasis was placed on the careful, systematic measurement of numerous physical and behavioral characteristics (Holden, in press). Subsequently, psychological testing became recognized as a screening mechanism having the potential both to identify a greater proportion of individuals with psychological problems and to do so at an earlier phase of problem development, thus reducing the total negative consequences. Within the domain of psychopathology, the origins of published structured test instruments date back to the assessment of emotional malaise by Heymans and Wiersma (1906). Following this, Woodworth's (1917) Personal Data Sheet is often regarded as the first published, English language instrument for the structured assessment of psychological dysfunctioning.

In the two decades following the publication of Woodworth's Personal Data Sheet, numerous psychological tests emerged that assessed various domains of individual differences (Goldberg, 1971). In 1940, Hathaway and McKinley published the Minnesota Multiphasic Personality Inventory (MMPI). The MMPI represented a landmark in the assessment of psychopathology. One critical asset of the MMPI's popularity came from the breadth of its focus. The rationale for the MMPI's development was to construct a new personality inventory that would be especially appropriate for medical and psychiatric settings. Therefore, an emphasis was placed on developing an inventory that spanned a wide range of psychiatrically relevant behavior. It is this bandwidth of purpose that has contributed to the popularity of the MMPI. Items for the MMPI were based on various sources: clinical experience, psychiatric textbooks, medical and neurological case-taking directions, psychiatric examination forms, and other personality and social attitude inventories. In general, these items reflected 25 areas: General Health; General Neurologic; Cranial Nerves; Motility and Coordination; Sensibility; Vasomotor, Trophic, Speech, Secretory; Cardiorespiratory; Gastrointestinal; Genitourinary; Habits; Family and Marital; Occupational; Educational; Sexual Attitudes; Religious Attitudes; Political Attitudes — Law and Order; Social Attitudes; Affect, Depressive; Affect, Manic; Obsessive, Compulsive; Delusions, Hallucinations, Illusions, Ideas of Reference; Phobias; Sadistic, Masochistic; Morale; and Lie. Scales for the MMPI were then constructed empirically, based on how item responses differentiated between a normative group and appropriate clinical criterion groups. Ultimately, the end result was a 566-item inventory whose standard profile included 10 clinical (Hypochondriasis, Depression, Hysteria, Psychopathic Deviate, Masculinity-Femininity, Paranoia, Psychasthenia, Schizophrenia, Mania, and Social Introversion) and four validity scales: $?$ (Cannot say), L (Lie), F (Infrequency), and K (Correction) scales. Over the past 60 years, the MMPI (or its descendant, the MMPI-2) has become the most commonly used structured test of adult personality or psychopathology (Piotrowski & Keller, 1984; 1989; Piotrowski & Lubin, 1990).

STRATEGIES OF TEST CONSTRUCTION

Strategies of test construction developed in parallel with advances in the study of individual differences, which included the domain of psychopathology. When the structured assessment of personality first began, the initial strategy of test construction emphasized a rational or correspondence point of view, advocating a one-to-one relationship between verbal reports and internal states (Goldberg & Slovic, 1967; Wiggins, 1973). Test item content was to be direct and self-report was to be accepted at face value. Rational approaches, however, became subject to challenge partly because they seemed overly susceptible to faking (Ellis, 1946) and partly because of a perception that theories of psychology were not sufficiently advanced to merit this more intuitive approach (Meehl, 1945). Subsequently, newer strategies of structured test construction, such as the empirical and construct methods, came to the forefront.

The empirical approach to test construction emphasized item selection on the basis of contrasted groups. In its extremity (Berg, 1957, 1967), this method indicated that any form of stimulus material (e.g., geometric shapes) could be appropriate content for a psychological test. This approach was atheoretical and, although supposedly capable of identifying legitimate, unrealized links between test items and relevant group distinctions (Meehl, 1945), it also seemed likely to produce spurious results associated with statistical error and non-generalizable findings (Jackson, 1971). The MMPI, despite the original development of its item pool being based on some rational, clinical grounds, is often regarded as a primary instrument that personifies this empirical approach to test construction.

During the middle of this past century, the construct approach to test construction has emerged as a major strategy for instrument development. This particular approach viewed that assessment instruments should be tools of psychological theory and indicated that, for tests, the "... dangers of pure empiricism must not be underestimated" (Loevinger, 1957, p. 657). Following from this perspective and from Cronbach and Meehl's (1955) classic article on construct validity, construct-based test development has come to emphasize intrascale, interitem homogeneity, the role of a substantive, theoretical link among test items' content, concern for response styles, and the use of multivariate techniques to uncover underlying structural bonds (Jackson, 1973; Jackson & Reddon, 1987). Jackson's (1984) Personality Research Form is an instrument whose development is a prototypical example of the construct approach to test construction.

JACKSON'S CONSTRUCT-BASED APPROACH TO TEST CONSTRUCTION

In advocating a construct strategy of test construction, Jackson (1970, 1971, 1973, 1984; Jackson & Reddon, 1987) has specifically described some critical components for its implementation:

1. Substantive definition of the dimensions of interest prior to developing item pools.
2. A concern for both scale internal consistency and generalizability.
3. Suppression of response biases.
4. The fostering of convergent and discriminant validity.

First, without appropriate, distinct definitions of the constructs of interest, the test constructor is like a traveler lost in the woods. There may or may not be some experience-based knowledge to guide the undirected person, but arriving at the destination, if it is ever reached, is likely to be in a sub-optimal fashion. A systematic plan for outlining the scope and independent nature of each dimension to be measured is essential for optimal test development. Jackson (1970) affirms that much has been learned about individual differences, that such knowledge should be applied to the measurement of these differences, and that "No longer is it necessary, or even desirable, to take refuge from our psychological ignorance ..." (p. 63). Further, "... measures will have broad import and substantial construct validity to the extent, and only to the extent, that they are derived from an explicitly formulated, theoretically based definition of a trait." (Jackson, 1971, p. 232). Thus, theory and definitions are seen as central aspects to construct-based test construction.

Second, there is an important, but delicate, balance to be struck between enhancing scale internal consistency reliability and ensuring that scale items sample adequately from the domain associated with the dimension of interest (Jackson, 1970). The development of scale homogeneity may promote the univocal, unconfounded interpretation of scales, but its overemphasis can produce either random errors in domain sampling or population-specific content validity. Up to a point, scale internal consistency is a highly desirable characteristic; beyond that point, it may yield a lack of representativeness whereby a particular scale is not a complete model of a broader construct. In indicating the importance of human judgment in test construction, Jackson et al. (1989) highlight that "although statistical criteria for item selection are important, they do not guarantee that the final scale possesses content validity in the sense that it represents an adequate sample of the domain..." (p. 49).

Third, consideration of response biases is essential for developing scales with unconfounded interpretations. Jackson (1971, p. 240) indicates "... that to construct psychological measures in disregard for sources of method variance is to court disaster." Common response biases that are of interest and thought to be prevalent include social desirability and acquiescence. If there is an intention to produce relatively independent scales of conceptually orthogonal constructs, then it would seem logical to minimize these pervasive, extraneous sources of variance and, in doing so, promote the distinct operationalizations of the dimensions of interest. The ignoring of construct-irrelevant commonalities in the initial formulation of measurement scales will produce individual scales that not only may have multiple interpretations, but that may also correlate excessively among themselves.

Fourth, in endorsing Campbell and Fiske's seminal article on convergent and discriminant validity, Jackson (1970) re-emphasizes and extends the requirement that a scale should not only relate to theoretically similar measures, but *should not* correlate with conceptually unrelated constructs. In particular, his view is that this focus on construct validity should be built directly into the test construction process rather than being employed just in the post hoc evaluation of a final scale. In incorporating this concern for construct validity, Jackson has been prominent in the development of multivariate item analytic and selection procedures designed to develop item and scale convergent and discriminant validity (Jackson, 1984; Jackson et al., 1989; Neill & Jackson, 1976).

GENEALOGY AND DEVELOPMENT OF THE HPSI

In some ways, the MMPI may be regarded as the great grandparent of the Holden Psychological Screening Inventory (HPSI). The MMPI begot the Differential Personality Inventory (DPI; Jackson & Messick, 1971) which parented the Basic Personality Inventory (BPI; Jackson, 1976) from which arose the Holden Psychological Screening Inventory (HPSI; Holden, 1996):

1940 ------ 566-item Minnesota Multiphasic Personality Inventory (Hathaway & McKinley)

1971 ------ 432-item Differential Personality Inventory (Jackson & Messick)

1976 ------ 240-item Basic Personality Inventory (Jackson)

1996 ------ 36-item Holden Psychological Screening Inventory (Holden)

More specifically, in reaction to some of the MMPI's shortcomings (see Faschingbauer, 1979; Helmes & Reddon, 1993), Jackson and Messick (1971) set out to develop a differentiated inventory that, like the MMPI, was meant to cover the major dimensions of psychopathology in a comprehensive fashion. The result was the Differential Personality Inventory whose 28 scales included:

Insomnia	Health Concern	Perceptual Distortion
Headache Proneness	Hostility	Rebelliousness

Broodiness	Hypochondriasis	Repression
Cynicism	Ideas of Persecution	Sadism
Depression	Impulsivity	Self Depreciation
Desocialization	Irritability	Shallow Affect
Disorganization of Thinking	Mood Fluctuation	Socially Deviant Attitudes
Familial Discord	Neurotic Disorganization	Somatic Complaints
Feelings of Unreality	Panic Reaction	Defensiveness
		Infrequency

Consistent with Jackson's (1970, 1971) construct-oriented approach to test construction, the DPI emphasized: (a) defining distinct dimensions of psychopathology; (b) formulating large item pools to represent each of the 28 constructs independently; (c) statistical item selection procedures designed to promote scale reliability and inter-scale orthogonality; (d) evaluation of scale convergent and discriminant validity.

The Basic Personality Inventory (BPI; Jackson, 1989) arose as an offspring of the DPI. As a starting point, based on a factor analysis of the MMPI and the DPI, there was an identification of a group of 11 broad, independent dimensions of psychopathology associated with a population of psychiatric patients (Hoffmann, Jackson, & Skinner, 1975; Jackson, 1975). With the addition of a critical item scale (Deviation), the 12 proposed components (and, subsequently, scales) of the BPI were then designated:

Hypochondriasis	Alienation	Impulse Expression
Depression	Persecutory Ideas	Social Introversion
Denial	Anxiety	Self Depreciation
Interpersonal Problems	Thinking Disorder	Deviation

Once these components had been identified, the construct-oriented method of test construction was employed: definitions were elucidated; new item pools were written; statistical item procedures for fostering scale reliability and inter-scale independence were implemented; convergent and discriminant validity of scales was evaluated (Jackson et al., 1989).

Progression from the DPI (28 scales) through the BPI (12 scales) to the HPSI (3 scales) involved moving up a hierarchy of dimensions of psychopathology. Accordingly, the HPSI is a more general screen than either the BPI or the DPI. The actual test construction for the HPSI began with the higher-order factors (Figure 1) associated with the BPI (Austin, Leschied, Jaffe, & Sas, 1986) and followed the procedure outlined in Table 1. Austin et al. factor analyzed the BPI scale scores of 1,232 young offenders and identified three factors: Psychiatric Symptomatology, Social Symptomatology, and Depression. This latent structure has been subsequently confirmed for the BPI with other populations (Bjorgvinsson & Thompson, 1994; Chrisjohn, Jackson, & Lanigan, 1984) and with other multiphasic measures, such as the MMPI-2 (Butcher, Morfitt, Rouse, & Holden,

1997). It is these three factors associated with the BPI and MMPI that then served as the foci of the HPSI.

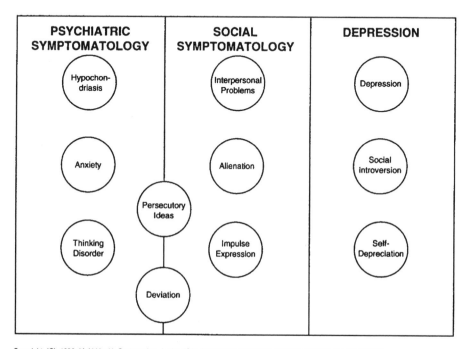

Figure 1. Domain of Psychopathology Based on Factor Analysis of Jackson's Basic Personality Inventory

Table 1. Steps in the Construction of the Holden Psychological Screening Inventory (HPSI)

Step 1- Identification of the HPSI constructs (i.e., Psychiatric Symptomatology, Social Symptomatology, Depression) from the higher-order factors of psychopathology associated with Jackson's (1976) BPI (Basic Personality Inventory).

Step 2 -Administration of BPI items and corresponding criterion scales to psychiatric patients and clinicians, respectively, and to university undergraduates and room-mates, respectively. For both the BPI and the criteria, the three higher-order factor scales (i.e., Psychiatric Symptomatology, Social Symptomatology, Depression) are scored.

Step 3 -Deletion from the item pool of those BPI items correlating more with an irrelevant self-report higher-order factor scale than a relevant self-report higher-order factor scale, in either psychiatric patient or university undergraduate samples.

Step 4 -Deletion from the item pool of those BPI items correlating more with an irrelevant criterion higher-order factor scale than a relevant criterion higher-order factor scale, in either psychiatric patient or university undergraduate samples.

Step 5 -Deletion from the item pool of those BPI items with endorsement frequencies less than .05 or greater than .95 in either the psychiatric patient or university undergraduate samples.

Step 6 -Preparation of a new item pool (HPSI items) to reflect the core content associated with BPI items remaining after Step 5. New items avoided direct overlap with the BPI, negations, outdated and sexist language, and reference to historical and biographical content. Items were written to be brief and direct, and to sample from all facets of their corresponding construct. To enhance item variance and scale reliability, a 5-point Likert scale response format is used.

Step 7 -Administration of new HPSI items to a large sample of university undergraduates. Based on a components analysis of item responses where three factors (i.e., Psychiatric Symptomatology, Social Symptomatology, Depression) are extracted, the 12 HPSI items loading most highly on each of the three components are retained for the HPSI.

Step 8 -Assembly of final form of the HPSI.

Step 9 -Undertaking of validation and norming studies.

Once the three constructs (Psychiatric Symptomatology, Social Symptomatology, Depression) had been designated as those of primary focus, an emphasis was placed on the systematic development of an inventory that would be appropriate for both clinical and nonclinical populations. Consequently, HPSI item development procedures included consideration of two primary data sets; one clinical, and one nonclinical. Holden, Fekken, Reddon, Helmes, and Jackson (1988) obtained BPI self-report item data and associated clinical criterion ratings for a sample of 112 psychiatric patients. Clinical criterion ratings for the 11 relevant BPI construct scales were collected from two clinical staff members per patient. Holden, Fekken, and Cotton (1991) obtained BPI self-reports and associated peer criterion ratings for 94 university undergraduates. These peer ratings were for the 11 relevant BPI construct scales and were provided by a roommate of the same sex who had lived with the respondent for at least three months.

The HPSI focuses on the three higher-order factors defined by the BPI. First, as a starting point for the HPSI, the three higher-order components of the BPI were scored. Psychiatric Symptomatology (sum of BPI measures of Hypochondriasis, Anxiety, Thinking Disorder, Persecutory Ideas, and Deviation), Social Symptomatology (sum of BPI measures of Interpersonal Problems, Alienation, Impulse Expression, Persecutory Ideas, and Deviation), and Depression (sum of BPI measures of Depression, Social Introversion, and Self Depreciation) scores were calculated for self-report and corresponding criteria in each of the clinical and nonclinical samples. Second, item-total correlations were calculated between each BPI item and each self-report higher-order score for each of the clinical and nonclinical samples. If a BPI item failed to show a higher item-total correlation with its relevant total than with an irrelevant total for both the clinical and nonclinical samples, it was deleted from further consideration. Third, item-criterion correlations were computed between each BPI item and each criterion self-report higher-order score for each of the clinical and nonclinical sample. If a BPI item did not demonstrate a higher item-criterion correlation with its relevant criterion than with an irrelevant criterion for both the clinical and nonclinical samples, it was removed from additional consideration. Fourth, for each of the two samples, item endorsement proportions were examined. If a BPI item did not have an endorsement proportion between .05 and .95 in both samples, it was deleted from further consideration. At this point, 50 BPI items had met these criteria for the two data samples. These items, then, represented the prototypical content of Psychiatric Symptomatology, Social Symptomatology, and Depression.

Subsequently, new HPSI items were constructed to assess the similar core content to those prototypical BPI items. HPSI items and their response format were written to: (a) avoid overlap with the BPI; (b) enhance item variance and scale reliability; (c) emphasize brief, direct, undisguised content; (d) avoid the use of negations and outdated and sexist content; and (e) minimize references to historical or biographical content that may restrict the ability to permit the assessment of change (e.g., "As a child, I was once caught shoplifting" is an item that once answered as true must always be true and, thus, is not amenable to detecting change). In addition, content validity was enhanced by ensuring that item pools for each of the HPSI constructs sampled from each construct's corresponding facets (Figure 1).

In total, 58 new items were formulated for the revised HPSI item pool. The response format for each of these items was also modified to be a 5-point Likert scale. These 58 items were then administered to a sample of 343 university undergraduates. Intercorrelations derived from responses to items were subjected to a principal components analysis whereby three components (reflecting HPSI scales of Psychiatric Symptomatology, Social Symptomatology, and Depression) were extracted and rotated to a varimax criterion. For each of these three rotated components, the 12 items loading most highly on their relevant component and loading less on each of the other two components were chosen to be on the associated final HPSI scale.

DOES THE HPSI CONFORM TO JACKSON'S CONSTRUCT-BASED APPROACH TO TEST CONSTRUCTION?

To a large degree, development of the HPSI followed the methods outlined by Jackson (1970, 1971, 1973). First, consider the HPSI constructs. The decision to focus on Psychiatric Symptomatology, Social Symptomatology, and Depression did not come out of any specific theory of psychopathology. The choice of constructs was based on empirical identification of those constructs associated with replicated findings of latent structures for the BPI and the MMPI. Definitions of these constructs and item writing were then guided mostly by the BPI scales and their corresponding definitions (Holden & Jackson, 1992; Jackson et al., 1989) which represent facets of the HPSI constructs. Thus, distinct from a more theoretically based application, such as an inventory based on Murray's (1938) theory of personality (e.g., the construct-based Personality Research Form; Jackson, 1984), the HPSI may be regarded as an inductive-hypothetico-deductive (Ozer & Reise, 1994; Tellegen & Waller, in press) version of the construct approach. That is, the HPSI is based on empirically derived and replicated factors for which constructs have subsequently been defined and for which items have been written, refined, and selected.

Second, development of the HPSI focused on balancing considerations of both scale homogeneity and generalizability. Although there was an intention to select items that loaded most strongly on appropriate rather than non-specified principal components, there was also an emphasis placed on the inclusion of all facets of respective dimensions in the final item pools for each scale. For each HPSI scale, items were selected both to promote generalizability as well as to enhance internal consistency reliability. Thus, final Psychiatric Symptomatology items include content pertaining to hypochondriasis, anxiety, *and* thinking disorder; final Social

Symptomatology items comprise content related to interpersonal problems, alienation, *and* impulse expression; and final Depression items have content representing depression, social introversion, *and* self depreciation.

Third, consider the issue of the suppression of response biases. Rather than explicitly minimizing the presence of social desirability on individual HPSI scales, the pervasive influence of this and other response styles was reduced by an emphasis on the promotion of scale orthogonality at the item selection stage. The logic here was that, if scales are developed to be minimally correlated, then they cannot all be reflective of a socially desirable response bias. Further, for the response style of acquiescence, direction of keying was not balanced within a scale. This is because the presence of negations within items will tend to reduce validity, the generation of negatively keyed, positively worded items is problematic for many dimensions of psychopathology, and the balancing of direction of item keying within a scale will only be an effective control for acquiescence when all items are equally acquiescence-inducing and when the scale normative mean occurs at approximately the mid-point of possible scale values. Therefore, within the entire scale, 24 items are keyed in one direction for psychopathology with 12 items keyed in the other direction. The assessment of the influence of response styles and of individual protocol validity is assisted by the presence of an empirically constructed validity index (Holden, 1995; Holden et al., 1999), designed to detect various sources of invalid responding (e.g., faking *and* random responding).

Fourth, the development of convergent and discriminant validity was heavily incorporated in the development of the HPSI. Item selection procedures stressed convergent and discriminant properties relative both to self-report and to the report of significant others. Further, these selection criteria were applied to data associated with both clinical and non-clinical respondents. This particular extreme emphasis on convergent and discriminant validity arose because of the documented presence of moderate to very large correlations among scales of many other existing multiphasic inventories of psychopathology. The presence of large correlations among scales indicates that they are not measuring distinct concepts and, consequently, should not offer differentiated interpretations.

In summary, therefore, the HPSI has implemented many of the specific features outlined by Jackson (1970, 1971, 1973) as pertinent for a construct-based approach to test construction. Although not entirely congruent with a more theoretically based construct approach, the HPSI may certainly be viewed as a variant of this construct strategy of test development.

EVALUATION OF THE CONSTRUCT VALIDITY OF THE HPSI

Psychometrically, construct validation is an ongoing process that is addressed at a number of levels. At the item level, the construct validity of the HPSI has been evaluated in terms of both internal consistency reliability and factor structure.

Internal consistency reliability, an index of the degree to which items correlate with one another, may be regarded as operationalizing one form of construct validity, convergent validity. Research studies have provided evidence as to the internal consistency reliability of HPSI scales and are summarized in Table 2. Data are drawn from 14 different university, high school, medical, military, forensic, and psychiatric samples. Across all samples, the median coefficient alpha reliability is .76 for Psychiatric Symptomatology, .71 for Social Symptomatology, and .82 for Depression. Although what constitutes an adequate level for coefficient alpha may be dependent on the purpose and context of the assessment (Nunnally & Bernstein, 1994), a value below .60 may be regarded as inadequate for any purpose (DeVellis, 1991). Therefore, in general, HPSI scales appear to possess appropriate levels of internal consistency reliability, one component of construct validity.

Although convergence among items represents one essential component for the construct validity of items, discriminant validity is also a crucial aspect of this validity. That is, items on a scale should not relate to other hypothetically independent constructs and measures. This form of construct validity, as well as convergent validity, may be examined through factor analytic procedures. For the HPSI, at an item level, factor analytic support for both the convergent and discriminant validity of items should be provided by demonstrating that items keyed for particular scales load on the same relevant factor (i.e., have convergent validity) and not on irrelevant (i.e., non-keyed) factors (i.e., have discriminant validity). A total of seven studies have examined the item factor structure of the HPSI. Included in these analyses are respondents sampled from university, high school, military, general normative, psychiatric, and offender populations. In these investigations, confirmatory principal components analysis has been used whereby three components are extracted from the HPSI item intercorrelation matrix and rotated orthogonally to a target matrix representing the HPSI scoring key. The fit between the rotated item factor loading matrix and the target matrix is then quantified using coefficients of congruence (Harman, 1976). Results from these studies are reported in Table 3. Observed congruence coefficients are all strong, indicating substantial support for the convergent and discriminant validity of the HPSI items.

As well as examining construct validity at the item level, the establishment of construct validity for scales is perhaps even more important. Although items represent the basic building blocks of scales, item construct validity may be a necessary but not sufficient condition for similar validity at the scale level.

Table 2. HPSI Scale Internal Consistency Reliability (Coefficient Alpha)

Sample	Psychiatric Symptomatology	Social Symptomatology	Depression
343 university students (Holden, 1991)	.74	.72	.83
150 university students (Holden, 1991)	.63	.68	.77
64 university students (Holden, 1992)	.75	.70	.87
64 psychiatric patients (Holden et al., 1992)	.81	.74	.90
61 male adolescents ˙ (Reddon, 1993)	.81	.81	.86
78 female adolescents (Reddon, 1993)	.69	.82	.82
84 psychiatric offenders (Holden & Grigoriadis, 1995)	.81	.79	.87
564 adults (Holden et al., 1996)	.73	.66	.82
265 offenders (Reddick, 1998)	.79	.76	.88
144 mature high school students (Reddon et al., 1998)	.73	.62	.81
33 male urology patients (Holden, 1999)	.78	.60	.80
29 wives of male urology patients (Holden, 1999)	.81	.52	.82
1709 military personnel (Magruder et al., in press)	.79	.81	.80
200 university students (Holden et al., 1999)	.75	.60	.86
Median	.76	.71	.82

Table 3. Congruence of HPSI Item Factor Loading Matrices Orthogonally Rotated to Target Matrix Based on Scoring Key

Sample	Psychiatric Symptomatology	Social Symptomatology	Depression
64 psychiatric patients (Holden et al., 1992)	.91	.79	.93
139 adolescents (Reddon, 1993)	.85	.89	.94
84 psychiatric offenders (Holden & Grigoriadis, 1995)	.91	.84	.92
564 adults (Holden et al., 1996)	.85	.85	.93
265 offenders (Reddick, 1998)	.90	.92	.95
1709 military personnel (Magruder et al., in press)	.81	.87	.90
200 university students (Holden et al., 1999)	.87	.81	.93
Median	.87	.85	.93

Furthermore, given that the focus of inventory interpretation is primarily for scales, the consideration of scale convergent and discriminant validity is a highly relevant aspect for evaluating the construct validity of the HPSI.

A first issue that arises is the relative independence of HPSI scales. Are the three scales of the HPSI statistically distinct from one another and, thus, capable of differential interpretation? Data for eight samples of students, general normative adults, offenders, and psychiatric patients all attest to the relative orthogonality of scales (Holden, 1996, p. 33). Correlations between Psychiatric Symptomatology and Social Symptomatology vary between -.01 and .42 (mean correlation = .28). For Psychiatric Symptomatology and Depression, correlations average .34 (range between .15 and .59). For Social Symptomatology and Depression, correlations vary between -.07 and .28 (mean correlation = .16). Although Holden indicates that scale intercorrelations do vary as a function of the nature of the sample of respondents, in general, the magnitudes of the associations indicate the appropriateness of interpreting three different dimensional scales for the HPSI.

The convergent validity of the HPSI scales has been evaluated by examining correlations between HPSI scales and other theoretically relevant ratings or scales.

This form of validity has been investigated with samples of students, military personnel, psychiatric patients, and offenders. For HPSI scales of Psychiatric

Table 4. Convergent Validities (Zero-order Correlations) for the HPSI Scale of Psychiatric Symptomatology

Sample	Criterion	Validity
150 students (Holden, 1991)	Peer Ratings	.28
64 psychiatric patients (Holden et al., 1992)	Clinician Ratings	.28
84 psychiatric offenders (Holden & Grigoriadis, 1995)	MMPI-2 Self-Report Scale: Hypochondriasis	
	Hysteria	.71
	Paranoia	.28
	Psychasthenia	.54
	Schizophrenia	.60
		.61
	BPI Self-Report Scale: Hypochondriasis	
	Anxiety	.67
	Thinking Disorder	.53
	Persecutory Ideas	.66
	Deviation	.42
		.58
144 mature high school students (Reddon et al., 1998)	BPI Self-Report Scale: Hypochondriasis	.63
	Anxiety	.54
	Thinking Disorder	.31
	Persecutory Ideas	.41
	Deviation	.49
277 psychiatric offenders (Lawrence, 1995)	Carlson (1981) Psychological Survey Self-Report Scale: Thought Disturbance	.62
1709 military personnel (Holden et al., 1999)	Q-SAD Self-Report Scale: Posttraumatic Stress Disorder	.34
	Panic Disorder	.32

Table 5. Convergent Validities (Zero-order Correlations) for the HPSI Scale of Social Symptomatology

Sample	Criterion	Validity
150 students (Holden, 1991)	Peer Ratings	.37
64 psychiatric patients (Holden et al., 1992)	Clinician Ratings	.40
84 psychiatric offenders (Holden & Grigoriadis, 1995)	MMPI-2 Self-Report Scale:	
	Psychopathic Deviate	.27
	Paranoia	.39
	Hypomania	.43
	BPI Self-Report Scale:	
	Interpersonal Problems	.50
	Alienation	.63
	Persecutory Ideas	.40
	Impulse Expression	.57
	Deviation	.45
144 mature high school students (Reddon et al., 1998)	BPI Self-Report Scale:	
	Interpersonal Problems	.51
	Alienation	.49
	Persecutory Ideas	.31
	Impulse Expression	.37
	Deviation	.38
277 psychiatric offenders (Lawrence, 1995)	Carlson (1981) Psychological Survey Self-Report Scale:	
	Chemical Abuse	.51
	Antisocial Tendencies	.51
200 university students (Holden et al., 1999)	Brief Symptom Inventory Self-Report Scale:	
	Hostility	.38
	Paranoid Ideation	.20
1709 military personnel (Holden et al., 1999)	Q-SAD Self-Report Scale:	
	Substance Abuse	.50

Table 6. Convergent Validities (Zero-order Correlations) for the HPSI Scale of Depression

Sample	Criterion	Validity
150 students (Holden, 1991)	Peer Ratings	.41
64 psychiatric patients (Holden et al., 1992)	Clinician Ratings	.75
84 psychiatric offenders (Holden & Grigoriadis, 1995)	MMPI-2 Self-Report Scale: Depression	.59
	Social Introversion	.55
	BPI Self-Report Scale: Depression	.73
	Social Introversion	.46
	Self-Depreciation	.57
144 mature high school students (Reddon et al., 1998)	BPI Self-Report Scale: Depression	.68
	Social Introversion	.49
	Self-Depreciation	.46
277 psychiatric offenders (Lawrence, 1995)	Carlson (1981) Psychological Survey Self-Report Scale: Self-Depreciation	.66
200 university students (Holden et al., 1999)	Brief Symptom Inventory Self-Report Scale: Depression	.38
1709 military personnel (Holden et al., 1999)	Q-SAD Self-Report Scale: Depression	.41

Symptomatology, Social Symptomatology, and Depression, convergent validities (zero-order correlations) from different studies are summarized in Tables 4, 5, and 6, respectively. For Psychiatric Symptomatology, reported validities range between .28 (correlation with corresponding ratings by peers or clinicians) and .71 (correlation with BPI Hypochondriasis scale scores). Validities for Social Symptomatology vary from .20 (correlation with Brief Symptom Inventory Paranoid Ideation scale) and .63 (correlation with BPI Alienation scale). For the HPSI Depression scale, validities range between .38 (correlation with the Brief Symptom Inventory Depression scale) and .75 (correlation with corresponding ratings by clinicians). Values generally provide substantial evidence for the convergent validity of the HPSI scales, one component of their construct validity.

Discriminant validity for the HPSI scales is also an important component of construct validity. Particularly for scales of psychopathology, convergence among scales may be enhanced by confounds associated with response styles such as social (un)desirability. Consequently, the evaluation of construct validity for measures of psychopathology demands not only that relevant scales group together appropriately, but also that supposedly distinct measures exist as separate entities. Discriminant (and convergent) validity of HPSI scales has been examined through two different types of multivariate analysis: factor analysis and canonical correlation. Two factor analytic results, one based on psychiatric offenders and one based on mature high school students, are displayed in Tables 7 and 8, respectively

Table 7. Varimax-Rotated Factor Loadings for HPSI, MMPI-2, and BPI Scales

	Factor		
Scale	I	II	III
Hypomania (MMPI-2)	.80		
Alienation (BPI)	.78		
Social Symptomatology (HPSI)	**.74**		
Impulse Expression (BPI)	.72		
Persecutory Ideas (BPI)	.69		
Schizophrenia (MMPI-2)	.66		
Deviation (BPI)	.63		
Interpersonal Problems (BPI)	.62		
Psychasthenia (MMPI-2)	.62	.56	
Thinking Disorder (BPI)	.61		.53
Paranoia (MMPI-2)	.58		.55
Anxiety (BPI)	.53		
Depression (HPSI)		**.85**	
Depression (BPI)		.83	
Social Introversion (MMPI-2)		.76	
Depression (MMPI-2)		.75	
Self Depreciation (BPI)		.74	
Social Introversion (BPI)		.60	
Psychopathic Deviate (MMPI-2)		.56	
Hypochondriasis (MMPI-2)			.84
Hypochondriasis (BPI)			.82
Hysteria (MMPI-2)			.70
Psychiatric Symptomatology (HPSI)			**.66**

Note. Adapted from Holden and Grigoriadis (1995). Only loadings above .50 are presented. HPSI scales are in boldface.

demonstrating that HPSI scales: (1)   load separate latent dimensions; (2) group together with theoretically relevant scales from the MMPI-2 and the BPI; and (3) are distinct from theoretically irrelevant MMPI-2 and BPI scales.

Table 8. Varimax-Rotated Factor Loadings for HPSI and BPI Scales

		Factor	
Scale	I	II	III
Self Depreciation (BPI)	.79		
Thinking Disorder (BPI)	.73		
Depression (BPI)	.69		
Social Introversion (BPI)	.67		
Depression (HPSI)	**.65**		
Persecutory Ideas (BPI)	.59		
Psychiatric Symptomatology (HPSI)		**.82**	
Hypochondriasis (BPI)		.81	
Anxiety (BPI)		.67	
Social Symptomatology (HPSI)			**.80**
Interpersonal Problems (BPI)			.76
Alienation (BPI)			.65
Denial			-.64
Deviation			
Impulse Expression			

Note. Adapted from Reddon, Willis, and Choldin (1998). Only loadings above .50 are presented. HPSI scales are in boldface.

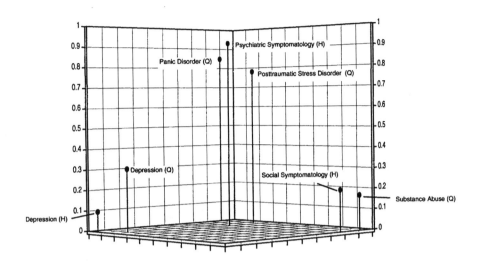

Note. - (H) and (Q) refer to HPSI and Q-SAD scales, respectively.

Figure 2.   Varimax-Rotated Canonical Loadings of HPSI and Q-SAD Scales

Canonical analyses have also supported the tri-dimensional nature of the HPSI and offered support for the convergent and discriminant validity of its scales. Figure 2 is a graphical display of how scales from the DSM-IV-based Questionnaire for Substance Abuse, Anxiety, and Depression (Q-SAD; First, Spitzer, Williams, & Gibbon, 1996) relate to HPSI scales for a large sample of U.S. military personnel. Figure 3 portrays the relationships between scales from the HPSI and those from the Brief Symptom Inventory (BSI; Derogatis, 1993) for a sample of university undergraduates. In both instances, three significant independent linear sets of scale variates emerged. Further, each HPSI scale loaded only on one rotated dimension, that specific dimension was also marked by hypothetically related scales from the other inventory, and that particular dimension was not loaded by theoretically unrelated scales from the other inventory.

APPLICATIONS OF THE HPSI

Although still a relatively new screening instrument, the HPSI has been used in various applied settings and use of the inventory continues to grow. Populations for which the HPSI has been employed include psychiatric patients (Holden, 1996; Holden, Mendonca, Mazmanian, & Reddon, 1992), psychiatric offenders (Holden & Grigoriadis, 1995; Reddick, 1998), young offenders (Reddon, Pope, Friel, & Sinha, 1996; Starzyk, Reddon, & Friel, in press), urology patients (Holden, 1999), the military (Holden, Magruder, Stein, Sitarenios, & Sheldon, 1999; Magruder, Holden, Stein, Harazin, Alonso, Sitarenios, & Sheldon, in press), university students (Holden, 1992), and the general public (Holden, Kerr, & Hill, 1996; Reddon, Willis, & Choldin, 1998). Purposes of HPSI use have included screening for psychopathology, examination of various psychological phenomena (e.g., faking; Holden, 1995), and both program evaluation and the measurement of patient improvement with psychological treatment (Reddon, Pope, Dorias, & Pullan, 1996; Reddon, Starzyk, Pullan, & Dorais, 1997; Waring, Holden, & Kimmons, 1994). Additional future research will serve to delineate more fully the extensiveness of the HPSI's applicability.

CONCLUSIONS

Overall, evidence supports the construct validity of the HPSI scales. Scales are internally consistent and items representatively sample from appropriate facets of psychopathology. Item factor analytic results support the convergent and discriminant validity of the items and the appropriateness of the inventory's scoring key. HPSI scales are relatively independent of each other and demonstrate convergent validity in terms of correlations with other corresponding scales and criterion ratings by significant others. Scale convergent and discriminant validity is also evident through factor analytic and canonical relationships between HPSI scales and other self-report scales of psychological dysfunctioning. To date, therefore, the HPSI appears to be a promising new self-report screening measure of psychopathology. The HPSI's promise, however, is largely predicated on its foundation in construct-based test development.

Few multiphasic inventories of psychopathology have been shown to generate discriminantly valid scale scores (Holden & Jackson, 1992). This shortcoming is partly attributable to the empirical approach to test construction having emerged earlier in time than the construct-based strategy. Particularly, with the rapid ascendance and dominance of the MMPI, an empirically based instrument, the construct strategy of test construction has been relatively slower to establish a major foothold in the practice of the assessment of psychopathology. In more recent years, however, construct-based inventories of psychopathology have begun to emerge, become accepted, and, in some instances, to outperform other, older inventories that were developed using alternative strategies of test construction. As this trend continues, future test developers and users will look back to the last half of the 20th century and more fully appreciate the pioneering efforts of advocates of the construct approach to test construction, such as Douglas N. Jackson.

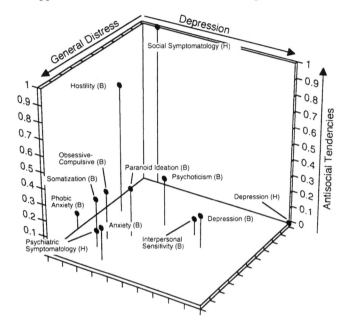

Note. - (H) and (B) refer to scales from the HPSI and BSI, respectively.

Figure 3. Varimax-Rotated Canonical Loadings of HPSI and BSI Scales

REFERENCES

Austin, G. W., Leschied, A. W., Jaffe, P. G., & Sas, L. (1986). Factor structure and construct validity of the Basic Personality Inventory. *Canadian Journal of Behavioural Science,* **18,** 238-247.

Berg, I. A. (1957). Deviant responses and deviant people: The formulation of the Deviation Hypothesis. *Journal of Counseling Psychology,* **4,** 154-161.

Berg, I. A. (1967). The Deviation Hypothesis. A broad statement of its assumptions and postulates. In I. A. (Ed.), *Response set in personality assessment* (pp. 146-190). Chicago: Aldine.

Bjorgvinsson, T., & Thompson, A. P. (1994). Psychometric properties of an Icelandic translation of the Basic Personality Inventory: Cross-cultural invariance of a three-factor solution. *Personality and Individual Differences,* **16,** 47-56.

Bowman, M. L. (1989). Testing individual differences in ancient China. *American Psychologist,* **44,** 576-578.

Butcher, J. N., Morfitt, R. C., Rouse, S. V., & Holden, R. R. (1997). Reducing MMPI-2 defensiveness: The effect of specialized instructions on retest validity in a job applicant sample. *Journal of Personality Assessment*, **68**, 385-401.

Campbell, D. T., & Fiske, D. W. (1959). Convergent and discriminant validation by the multitrait-multimethod matrix. *Psychological Bulletin*, **56**, 81-105.

Carlson, K. A. (1981). *Carlson Psychological Survey*. Port Huron, MI: Sigma Assessment Systems.

Chrisjohn, R. D., Jackson, D. N., & Lanigan, C. B. (1984, June). *The stability of the factor structure of the Basic Personality Inventory*. Paper presented at the Canadian Psychological Association Annual Convention, Ottawa, Canada.

Cronbach, L. J., & Meehl, P. E. (1955). Construct validity in psychological tests. *Psychological Bulletin*, **52**, 281-302.

Derogatis, L. R. (1993). *Brief Symptom Inventory (BSI): Administration, scoring, and procedures manual*. Minneapolis, MN: National Computer Systems.

DeVellis, R. F. (1991). *Scale development: Theory and applications*. Newbury Park, CA: Sage.

Dubois, P. H. (1970). *A history of psychological testing*. Boston: Allyn & Bacon.

Ellis, A. (1946). The validity of personality questionnaires. *Psychological Bulletin*, **43**, 385-440.

Faschingbauer, T. R. (1979). The future of the MMPI. In C. S. Newmark (Ed.), *MMPI clinical and research trends* (pp. 373-398). New York: Praeger.

First, M. B., Spitzer, R. L., Williams, J. B. W., & Gibbon, M. (1996). *Q-SAD*. North Tonawanda, NY: Multi-Health Systems.

Goldberg, L. R. (1971). A historical survey of personality scales and inventories. In P. McReynolds (Ed.), *Advances in psychological assessment* (Vol. 2, pp. 293-336). Palo Alto, CA: Science and Behavior Books.

Goldberg, L. R., & Slovic, P. (1967). Importance of test item content: An analysis of a corollary of the Deviation Hypothesis. *Journal of Counseling Psychology*, **14**, 462-472.

Harman, H. H. (1976). *Modern factor analysis* (3rd ed.). Chicago: University of Chicago Press.

Hathaway, S. R., & McKinley, J. C. (1940). A multiphasic personality schedule (Minnesota): I. Construction of the schedule. *Journal of Psychology*, **10**, 249-254.

Helmes, E., & Reddon, J. R. (1993). A perspective on developments in assessing psychopathology: A critical review of the MMPI and MMPI-2. *Psychological Bulletin*, **113**, 453-471.

Heymans, G., & Wiersma, E. (1906). Beitrage zur speziellen psychologie auf grund einer massenuntersuchung. *Zeitschrift fur Psychologie*, **43**, 81-127, 158-301.

Hoffmann, H., Jackson, D. N., & Skinner, H. A. (1975). Dimensions of psychopathology among alcoholic patients. *Journal of Studies on Alcohol*, **36**, 825-837.

Holden, R. R. (1991, June). *Psychometric properties of the Holden Psychological Screening Inventory (HPSI)*. Paper presented at the Canadian Psychological Association Annual Convention, Calgary, Canada.

Holden, R. R. (1992). Associations between the Holden Psychological Screening Inventory and the NEO Five-Factor Inventory in a nonclinical sample. *Psychological Reports*, **71**, 1039-1042.

Holden, R. R. (1995). Faking and its detection on the Holden Psychological Screening Inventory. *Psychological Reports*, **76**, 1235-1240.

Holden, R. R. (1996). *Holden Psychological Screening Inventory (HPSI)*. North Tonawanda, NY: Multi-Health Systems.

Holden, R. R. (1999). The Holden Psychological Screening Inventory and sexual efficacy in urological patients with erectile dysfunction. *Psychological Reports*, **84**, 255-258.

Holden, R. R. (in press). Psychometrics. In A. E. Kazdin (Ed.), *Encyclopedia of psychology*. Washington: American Psychological Association.

Holden, R. R., Fekken, G. C., & Cotton, D. H. G. (1991). Assessing psychopathology using structured test-item response latencies. *Psychological Assessment*, **3**, 111-118.

Holden, R. R., Fekken, G. C., Reddon, J. R., Helmes, E., & Jackson, D. N. (1988). Clinical reliabilities and validities of the Basic Personality Inventory. *Journal of Consulting and Clinical Psychology*, **56**, 766-768.

Holden, R. R., & Grigoriadis, S. (1995). Psychometric properties of the Holden Psychological Screening Inventory for a psychiatric offender sample. *Journal of Clinical Psychology*, **51**, 811-819.

Holden, R. R., & Jackson, D. N. (1992). Assessing psychopathology using the Basic Personality Inventory: Rationale and applications. In J. C. Rosen & P. McReynolds (Ed.), *Advances in psychological assessment* (Vol. 8, pp. 165-199). New York: Plenum.

Holden, R. R., Kerr, P. S., & Hill, S. A. (1996, August). *The Holden Psychological Screening Inventory: Canadian normative data and demographic correlates.* Paper presented at the XXVI International Congress of Psychology, Montreal, Canada.

Holden, R. R., Magruder, C. D., First, M. B., Stein, S. J., Sitarenios, G., & Sheldon, S. (1999, August). *Validity of the Holden Psychological Screening Inventory in the military.* Paper presented at the American Psychological Association Annual Convention, Boston, MA.

Holden, R. R., Magruder, C. D., Stein, S. J., Sitarenios, G., & Sheldon, S. (1999). The effects of anonymity on the Holden Psychological Screening Inventory. *Personality and Individual Differences, 27*, 737-742.

Holden, R. R., Mendonca, J. D., Mazmanian, D., & Reddon, J. R. (1992). Clinical construct validity of the Holden Psychological Screening Inventory (HPSI). *Journal of Clinical Psychology, 48*, 627-633.

Holden, R. R., Starzyk, K. B., McLeod, L. D., & Edwards, M. J. (1999). *Comparisons among the Holden Psychological Screening Inventory (HPSI), the Brief Symptom Inventory (BSI), and the Balanced Inventory for Desirable Responding (BIDR).* Manuscript submitted for publication.

Jackson, D. N. (1970). A sequential system for personality scale development. In C. D. Spielberger (Ed.), *Current topics in clinical and community psychology* (Vol. 2, pp. 61-96). New York: Academic Press.

Jackson, D. N. (1971). The dynamics of structured personality tests: 1971. *Psychological Review, 78*, 229-248.

Jackson, D. N. (1973). Structured personality assessment. In B. B. Wolman (Ed.), *Handbook of general psychology* (pp. 775-792). Englewood Cliffs, NJ: Prentice-Hall.

Jackson, D. N. (1975, November). *Orthogonal components of psychopathology: A fresh approach to measuring the constructs underlying MMPI clinical scales.* Paper presented at the Society of Multivariate Experimental Psychology, Eugene, Oregon.

Jackson, D. N. (1984). *Personality Research Form manual (3rd ed.).* Port Huron, MI: Sigma Assessment Systems.

Jackson, D. N. (1989). *Basic Personality Inventory.* Port Huron, MI: Sigma Assessment Systems.

Jackson, D. N., Helmes, E., Hoffmann, H., Holden, R. R., Jaffe, P., Reddon, J. R., & Smiley, W. C. (1989). *Basic Personality Inventory manual.* Port Huron, MI: Sigma Assessment Systems.

Jackson, D. N., & Messick, S. (1971). *The Differential Personality Inventory.* London, Ontario: Authors.

Jackson, D. N., & Paunonen, S. V. (1980). Personality structure and assessment. *Annual Review of Psychology, 31*, 503-551.

Jackson, D. N., & Reddon, J. R. (1987). Construct interpretation of Minnesota Multiphasic Personality Inventory (MMPI) clinical scales: An orthogonal transformation. *Journal of Psychopathology and Behavioral Assessment, 9*, 149-160.

Lawrence, P. G. (1995). [The HPSI in a psychiatric prison]. Unpublished raw data.

Loevinger, J. (1957). Objective tests as instruments of psychological theory. *Psychological Reports, 3*, 635-694.

Magruder, C. D., Holden, R. R., Stein, S. J., Harazin, J. S., Alonso, R. A., Sitarenios, G., & Sheldon, S. (in press). Psychometric properties of the Holden Psychological Screening Inventory (HPSI in the U.S. military. *Military Psychology.*

Meehl, P. E. (1945). The dynamics of "structured" personality tests. *Journal of Clinical Psychology, 1*, 296-303.

Murray, H. A. (1938). *Explorations in personality.* New York: Oxford University Press.

Neill, J. A., & Jackson, D. N. (1976). Minimum redundancy item analysis. *Educational and Psychological Bulletin, 36*, 123-134.

Nunnally, J. C., & Bernstein, I. H. (1994). *Psychometric theory (3rd ed.).* New York: McGraw-Hill.

Ozer, D. J., & Reise, S. P. (1994). Personality assessment. *Annual Review of Psychology, 45*, 357-388.

Piotrowski, C., & Keller, J. W. (1984). Psychodiagnostic testing in APA-approved clinical psychology programs. *Professional Psychology: Research and Practice, 15*, 450-456.

Piotrowski, C., & Keller, J. W. (1989). Psychological testing in outpatient mental health facilities: A national study. *Professional Psychology: Research and Practice, 20*, 423-425.

Piotrowski, C., & Lubin, B. (1990). Assessment practices of health psychologists: Survey of APA Division 38 clinicians. *Professional Psychology: Research and Practice, 21*, 99-106.

Reddick, R. D. (1998). *The relationship between patient satisfaction and psychosocial adjustment in a forensic psychiatric outpatient population.* Unpublished master's thesis, University of Alberta, Edmonton, Alberta, Canada.

Reddon, J. R. (1993). [HPSI high school norms]. Unpublished raw data.

Reddon, J. R., Pope, G. A., Dorais, S., & Pullan, M. D. (1996). Improvement in psychosocial adjustment for psychiatric patients after a 16-week life skills education program. *Journal of Clinical Psychology, 52*, 165-168.

Reddon, J. R., Pope, G. A., Friel, J. P., & Sinha, B. K. (1996). Leisure motivation in relation to psychosocial adjustment and personality in young offender and high school samples. *Journal of Clinical Psychology, 52*, 679-685.

Reddon, J. R., Starzyk, K.B., Pullan, M. D., & Dorais, S. (1997, February). *Psychosocial adjustment in 44 psychiatric patients following a 16-week life skills education course: A replication and extension.* Pater presented at the Annual Royce Research Conference, Edmonton, Alberta, Canada.

Reddon, J. R., Willis, S. D., & Choldin, S. (1998). Relationship between the Holden Psychological Screening Inventory (HPSI) and the Basic Personality Inventory (BPI) in a community sample. *Journal of Psychopathology and Behavioral Assessment, 20*, 295-306.

Starzyk, K. B., Reddon, J. R., & Friel, J. P. (In press). Need structure, leisure motivation, and psychosocial adjustment among young offenders and high school students. *Journal of Offender Rehabilitation.*

Tellegen, A., & Waller, N. G. (in press). Exploring personality through test construction: Development of the Multidimensional Personality Questionnaire. In S. R. Briggs & J. M. Cheek (Eds.), *Personality measures: Development and evaluation (Vol. 1).* Greenwich, CT: JAI Press.

Waring, E. M., Holden, R. R., & Kimmons, G. (1994, April). *Holden Psychological Screening Inventory (HPSI) as a measure of impact of brief psychiatric hospitalization.* Paper presented to the Department of Psychiatry, Hotel Dieu Hospital, Kingston, Ontario, Canada.

Wiggins, J. S. (1973). *Personality and prediction: Principles of personality assessment.* Reading, MA: Addison-Wesley.

Woodworth, R. S. (1917). *Personal Data Sheet.* Chicago: Stoetling.

6 CONSTRUCT VALIDITY AND THE SEARCH FOR CROSS-CULTURAL CONSISTENCIES IN PERSONALITY

Sampo V. Paunonen[1]

Personality psychologists have long been interested in the issue of the consistency of human behavior across cultures. Research and theorizing in this area has typically addressed questions of the following type. Do people engage in the same behaviors in different cultures? If certain behaviors can be categorized as manifestations of so-called personality traits, are those traits themselves consistent or universal across cultures? If such traits are organized in a structured personality network, is that organization a universal one? Answers to such questions are important for obvious theoretical reasons. They are also important for practical reasons – assuming there is some generality to personality and behavior, the expedient may exist of using personality measures developed in one culture with respondents from another culture.

Although definitive answers to questions like those above are notably lacking in the current state of the art, not lacking are recommendations on how to tackle the problems empirically. The purpose of this chapter is to evaluate some of these recommendations critically. I will point out that a certain amount of confusion exists in the literature regarding prescriptions for empirical methods of identifying cross-cultural consistencies in human behavior. Moreover, I will propose that much of this confusion could have been precluded had cross-cultural psychologists made reference to seminal works in the area of psychological measurement by Cronbach and Meehl, Jackson, Loevinger, Messick, and others. Those works pertain to the principle of construct validation.

I will begin my thesis by describing a model of personality that is generally accepted as an accurate representation of human behavior, at least in Western cultures. The model posits a hierarchical arrangement to the components of personality. I will then delineate some issues that arise when applying that model of personality to other cultures. Those issues pertain to the fact that some of the hierarchy's components may be general across cultures whereas others may not. Next, I will evaluate critically some of the empirical procedures that have been offered as methods of testing one culture's model of personality and behavior in another culture. I will show that those methods are problematic in many respects, primarily in harboring a bias toward the identification of behavioral specificity across cultures. Finally, I will offer my own recommendations for conducting a search for cross-cultural consistencies in personality. My recommendations are based on fundamental psychometric propositions involving the notion of construct validity.

A HIERARCHICAL MODEL OF PERSONALITY

As early as 1947, personality in Western cultures was conceptualized as having a formal hierarchical organization. The basis of one such hierarchy, shown in Figure 1 (see Paunonen, 1998), was the breadth of behaviors involved. As illustrated at the very bottom of that hierarchy, various specific behavioral acts are thought to define a person's habitual response pattern. Several such response patterns, or characteristic modes of behavior, combine to form what is commonly called a personality trait. Those personality traits then combine to form a personality factor at the top of the hierarchy. One can see that the behavior domains represented in Figure 1 increase in breadth as one moves from the lower levels of the hierarchy to the higher levels.

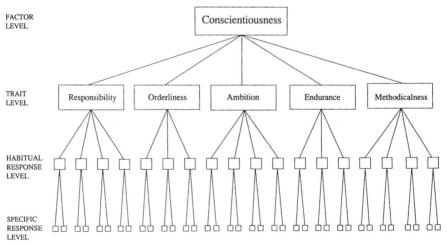

Figure 1. A hierarchical model of personality organization.

The hierarchy as illustrated in Figure 1 is, of course, a simplification. It is a simplification because only one personality factor is illustrated. Many personality factors are presumed to exist, factors that either are independent of one another or are correlated. The figure is also a simplification because each trait is shown to have an exclusive link to a single factor. In actuality, most traits probably have associations with more than one personality factor in varying degrees. Even the individual behavioral acts shown at the lowest level of the hierarchy can be differently construed. Whereas each behavior is illustrated as an exemplar or manifestation of a particular trait and factor, those behaviors might each represent multiple higher-order constructs, again in varying degrees.

The notion of a hierarchical organization to personality has long been appealing to psychologists. It is only recently, however, that the specific components of the hierarchy have been identified with some degree of empirical consensus. Some of those components are evident in the so-called Five-Factor Model of personality structure. That model maintains that there are exactly five personality factors at the top of the hierarchy that account for the majority of variations in human behavior. Those factors, often referred to as the Big Five factors, have been labeled as Extraversion, Agreeableness, Conscientiousness, Neuroticism, and Openness to Experience (e.g., see Digman, 1990; John, 1990; McCrae & John, 1992). Some of the specific personality traits and behaviors that feed into the Big Five at lower levels of the hierarchy have been identified concurrently, although there is less than a perfect consensus over the details (e.g., see Ashton, Jackson, Helmes, & Paunonen, 1998; Ashton, Paunonen, Helmes, & Jackson, 1998; Block, 1995; Jackson, Paunonen, Fraboni, & Goffin, 1996; Paunonen & Jackson, 1996; Saucier & Ostendorf, 1999).

Although the Big Five factors have been quite consistently found in personality data, those data have been mostly from North American and European respondents (Paunonen & Ashton, 1998), with some corroborative data from non-Western respondents (Church & Katigbak, 1989; Church & Lonner, 1998). Nonetheless, the factors have been proposed by some as being universal (McCrae, Costa, del Pilar, Rolland, & Parker, 1998). As will be pointed out later, however, this question of the generality of personality structure is only one of many questions that can be asked regarding cross-cultural consistencies in human behavior.

THE EMIC/ETIC DISTINCTION OF CROSS-CULTURAL PSYCHOLOGY

It has long been recognized by psychologists and anthropologists alike that there are particular problems that arise when one attempts to evaluate cross-cultural generalities in human behavior. One of these problems concerns the instruments used to record behavior and personality in the different cultures. A measure of, say, achievement motivation developed in one culture might not be appropriate for use in another culture. More important, the personality trait itself might not be relevant to the people of the other culture. The issue raised here concerns the so-called emic vs. etic distinction of cross-cultural psychology.

Berry (1969) has discussed at length some of the problems of comparative research in cross-cultural psychology. In that article, he highlighted and formalized Pike's (1966) distinction between emics and etics: "emics apply in only a particular society, while etics are culture-free or universal aspects of the world" (Berry, 1969, p. 123). A personality construct, for example, known to exist in one culture, might or might not exist in all cultures. In the latter case, in which the construct is relevant to only one or a few cultures, one would class it as an emic concept. In the former case, in which the trait is a universal one, it would be called an etic concept. This particular emic/etic distinction is summarized in the upper half of Figure 2.

PERSONALITY CONSTRUCT
   Emic: The personality construct or trait is regional and is
            relevant only to specific cultures
   Etic: The personality construct is universal and is
            relevant to all cultures

RESEARCH STRATEGY
   Emic: To use indigenous personality measures developed
            locally in each culture
   Etic: To use imported personality measures developed
            in other cultures

Figure 2.   Emic/etic distinctions of cross-cultural psychology.

The emic/etic distinction referred to above, regarding the underlying nature of personality traits and behaviors, is not the only distinction. As noted by Berry (1969), the terms emic and etic can also be applied to the research strategy used to evaluate personality cross-culturally. An emic research strategy involves the use of indigenous personality measures in each culture studied. That is, no assumption is made that an indicator of personality in one culture will be such an indicator in some other culture. An etic research strategy, also called the "imposed etic" strategy by Berry (1969), involves using measures of personality that have been developed and evaluated in one culture with people from another culture. The assumption here, of course, is that the measuring device is equally relevant to the different cultures being assessed. This second emic/etic distinction is summarized in the lower half of Figure 2.

Cross-cultural psychologists have, in general, recommended against using an etic, or imposed etic, approach to the study of personality in very different populations. One might easily arrive at the conclusion, for instance, that the cultures differ in terms of their personality characteristics when those differences are due merely to the fact that the personality measures used are not equally valid across the cultures assessed. As might be imagined, there are many reasons why a foreign or imported measure might not be valid in a culture, not the least of which are problems that can arise due to the improper translation of verbal materials (see also Paunonen & Ashton, 1998).

Another reason why an etic research strategy is generally eschewed in the study of personality can be gleaned from a consideration of the top half of Figure 2, and that is the fact the personality construct itself may not be etic. Therefore, the personality assessment device, which may be relevant for the culture in which it was constructed, may not be at all relevant for another culture. To put it another way, if a construct is truly emic to a particular culture, then only an emically-based measure of that construct will be appropriate for its assessment.

EMIC/ETIC COMPONENTS OF THE PERSONALITY HIERARCHY

If one considers Figure 1 in juxtaposition with Figure 2, something becomes immediately apparent – the emic/etic distinctions referred to in the latter are too coarse and simplistic to provide satisfying recommendations for the cross-cultural study of the personality components shown in the former. For example, one could argue that the emic/etic distinction applies to each of the different levels of the personality hierarchy separately. Moreover, one could argue that the very structure of the personality network might have emic/etic properties as well. I elaborate below.

Emic/Etic Behaviors

Consider the lowest level of the personality hierarchy, representing a person's specific behavioral acts. No one has ever questioned the fact that some personality-relevant acts are purely etic or universal (e.g., smiling) and some are purely emic or culturally specific. In the latter case, behaviors may be emic for cultural reasons. Or, they may be specific to a group for political, geographic, or economic reasons as well. Consider the practice of body-surfing as indicative of risk-taking tendencies. For reasons mostly related to climate, even the most adventurous Inuit resident of northern Canada is unlikely to practice this sport. Thus, body-surfing would be unlikely to be considered a universal or etic exemplar of thrill-seeking behavior.

But even when the same behavior exists in two or more cultures, it may have a different meaning in those cultures. This refers to the concept of functional equivalence as discussed by Berry (1969) and Frijda and Jahoda (1966). In Figure 1, for example, a single behavior is shown to be part of a characteristic pattern of behaviors, which in turn is considered a manifestation of a particular personality trait. But it is possible that the same behavior is an exemplar of a different trait in a different culture. To illustrate, attending a large party may be an indication of affiliation in an individualist culture whereas the same behavior may indicate dependence in a collectivist culture. Furthermore, the behaviors that represent affiliation in the collectivist culture may be different than the affiliation-related behaviors of the individualist culture.

Emic/Etic Traits

Although most will probably agree that specific behaviors can differ across cultures, and the meaning of those behaviors can also differ as far as their trait referents are concerned, can the traits themselves differ? Perhaps. An emic or culturally specific personality trait in Figure 1 might be ambition or achievement motivation, as an example. That trait simply might not be relevant to the people of some non-Western culture. Or, in that culture there might be other unique traits that exist, traits unheard of in Western cultures. Several putative examples of emic personality constructs have been compiled by Church and Katigbak (1988, p. 143), a couple of which are referred to later in this chapter. [2]

Now, assuming that common personality traits do in fact exist in two or more cultures, their organization within the presumed personality hierarchy could be different in those cultures. This means that the links represented in Figure 1 between the personality traits and the higher level factor could be culturally specific (emic) whereas the traits themselves are universal (etic). Consider the trait of ambition once again. Whereas it is shown in Figure 1 as indicating Conscientiousness, in some other culture that trait might better represent, say, Openness to Experience.

Emic/Etic Factors

Last but not least, one might find an emic or culturally specific aspect to the factors residing at the highest level of the personality hierarchy. Whereas five personality factors have been found in Western cultures as representing most of the variation in human behavior, other cultures might have only four of those five factors, or six factors, or five factors that do not resemble the traditional Big Five. It is even possible that the factors found in a culture are substantially intercorrelated, suggesting a second-order factor level as a superstratum to the personality hierarchy of Figure 1.

In summary, I maintain that the emic/etic distinction in cross-cultural psychology has been used rather loosely in general. Instead of simply referring to the specificity/universality of latent personality traits and their behavioral indicators or exemplars, it means much more. Not only can behaviors be emic or etic, their relations to lower-level personality traits can also be emic or etic. Those traits themselves could also be emic or etic, as could their relations to their overlying personality factors. And finally, the factors themselves, and the factors' interrelations, can be emic or etic.

The present analysis of emics and etics should not be interpreted as implying that the distinctions I have made are necessarily independent ones. For instance, it may be theoretically possible to find personality traits that are etic across cultures but that define a personality structure that is emic to a particular culture. It would be nonsense, however, to propose that a set of personality constructs are emic to a culture but have an etic or universal organization to them.

THE SEARCH FOR EMIC/ETIC PERSONALITY CONSTRUCTS

Cross-cultural consistencies in human behavior cannot simply be assumed; they must be demonstrated empirically. This means evaluating the generality of individual behaviors, personality traits, personality factors, and their relations separately across the cultures of interest. As a first step, one could apply an etic research strategy, which involves using personality instruments developed in one culture with respondents from the other cultures. As has been argued elsewhere (Paunonen & Ashton, 1998), if acceptable psychometric properties are found in all the cultures for those personality instruments, it is unlikely that the constructs measured by them are emic to only one culture. The psychometric properties to consider include, among others, scale means, variances, reliabilities, criterion validities, and factor structures.

But what is one to conclude if one finds that the psychometric properties of the personality instruments are different in the different cultures? Does that mean that the personality variables assessed are emic to some of those cultures? Not necessarily. There are many reasons why a personality inventory will yield different psychometric properties in different samples, even within the same culture. These reasons include item translation problems, response style involvement, test format issues, and more (see Paunonen & Ashton, 1998, pp. 152-154). But if such methodological reasons can be discounted as the cause of the psychometric differences, then perhaps there may be some basis for the claim that the personality measuring instruments are not equally appropriate for use in each culture assessed. Perhaps the behaviors or latent traits being evaluated are not equally relevant to the cultures; that is, perhaps they are emic.

Using an etic research strategy to discover emic personality constructs is certainly not an optimal way to conduct such a search. Another, less serendipitous, way to isolate emic personality constructs is to look for them purposely. How would such a guided empirical search take place? In the section that follows, I describe one proposal to achieve this end, offered by Church and Katigbak (1988).

Their method is based on subjective lay judgments about personality constructs and on factor analysis of cross-cultural personality data. I then offer my own proposal for finding emic personality traits. That method is based on the well-known principles and methods of construct validation.

Factor Analysis and the Search for Emic Traits

Church and Katigbak (1988) have illustrated their research strategy for the identification of emic personality constructs and for the generation of emic items to assess those constructs. Their method proceeds as follows. Interviews with cultural informants first serve as a source for the identification of culture-relevant dimensions of personality. Those same lay informants are then asked to specify critical behaviors that best reflect the constructs. The obtained critical behaviors are edited and written in the form of standard personality inventory items, which are then administered to respondents in that culture and factor analyzed. The resulting factors are said to reveal the personality constructs of importance to that culture, constructs to be later identified as emic or etic. (See related methods, also based on factor analysis, proposed by Leung & Bond, 1989, and used by Triandis et al., 1993.)

Using their interview method in a Filipino population, Church and Katigbak (1988) developed a preliminary pool of 315 personality statements. Subsequent factor analyses of Philippine response data showed nine dimensions underlying those personality items. That factor solution was then used as a basis for selecting about half of the items to create nine personality scales corresponding to the factors found (e.g., self-assurance, affective well-being, proper behavior, etc.). This statistical method of developing unidimensional personality measures follows the traditional factor analytic method of test construction used by Cattell, for example, in the development of the 16PF (Cattell, Eber, & Tatsuoka, 1970).

Church and Katigbak's (1988) informant interview method ensures that the constructs assessed will have some degree of relevance to the culture, at least in the eyes of the lay public. But, are those constructs purely emic? One way to answer that question, according to those authors, is to factor the items of the resultant personality measures in combination with items from similarly-derived personality measures developed in another culture. If the combined set of items contains etic dimensions common to the cultures, then separate factor analyses of each culture's response data will result in common factor dimensions that are congruent across those cultures. If the combined set of items contains emic dimensions specific to a single culture, then the analysis will result in unique factor dimensions found in only one culture. It is worth repeating Church and Katigbak's (1988) method here verbatim.

In one ideal design, a comprehensive set of scales of emic personality dimensions in two or more cultures would be administered as a single item pool to a large sample in each culture. Separate factor analyses of the combined-culture item pool would be conducted in each culture. Dimensions (factors) that emerge in all cultures are etic or universal. Items that load on these dimensions in all cultures are etic exemplars of the etic dimensions; items that load on these dimensions in only one culture are emic exemplars of the etic dimensions. In contrast, dimensions that emerge in only one culture are emic or culture-specific. (pp. 152-153)

Church and Katigbak (1988) viewed personality item factors that are cohesive in one culture, but that break apart in another culture, as indicating the fact that the construct assessed by those items cannot be an etic or universal one (see also Leung & Bond, 1989; Triandis et al., 1993). However, there are many reasons why the factor structures of the two analyses could appear to be different. I will describe such reasons below and will argue that the accumulation of them serves to imbue a considerable bias to Church and Katigbak's method, a bias in the direction of cross-cultural behavior specificity.

The factor structures underlying personality inventory items in two cultures can differ for many reasons including, but not limited to, the following. (a) The first and most obvious reason is simple measurement error. Even a personality measure administered twice to the same sample of respondents can produce different item-factor structures on the two occasions. (b) As is well understood, if the items are worded in different languages, translation accuracy becomes a concern. A group of unidimensional items that defines a homogeneous composite in one language can easily describe a different structure if translated improperly. (c) As noted by Church and Katigbak (1988), particular items might elicit little response variability in particular cultures and, thus, would not correlate with other exemplars of the same trait. The item "I often walk in the snow just to hear it crunching under my feet" would have little relevance to Samoan respondents and would contribute little to the internal consistency of a measure of sentience. (d) Related to the preceding point, a whole culture might lack variability on an entire trait dimension. If such were the case (not that I have ever seen evidence of this phenomenon), all of the items in the trait scale would lack variability and would be only randomly correlated with one another, resulting in a spurious item-factor structure. (e) There may be cultural differences in the tendency to respond desirably to personality inventory items (see Chapter 2 of this volume by Helmes). A scale containing items having both neutral and desirable items could show a unidimensional construction if the respondents in one culture endorsed the items according to their trait content, but a multidimensional construction if respondents in another culture endorsed the items according to their levels of desirability. (f) Sex differences in mean scores on personality trait scales can readily affect the levels of correlation among those sex-linked scales and their factor structure when mixed-sex samples are analyzed. A substantial disparity in the ratio of men to women in two samples from two cultures, therefore, can result in a substantial disparity in the corresponding item-factor structures. (g) With factor analysis of a personality item pool, a cultural difference in factor structure can signify a real difference in personality structure, but it does not immediately follow that the traits so assessed are differentially relevant to those cultures. For instance, if the items on a particular scale fall onto different factors in different cultures, the trait measured by those items could be equally relevant to the cultures (i.e., an etic personality construct) but placed differently within each cultural network of traits (i.e., an emic personality organization). (h) The inherent indeterminacy of factor rotations means that two independent factor solutions may look quite different on the surface, but actually be different mathematical transformations of the same item structure (see Chapter 3 of this volume by Velicer, Eaton, & Fava). I recommend confirmatory factoring procedures to deal with this problem (see McCrae, Zonderman, Costa, Bond, & Paunonen, 1996; Paunonen, Keinonen, Trzebinski, Forsterling, Grishenko-Rose, Kouznetsova, & Chan, 1996; Paunonen, Zeidner, Engvik, Oosterveld, & Maliphant, in press).

There is yet another reason why item factor analyses in two different cultures might lead to different factor solutions for a personality inventory. (i) Personality scales that are comprised of facets (and, therefore, are not truly unidimensional) may show different structures at the item level due to cross-cultural differences in the associations among those facets. A study by Jackson, Hourany, and Vidmar (1972), for example, found the trait of risk-taking to be defined with respect to four areas of behavior: physical activity, monetary investment, social involvement, and ethical conduct. Items measuring these facets were found, in a North American sample, to be all mutually correlated but nonetheless distinct, producing four first-order factors that collapsed into one second-order factor. In another culture, however, it is conceivable that, say, the ethical risk-taking items are orthogonal to the other three facets' items, defining a separate factor even in a higher-order analysis.

In short, I conclude that Church and Katigbak's (1988) factor analytic method of identifying emic personality constructs is biased in the direction of finding culture specificity in behavior (see also Leung & Bond, 1989; Triandis et al., 1993). Given the myriad possible causes of cross-cultural differences in personality item factor results, I would be quite surprised if their method did *not* result in the declaration of at least some personality variables as being emic in almost any cross-cultural comparison. Some of those declarations, however, would in all likelihood be erroneous.

Construct Validation and the Search for Emic Traits

Church and Katigbak's (1988) proposed emic research strategy, which uses interviews of cultural informants, is useful for identifying culture-specific behavior exemplars of personality traits. It may also be useful for identifying a culture-specific organization to those personality traits. But a different strategy is required to support, with conviction, the proposition that a particular unidimensional construct is truly emic. I describe such a method below, a method based in large part on important works by Jackson and his colleagues.

In order to conclude that a hypothesized personality construct is not relevant to a culture, a reasonable attempt must be made in that culture to find it. One must endeavor to develop an internally consistent and construct valid measure of the behavior domain under consideration, ideally one that is psychometrically parallel to such a measure in some other culture in which the construct has been established. Notice that, for good reasons, one cannot trust the factor analytic or the empirical methods of test construction to yield successful results on that task. The factor analytic method is an exploratory post hoc procedure, the trait dimensions measured generally not being known until after the item data have been analyzed. The empirical method has its applications in criterion prediction, but it is not particularly optimized for the purpose of developing measures of predetermined psychological attributes.

In order to create a measure of a putative psychological attribute, the construct-oriented approach to test construction must be implemented, an approach most eloquently advocated by D. N. Jackson (1971, 1979) and best exemplified by his renowned achievements in personality test construction (e.g., Jackson, 1984, 1994). Using his method, the behavior domain to be measured is not only postulated at the outset, but it is defined explicitly with regard to the culture-relevant behaviors and situations thought to reflect it. Items are written that are unidimensional and domain representative, and that bear logical relations to the latent trait of interest. The items in the pool are then evaluated for their internal consistency and their convergent and discriminant properties. Those data are used to select the best exemplars for the final form of the scale, which is then submitted to an extensive program of construct validation (see also Chapter 5 of this volume by Holden).[3]

Note that there is no one coefficient of construct validity. Construct validation involves a programmatic evaluation of hypotheses about the behavior of one's test in various situations (Cronbach & Meehl, 1955; Jackson, 1971, 1979; Loevinger, 1957). For example, the test scores should correlate with established measures of the same construct, assuming such criteria exist. Those scores should show predictable mean differences in groups known to differ on the measured trait. The scores should vary as a function of experimental interventions designed to increase or decrease the level of the trait. And, the personality measure should predict important life-criteria in which personality factors are strongly suspected to play a role (e.g. see Mershon & Gorsuch, 1988; Paunonen, 1998; Yik & Bond, 1993).

Cronbach and Meehl (1955) knew well the meaning of the words construct validity. When a researcher postulates the existence of a psychological construct, develops an instrument to measure that construct, and finds that the test's scores behave in a theoretically predictable manner in a variety of situations, then he or she has acquired demonstrable evidence of construct validity. But construct validity does not just describe the measuring instrument alone; it also describes the theory that gave rise to the measure in the first place. In other words, construct validity represents a validation of both the measure of the construct *and* the construct itself. For how could a measure of a construct be valid if that construct does not exist?

If the behavior domain under consideration is not etic, then the attempt at test construction will fail in a culture. It will fail in the initial moments of construct definition, or it will fail at the item writing stage, or it will fail during item analysis. Alternatively, the effort will fail in the course of construct validation. In order to conclude that a personality construct is not etic, a fair effort must have been made to find it by developing a construct valid measure of the putative personality trait using items relevant to the culture of interest.[4]

In summary, Church and Katigbak's (1988) informant interview procedure is a good way to identify possible candidates for emic personality traits. But their factor analytic method for empirically evaluating the emic/etic properties of such traits is found wanting. Instead, by applying the principles and techniques of construct validation one is better able to support a claim for the existence, or lack thereof, of a hypothetical domain of behavior.

THE PERSONALITY HIERARCHY REVISITED

Consider once again the hierarchical Five-Factor Model of personality partially illustrated in Figure 1. What components of that model are etic and what components are emic? Although it would be foolhardy to make any definite statements at this point, primarily because the relevant empirical data are noticeably lacking, some probabilistic statements may be warranted.

Starting at the bottom of the hierarchy, there is little question, as already maintained, that some human behaviors are universal whereas others are not. Classifying observable behaviors as etic or emic is relatively straightforward and noncontroversial. Nominations by members of a particular culture could serve well in identifying normative behavioral acts that might be indicators of some broader personality dispositions (e.g., Church & Katigbak, 1988). A cross-cultural comparison of such behaviors would then suggest those that are specific and those that are general.

As one moves up the hierarchy to the trait stratum, the current thinking about specific traits as emic or etic is not so straightforward, nor is it without controversy. Certainly some personality traits are probably etic or universal. I say this because many personality questionnaires developed (mostly) in North America seem to maintain their psychometric properties well when administered to respondents in other cultures (Paunonen & Ashton, 1998). But saying that some personality dimensions are etic is not the same as saying that no personality dimensions are emic.

A few trait-like constructs have been proposed in the past as possibly representing culturally-specific dimensions of personality (see Church & Katigbak, 1998, p. 143). Two examples are the Japanese construct of *on* (Lebra, 1969) and the Filipino construct called *utang na loob* (Kaut, 1961). (Both of these concepts, coincidentally, refer to feelings of obligation and indebtedness for favors rendered by others.) My own view, however, is that many claims of culture specificity may be premature for two reasons. First, it is relatively easy to find idiosyncratic empirical dimensions of behavior in a particular sample of people – simply ensure that there is a large component of random error in the personality data. Poorly developed measures of personality characteristics are, in fact, replete with error variance and wanting in true score variance. Such measures will tend to show spurious correlations with themselves and with other variables, perhaps leading to the conclusion that the constructs assessed are unique to the culture observed.

My second reason for discounting claims of the discovery of emic personality dimensions is that little attempt is generally made to find those dimensions in other cultures using the methods of construct validation as described above. I would wager that most of those supposedly emic traits, including *on* and *utang na loob*, would reveal themselves in almost all cultures if a decided and proper effort was made to find them. (To my knowledge, no one has yet to report *not* finding these two particular traits in a culture.) Moreover, simply because operational difficulties might arise in the measurement of a construct does not mean that it is nonexistent. Berry (1969), for example, discussed the still unsolved problem of deriving an adequate common metric for the cross-cultural comparison of intelligence, leading him to lament "Of what use, then, is the global term intelligence if only a scrap of the emic can be used from each component culture in the comparison"? (p. 126). But the criticisms he leveled at research in this area are entirely related to the failure to recognize the emic expressions of intelligence and the (possibly) emic structure of intelligence. Berry's quote notwithstanding, his criticisms should not be interpreted as supporting the argument that the concept of intelligence itself is emic or culturally specific, which it almost certainly is not (Jensen, 1980).[5]

What about the generality of the factors of personality, residing at the top of the personality hierarchy? As I mentioned earlier, some researchers consider the Big Five to be essentially universal (McCrae et al., 1998), because of their apparent consistency in empirical data. But most cross-cultural studies of those factors to date have been carried out with personality measures originally derived in North America. Does this raise the possibility that any common personality factor structure found across the different cultures has been, in part, imposed by the assessment tools used, tools that reflect the behavioral and semantic peculiarities of the English-speaking Western population (Church & Lonner, 1998; Yang & Bond, 1990)? One might further ask, if the measures used to assess personality characteristics were constructed locally in each culture being evaluated, is it possible that different, culture-specific, personality constructs would be found, constructs that could then define a structure of personality that is also different and culture-specific (Cheung & Leung, 1998; Church & Katigbak, 1989)?

I make three comments regarding the considerable cross-cultural generality of Big Five personality data. First, using a personality measure developed in North America with respondents from very different cultures will, in my opinion, be more likely to impose differences in factor structures rather than similarities. It is in fact quite remarkable that, considering all the potential causes operating to subvert factor structure invariance, some of which were described earlier in this paper (see also Paunonen & Ashton, 1998), larger differences across cultures have not been found. Second, cross-cultural linguistic analyses of the structure underlying the language of personality and behavior have tended to corroborate the omnipresence of most of the Big Five (De Raad, Perugini, Hrebícková & Szarota, 1998) or all of them (Goldberg, 1993; John, 1990). That structure, of course, cannot have been imposed on the cultures via the mechanism of imported personality measurement devices because such devices are not used in such linguistic studies.

My third comment with regard to the generality of cross-cultural evaluations of factor structure is this – the Big Five personality factors and the Five-Factor Model of personality are not the same things. Thus, finding the Big Five personality factors (in any culture) is not exclusive evidence for the Five-Factor Model of personality structure. Such a finding is not be inconsistent with, say, a six-factor model in a culture, where the sixth personality factor may be emic to that culture (e.g, the Chinese Tradition factor discussed by Cheung & Leung, 1998) or etic across cultures (e.g., the Honesty factor proposed by Ashton & Lee, 1999). In other words, finding evidence for the Big Five factors in a culture does not automatically falsify all other competing models of personality structure (see also Paunonen & Jackson, 1999).

SUMMARY AND CONCLUSIONS

The emic/etic distinction of cross-cultural psychology is typically used in referring to the cultural specificity/generality of trait dimensions and their behaviors. The concept is frequently invoked to support criticisms of the practice of using personality measures developed in one culture with respondents from another culture. The putative problem is that, if the construct being assessed is emic, or specific to a culture, its measurement in other cultures may be meaningless.

In this chapter, I proposed that the distinction between emics and etics usually referred to in the literature is poorly circumscribed. I first described the presumed hierarchical organization of human behavior, making particular reference to the Five-Factor Model of personality structure. I then argued that the emic/etic distinction can be applied separately to the different components of the personality hierarchy, including trait exemplary behaviors, the traits themselves, and the factors comprising the traits. Moreover, the distinction can be applied to different aspects of the organization or interrelatedness of the components of the hierarchy. I then maintained that some empirical methods of identifying emic personality constructs are biased toward the finding that behavior is culturally-specific. More important, I noted that proper methods of determining whether personality constructs exist in a culture have long existed, and they are to be found in the psychometric procedures of construct validation. For to acquire evidence of construct validity with a particular personality measuring device in a particular culture is to demonstrate, contemporaneously, the validity of that instrument *and* the validity of the construct it purports to measure.

I agree with proponents of an emic strategy for cross-cultural research when they urge caution in the thoughtless adoption of foreign measurement devices in a culture. But my reasons pertain more to the problem of the cultural relevance of the test items used, rather than to questions about the cultural relevance of the personality construct underlying those items. It is my hunch that a proper search, following a rigorous program of construct validation in the tradition of D. N. Jackson (1971, 1979, 1984, 1994), would reveal that there are relatively few, if any, unidimensional domains of human behavior that are relevant only to particular cultures.

NOTES

[1] Supported by the Social Sciences and Humanities Research Council of Canada grant 410-98-1555.

[2] A complete analysis of the meaning of the emic trait concept could form the basis for a separate essay. Whereas it is relatively easy to grasp the idea of an observable behavior never occurring in a culture, the idea of a personality trait being nonexistent, or a whole domain of behavior not being relevant or important to a culture's population, is infinitely more elusive. Personality traits can be viewed as latent causes of behavior, or as mere summary descriptions of behavior. Either way, an emic trait must mean that either (a) no postulated trait-relevant behaviors exist in a culture, a highly improbable circumstance, or (b) some of those

behaviors exist, but they are not manifestations of the trait in question. In either case, any empirical attempt to measure the nonexistent personality construct with an imported assessment device would in all likelihood find no reliable individual differences in the respondents' scores. This lack of variance might serve as an empirical indicator of the lack of relevance of the trait to the culture (but see Footnote 4).

[3]I use the terms items and scales in a generic sense in this discussion. Any instrument purporting to measure a psychological attribute, be it a questionnaire, an electro-mechanical device, an experimental manipulation, a performance task, or a subjective judgment can be evaluated from the point of view of construct validity.

[4]I say a fair effort is required because shoddy workmanship can easily undermine the psychometric characteristics of the local instrument, possibly leading to the premature conclusion that the construct is unmeasurable and therefore nonexistent in that culture.

[5]Relevant to the etic/emic trait distinction is the question of whether a trait can be etic, or universal, if trait-relevant behaviors exist in a culture but the members of that population all engage in those behaviors to the same extent. To illustrate, a trait might show no individual difference variance in a culture because its people are all high, all moderate, or all low on that dimension (cf. Footnote 1). Leung and Bond (1989) have maintained that such a trait might qualify as a pancultural or cross-cultural dimension (because it shows variation across cultures) but not as an intracultural dimension (because it shows no variation within a culture), further claiming that such dimensions are "cultural but not etic" (p. 147). But, surely, the uniformly high levels of aggression in the Yanomamo Indians of South America, as an example, indicate a trait that is conspicuously relevant to the people of that culture – and such a finding by itself should not preclude the possibility that aggression is an etic trait.

REFERENCES

Ashton, M. C., Jackson, D. N., Helmes, E., & Paunonen, S. V. (1998). Joint factor analysis of the Personality Research Form and the Jackson Personality Inventory? *Journal of Research in Personality*, 32, 243-250.
Ashton, M. C., & Lee, K. (1999). *Evidence of a sixth lexical personality factor*. Manuscript submitted for publication.
Ashton, M. C., Paunonen, S. V., Helmes, E., & Jackson, D. N. (1998). Kin altruism, reciprocal altruism, and the Big Five personality factors. *Evolution and Human Behavior*, 19, 243-255.
Berry, J. W. (1969). On cross-cultural comparability. *International Journal of Psychology*, 4, 119-128.
Block, J. (1995). A contrarian view of the Five-Factor Approach to personality description. *Psychological Bulletin*, 117, 187-215.
Cattell, R. B., Eber, H. W., & Tatsuoka, M. (1970). *Handbook for the Sixteen Personality Factor Questionnaire*. Champaign, IL: Institute for Personality and Ability Testing.
Cheung, F. M., Leung, K. (1998). Indigenous personality measures: Chinese examples. *Journal of Cross-Cultural Psychology*, 29, 233-248.
Church, A. T., & Katigbak, M. S. (1988). The emic strategy in the identification and assessment of personality dimensions in a non-western culture. *Journal of Cross-Cultural Psychology*, 19, 140-163.
Church, A. T., & Katigbak, M. S. (1989). Internal, external, and self-report structure of personality in a non-western culture: An investigation of cross-language and cross-cultural generalizability. *Journal of Personality and Social Psychology*, 57, 857-872.
Church, A. T., & Lonner, W. J. (1998). The cross-cultural perspective in the study of personality: Rationale and current research. *Journal of Cross-Cultural Psychology*, 29, 32-62.
Cronbach, L. J., & Meehl, P. E. (1955). Construct validity in psychological tests. *Psychological Bulletin*, 52, 281-302.
De Raad, B., Perugini, M., Hrebícková, M., & Szarota, P. (1998). Lingua franca of personality: Taxonomies and structures based on the lexical approach. *Journal of Cross-Cultural Psychology*, 29, 212-232.
Digman, J. M. (1990). Personality structure: Emergence of the five-factor model. *Annual Review of Psychology*, 41, 417-440.
Frijda, N., & Jahoda, G. (1966). On the scope and methods of cross-cultural research. *International Journal of Psychology*, 1, 109-127.

Goldberg, L. R. (1993). The structure of personality traits: Vertical and horizontal aspects. In D. C. Funder, R. D. Parke, C. Tomlinson-Keasey, & K. Widaman (Eds.), *Studying lives through time: Personality and Development* (pp. 169-188). Washington, DC: American Psychological Association.

Jackson, D. N. (1971). The dynamics of structured personality tests: 1971. *Psychological Review, 78*, 229-248.

Jackson, D. N. (1979, October). *Construct validity and personality assessment.* Proceedings of a colloquium on theory and application in education and employment, Educational Testing Service, Princeton.

Jackson, D. N. (1984). *Personality Research Form manual.* Port Huron, MI: Research Psychologists Press.

Jackson, D. N. (1994). *Jackson Personality Inventory-Revised manual.* Port Huron, MI: Research Psychologists Press.

Jackson, D. N., Hourany, L., & Vidmar, N. J. (1972). A four-dimensional interpretation of risk taking. *Journal of Personality, 40*, 483-450.

Jackson, D. N., Paunonen, S. V., Fraboni, M., & Goffin, R. G. (1996). A five-factor versus a six-factor model of personality structure. *Personality and Individual Differences, 20*, 33-45.

Jensen, A. R. (1980). *Bias in mental testing.* New York: The Free Press.

John, O. P. (1990). The "Big Five" factor taxonomy: Dimensions of personality in the natural language and in questionnaires. In L. A. Pervin (Ed.), *Handbook of personality: Theory and research* (pp. 66-100). New York: Springer-Verlag.

Kaut, C. R. (1961). *Utang na loob*: A system of contractual obligation among Tagalogs. *Southwestern Journal of Anthropology, 17*, 256-272.

Lebra, T. S. (1969). Reciprocity and the asymmetric principle: An analytical reappraisal of the Japanese concept of *on. Psychologia, 12*, 129-138.

Leung, K., & Bond, M. H. (1989). On the empirical identification of dimensions for cross-cultural comparisons. *Journal of Cross-Cultural Psychology, 20*, 133-151.

Loevinger, J. (1957). Objective tests as instruments of psychological theory [Monograph]. *Psychological Reports, 3*, 635-694.

McCrae, R. R., Costa, P. T., Jr., del Pilar, G. H., Rolland, J.-P., & Parker, W. D. (1998). Cross-cultural assessment of the Five-Factor Model: The revised NEO Personality Inventory. *Journal of Cross-Cultural Psychology, 29*, 171-188.

McCrae, R. R., & John, O. P. (1992). An introduction to the five-factor model and its applications. *Journal of Personality, 60*, 175-215.

McCrae, R. R., Zonderman, A. B., Costa, P. T., Bond, M. H., & Paunonen, S. V. (1996). Evaluating replicability of factors in the Revised NEO Personality Inventory: Confirmatory factor analysis and Procrustes rotation. *Journal of Personality and Social Psychology, 70*, 552-566.

Mershon, B., & Gorsuch, R. L. (1988). Number of factors in the personality sphere: Does increase in factors increase predictability of real-life criteria? *Journal of Personality and Social Psychology, 55*, 675-680.

Paunonen, S. V. (1998). Hierarchical organization of personality and prediction of behavior. *Journal of Personality and Social Psychology, 74*, 538-556.

Paunonen, S. V., & Ashton, M. C. (1998). The structured assessment of personality across cultures. *Journal of Cross-Cultural Psychology, 29*, 150-170.

Paunonen, S. V., & Jackson, D. N. (1996). The Jackson Personality Inventory and the Five-Factor Model of personality. *Journal of Research in Personality, 30*, 42-59.

Paunonen, S. V., & Jackson, D. N. (1999). *What is beyond the Big Five? Plenty!* Manuscript submitted for publication.

Paunonen, S. V., Keinonen, M., Trzebinski, J., Forsterling, F., Grishenko-Rose, N., Kouznetsova, L., & Chan, D. W. (1996). The structure of personality in six cultures. *Journal of Cross-Cultural Psychology, 27*, 339-353.

Paunonen, S. V., Zeidner, M., Engvik, H., Oosterveld, P., & Maliphant, R. (in press). The nonverbal assessment of personality in five cultures. *Journal of Cross-Cultural Psychology.*

Pike, K. L. (1966). *Language in relation to a unified theory of the structure of human behavior.* The Hague: Mouton.

Saucier, G. & Ostendorf F. (1999). Hierarchical subcomponents of the Big Five personality factors: A cross-language replication. *Journal of Personality and Social Psychology, 76*, 613-627.

Triandis, H. C., McCusker, C., Betancourt, H., Iwao, S., Leung, K., Salazar, J. M., Setiadi, B., Sinha, J. B. P., Touzard, H., & Zaleski, Z. (1993). An etic-emic analysis of individualism and collectivism. *Journal of Cross-Cultural Psychology, 24*, 366-383.

Yang, K. S., & Bond, M. H. (1990). Exploring implicit personality theories with indigenous or imported constructs: The Chinese case. *Journal of Personality and Social Psychology, 58*, 1087-1095.

Yik, M. S. M., & Bond, M. H. (1993). Exploring the dimensions of Chinese person perception with indigenous and imported constructs: Creating a culturally balanced scale. *International Journal of Psychology, 28*, 75-95.

7 THE CHALLENGE OF CONSTRUCT VALIDITY IN THE ASSESSMENT OF PSYCHOPATHOLOGY

Leslie C. Morey

It is a great pleasure to contribute to this volume honoring Douglas Jackson, as his seminal work in assessment has influenced my thinking in many ways. The most direct influence, of course, has been the large number of essential writings on the construct validation approach to assessment theory and research, and in this way he has served as a guide and inspiration not only for me, but for the entire discipline. But there are two other, more personal, influences that operated quite early on the development of my career as an assessment researcher, and both had a considerable role in pointing me in the direction that I have taken ever since.

The first of these dates back to my undergraduate class in psychological assessment, one of the first courses that I took after completing the introductory course. It soon became obvious that I was an outlier in this class, in that I seemed to be the only student who actually enjoyed the material! While the other students scattered for cover at the first sign of a regression equation, I was (apparently idiosyncratically) excited by the field and the opportunities for the advancement of knowledge therein. I was particularly intrigued by the area of personality assessment, and discovered to my amazement that the most popular instruments of the time (the MMPI and the Rorschach) both impressively violated many of the most basic psychometric doctrines with which my classmates had struggled so mightily during the beginning sections of the class. I could not understand how instruments with such shortcomings could see such widespread use. Then, the text provided a ray of hope: a brief section on a then "new" personality instrument, one that seemed to incorporate many of the important developments in the assessment field-the Personality Research Form (PRF: Jackson, 1967). The PRF was cited as a promising new state-of-the-art instrument that avoided many of the pitfalls of earlier measures through the use of the novel "construct validation" approach to test development. That early exposure convinced me that *this* was the way to progress in personality assessment, a conviction that I retain to this day even with a more complex understanding of the approach.

The second sphere of influence began in my first year of graduate school, when I attended the meetings of the Classification Society and had arranged a meeting with a young researcher named Harvey Skinner, who had worked with Douglas Jackson himself as a graduate student. Jackson's influence on Skinner can be seen in the latter's groundbreaking work in the application of the construct validation approach to psychiatric classification (e.g., Skinner, 1981, 1986). This evolved into an ongoing relationship, and ultimately I had the good fortune to have Harvey serve as my doctoral co-mentor. The impact on my thinking will be obvious to anyone familiar with my research, and although I have probably had less direct contact with Douglas Jackson than any of the other participants in this volume, his role as my "academic grandfather" should be unmistakable.

Armed with this belief in the construct validation approach as a foundation, I have pursued issues in the assessment and classification of constructs related to mental disorder for my entire career. After a few decades of working within the paradigm, I retain my enthusiasm for the approach while I am humbled by its complexity and subtlety. I now teach psychological assessment myself, although I believe that one of the best learning experiences is to actually undertake the development of a multiscale instrument, where many of the aforementioned complexities become pragmatic obstacles. To that end, the purpose of this chapter is to detail some of what I have learned in developing my own instrument for the assessment of mental disorder, the Personality Assessment Inventory (PAI; Morey, 1991a). The development of the PAI was based upon a construct validation framework, and throughout the chapter I will use issues that arose in the development and validation of the PAI to illustrate various points. Hopefully, some of the lessons I have learned along the way may in some way help to elaborate our understanding of the construct validation approach.

THE CONSTRUCT VALIDATION APPROACH

In working within a construct validation framework, it is essential to understand that each of the two words – *construct* and *validation* – is there for a reason. Neither is very useful without the other. Constructs without validation tend to be abstractions that typically have little utility in an empirical or in a pragmatic sense; validation in the absence of a construct tends to yield specific-use applications that have little generalizability and do little to further an understanding of what is being measured. The construct validation approach emphasizes the interplay between the theoretical elaboration of the construct and its methodological validation, and both elements deserve some further consideration.

Constructs

Within the construct validation framework, test development cannot proceed without a specification and elaboration of the construct to be measured. While this may seem obvious to many, the history of psychological assessment is replete with examples to the contrary (see Holden, this volume, for an overview of this history). The differences can be seen in as basic a level as the names of scales on instruments. Construct validation requires that the scale name reflect the construct being measured; this contrasts with instruments where scale names are task descriptions (such as the subscales on the Wechsler intelligence scales), factor names (as on the 16PF), or even numerals (such as the MMPI).

In designing a scale to measure a particular construct, the scale must be evaluated within the context of a theoretically informed network that makes explicit hypotheses about interrelationships among indicators of various constructs. I have advocated (e.g., Morey, 1991b) that our classifications in psychopathology be viewed simply as a collection of hypothetical constructs that are themselves subject to construct validation procedures. In recent years, there has been increasing recognition that psychopathological constructs are best represented by rules that are probabilistic rather than classical (i.e., the use of necessary and sufficient features) in nature. The resulting fuzzy quality of critical constructs in mental health weighs against the success of criterion-referenced approaches (e.g., those tied to specific etiology in a strong sense) to the development and validation of construct indicators. Despite recent efforts to increase the rigor with which certain clinical constructs are identified, the fact remains that no "gold standard" has been discovered for use as a criterion for membership in any of the major categories of mental disorder since the discovery of the specific qualitative etiology of general paresis around the turn of the 20th century. Most constructs in psychiatric classification are "open concepts" (Meehl, 1977) with little known about their inner nature. As such, the construct validational approach is perhaps the only viable strategy with which to tackle this type of measurement problem.

Cronbach and Meehl (1955) suggested that assigning variability in observable behavior to a hypothetical construct requires a theory with respect to that construct that is comprised of an interconnected system of laws (which Cronbach and Meehl called a "nomological network") relating hypothetical constructs to one another and to behavior observable in the environment. Skinner (1981, 1986) has described a three stage framework for the elaboration of psychopathological constructs that follows Loevinger's (1957) and Jackson's (e.g., 1971) construct validation frameworks in psychometrics. The stage of *theory formulation* involves an explication of the content domain of the construct, a delineation of the nature of the classification model and the linkages between constructs in the model, and a specification of the relationship of constructs to external variables, such as etiology or treatment outcome. The second stage of *internal validation* involves the operationalization of the constructs and examining various internal properties of the classification; specific properties to be emphasized would depend on the theory elaborated in the initial stage. These properties might include interrater reliability, coverage of the classification, stability of measurement over occasions, internal correlation matrices, internal consistency of features assumed to be indicators of the same construct, or the replicability of classification or factorial structures across different samples. The third stage of construct validation described by Skinner (1981) involves *external validation*. At this stage, links of the constructs to other variables related to etiology, course, or prediction must be tested. This process will be involve both convergent and discriminant validation (Campbell & Fiske, 1959). That is, in addition to showing that expected relationships prevail between the construct and to conceptually similar constructs, the process must also involve efforts to demonstrate that observed relationships are not attributable to constructs presumed not to be operating within the theoretical network. As empirical evidence is gathered, the theoretical formulation will likely be revised to accommodate new and unexpected information.

It should be noted that the links among constructs in the theoretical network may be of many types. Historically, classification in medicine has given prominence to etiology as a basis for organization, but there is no reason to presume that theoretically-based construct validation research must begin and end with investigations into etiology. Meehl (1977) points out that the complexity of causation of most phenomena in the biological and social sciences does not seem compatible with the notion of "specific etiology." As such, specific etiology may not be a particularly promising candidate to serve as the basis of a scientific classification of mental disorders. Even with the presumption of multiple etiological pathways there seems to be a need to provide a theoretical link between the observed phenomena and some etiologically proximal "final common pathway" if the taxonomic construct is to achieve scientific coherence. Thus, efforts directed at establishing theoretical links between constructs and other external validator variables such as treatment response or course may have as much promise for clarifying psychiatric classification as do etiological investigations. As with etiological research, there is little reason to presume to find specificity (in other words, that disorders should respond specifically to particular treatments) as treatment response may involve variables fairly distal to the core of the construct. Nonetheless, more proximal links between certain, presumably malleable, elements of the construct and theoretical mechanisms of treatment are reasonable objects of investigation for construct validation. Ultimately, those constructs that are central in a theory that provides such linkages to etiology, description, and treatment should be those that emerge as superordinate in a taxonomy of psychopathology.

It was thus my aim to construct an inventory that would focus upon these constructs. The scales included on the PAI, shown in Tables 1 and 2, represent constructs selected on the basis of the depth of their elaboration in the theoretical and empirical literature, as well as the stability of their importance within the conceptualization and nosology of mental disorder, and their significance in contemporary clinical practice. These criteria were assessed through a review of the historical and contemporary literature, and constructs which failed to meet these criteria were not candidates to be included as PAI scales. Given my continuing interest in the field of personality disorders, I am often asked why the PAI includes only two scales (Borderline Personality, or BOR, and Antisocial Personality, or ANT) that are targeted directly at personality disorders. The reason is that the remaining disorders simply do not adequately meet these criteria for adequate construct articulation. First, the two disorders included on the PAI account for the majority of all research on personality disorders; Borderline Personality alone accounts for over half of all studies on Axis II (Blashfield & McElroy, 1987). Second, the well-documented lack of discriminant validity among the personality disorders is quite problematic from a construct validity perspective. For example, individuals meeting criteria for only one personality disorder (as opposed to two or more) are a small minority of personality disordered patients (Morey, 1988). Given such marked diagnostic overlap, the task of constructing conceptually independent scales is greatly hampered. Under such circumstances, it was deemed more useful to focus only on personality constructs that were empirically supported and clinically relevant (such as BOR, ANT, and the interpersonal dimensions), and to use these constructs to inform the user about personality disorder phenomena.

In contrast to some of the personality disorder diagnoses, "depression" is useful as an example of a well-articulated construct. Of all mental disorder concepts, its description is perhaps the most stable as it has been described consistently at least since the time of the classical Greek physicians (Menninger, 1963). The construct has also received a great deal of theoretical and empirical attention, with a host of instruments available for assessing depression, including the self-report Beck Depression Inventory (BDI: Beck & Steer, 1987), Zung (1965) Depression Scale, and MMPI D scale, as well as the observer rating scales such as the Hamilton Rating Scale for Depression (HAM-D: Hamilton, 1960). Despite the fact that these scales are widely used and tend to be positively correlated, they each have somewhat different characteristics (Lambert, Hatch, Kingston, & Edwards, 1986). For example, the HAM-D is one of the most commonly used instruments in psychopharmacologic trials of antidepressants, perhaps because it emphasizes the measurement of physiological symptoms of depression that are reasonably responsive to such medications (a nomological link to treatment). As an example, there are three distinct items of the 17 items on the original scale that inquire about sleep disturbances, but none asking about negative cognitions or expectancies. In contrast, the Beck Depression Inventory tends to emphasize cognitive features of depression, such as beliefs about helplessness and negative expectations about the future (Louks, Hayne, & Smith, 1989). This emphasis is not surprising, given Beck's theoretical elaboration (e.g., Beck, 1967) of the role of these factors in the development and maintenance of depression (a nomological link to etiology). Empirically, factor analyses of the BDI support the conclusion that such cognitive elements of depression are a major source of variance on this instrument, with somatic and affective elements relatively undifferentiated (Steer, Ball, Ranieri, & Beck, 1999). In contrast, other commonly used instruments, such as the MMPI D scale, focus upon affective features such as unhappiness and psychological discomfort, with limited assessment of either the cognitive or physiological features of depression. As a result, these instruments tap more generalized distress and have little specificity in the diagnosis of depression.

The construction of the Depression (DEP) scale of the PAI proceeded with the goal of representing these empirically related, but conceptually independent, components of the depression construct, as the empirical and theoretical significance of each had been established in the literature. The initial item pool for these components was generated by examining the literature in each area to identify those characteristics of each that were most central to the definition of the concept. The content of these items was assumed to be crucial to its success, as each item was carefully constructed to measure a reasonably well-articulated facet of a complex construct.

Table 1. The 22 full scales of the PAI.

Scale (designation)	Description
Validity Scales	
Inconsistency (ICN)	Determines if client is answering consistently throughout inventory. Each pair consists of highly correlated (positively or negatively) items.
Infrequency (INF)	Determines if client is responding carelessly or randomly. Items are neutral with respect to psychopathology and have extremely high or low endorsement rates.
Negative Impression (NIM)	Suggests an exaggerated unfavorable impression or malingering. Items have relatively low endorsement rates among clinical subjects
Positive Impression (PIM)	Suggests the presentation of a very favorable impression or reluctance to admit minor flaws.
Clinical Scales	
Somatic Complaints (SOM)	Focuses on preoccupation with health matters and somatic complaints associated with somatization and conversion disorders.
Anxiety (ANX)	Focuses on phenomenology and observable signs of anxiety with an emphasis on assessment across different response modalities
Anxiety-Related Disorders (ARD)	Focuses on symptoms and behaviors related to specific anxiety disorders, particularly phobias, traumatic stress, and obsessive-compulsive symptoms.
Depression (DEP)	Focuses on symptoms and phenomenology of depressive disorders.

Table 1. (continued)

Mania (MAN)	Focuses on affective, cognitive, and behavioral symptoms of mania and hypomania
Paranoia (PAR)	Focuses on symptoms of paranoid disorders and more enduring characteristics of paranoid personality.
Schizophrenia (SCZ)	Focuses on symptoms relevant to the broad spectrum of schizophrenic disorders.
Borderline Features (BOR)	Focuses on attributes indicative of a borderline level of personality functioning, including unstable and fluctuating interpersonal relations, impulsivity, affective lability and instability, and uncontrolled anger.
Antisocial Features (ANT)	Focuses on history of illegal acts and authority problems, egocentrism, lack of empathy and loyalty, instability, and excitement-seeking.
Alcohol Problems (ALC)	Focuses on problematic consequences of alcohol use and features of alcohol dependence.
Drug Problems (DRG)	Focuses on problematic consequences of drug use (both prescription and illicit) and features of drug dependence.
Treatment Scales	
Aggression (AGG)	Focuses on characteristics and attitudes related to anger, assertiveness, hostility, and aggression.
Suicidal Ideation (SUI)	Focuses on suicidal ideation, ranging from hopelessness to thoughts and plans for the suicidal act.
Stress (STR)	Measures the impact of recent stressors in major life areas.
Nonsupport (NON)	Measures a lack of perceived social support, considering both the level and quality of available support.
Treatment Rejection (RXR)	Focuses on attributes and attitudes theoretically predictive of interest and motivation in making personal changes of a psychological or emotional nature.
Interpersonal Scales	
Dominance (DOM)	Assesses the extent to which a person is controlling and independent in personal relationships. A bipolar dimension with a dominant style at the high end and a submissive style at the low end.
Warmth (WRM)	Assesses the extent to which a person is interested in supportive and empathic personal relationships. A bipolar dimension with a warm, outgoing style at the high end and a cold, rejecting style at the low end.

The above discussion makes it clear that the construct validation method of test construction differs markedly from atheoretical methods, such as the empirically-keyed method of item selection employed in instruments such as the MMPI.   In the construct validation view, theory and measurement are inextricably interlinked, and an instrument is viewed as a scientific theory that is open to empirical falsification.   Thus, not even instruments such as the MMPI or even the DSM-IV are truly "atheoretical" (e.g., Faust & Miner, 1986; Schwartz & Wiggins, 1987), as each represents an implicit theory about the representation of the constructs and the boundaries between them. However, in such methods the theoretical networks underlying the constructs are typically poorly articulated and measurement problems invariably result. Thus, the PAI representation of constructs does *not* attempt to adhere to DSM definitions of disorders, but rather attempts to instantiate contemporary knowledge about the constructs. Where it appeared warranted, the PAI departs from the DSM representation of constructs, including such areas as depression (with a greater emphasis on cognitive features), schizophrenia (emphasizing a positive-negative symptom distinction rather than a Kraepelinian structure), and antisocial personality (which attempts to measure the full construct of psychopathy rather than the DSM's more behavior-based focus).

In the context of discussing the utility of theory-based assessment, some mention should be made of the nature of the theories from which assessments may be derived. In general, the nomological network for one construct may look quite different than that for another; for example, it is unlikely that the same set of explanatory principles will hold for bipolar affective disorder, post-traumatic stress disorder, and dependent personality disorder. As such, many of the theories that most help to elaborate psychopathologic constructs tend to be restricted in scope. Theories that are intended to be applicable across the broad expanse of psychopathology (such as early applications of psychoanalytic theory, or Millon's 1969 model of syndromes) tend to achieve their expansive coverage at the expense of specificity, and hence falsifiability. Thus, it should be understood that there is no one theoretical subtext for the PAI; rather, the instrument draws from more circumscribed theoretical models that have shown promise for specific constructs, whether they be psychodynamic (as for borderline personality), interpersonal (as for the interpersonal scales), cognitive (as for depression), or psychopathologic (as for schizophrenia) in nature.

Table 2. PAI subscales and their descriptions.

Subscale (designation)	Description
Somatic Complaints	
Conversion (SOM-C)	Focuses upon symptoms associated with conversion disorder, particularly sensory or motor dysfunctions.
Somatization (SOM-S)	Focuses upon the frequent occurrence of various common physical symptoms and vague complaints of ill health and fatigue.
Health Concerns (SOM-H)	Focuses upon a preoccupation with health status and physical problems.
Anxiety	
Cognitive (ANX-C)	Focuses upon ruminative worry and concern about current issues that results in impaired concentration and attention.
Affective (ANX-A)	Focuses upon the experience of tension, difficulty in relaxing, and the presence of fatigue as a result of high perceived stress.
Physiological (ANX-P)	Focuses upon overt physical signs of tension and stress, such as sweaty palms, trembling hands, complaints of irregular heartbeats and shortness of breath.

Table 2. (continued)

Anxiety-Related Disorders

Obsessive-Compulsive (ARD-O) Focuses on intrusive thoughts or behaviors, rigidity, indecision, perfectionism, and affective constriction.

Phobias (ARD-P) Focuses on common phobic fears, such as social situations, public transportation, heights, enclosed spaces, or other specific objects.

Traumatic Stress (ARD-T) Focuses upon the experience of traumatic events that cause continuing distress and that are experienced as having left the client changed or damaged in some fundamental way.

Depression

Cognitive (DEP-C) Focuses on thoughts of worthlessness, hopelessness, and personal failure, as well as indecisiveness and difficulties in concentration.

Affective (DEP-A) Focuses on feeling of sadness, loss of interest in normal activities, and anhedonia.

Physiological (DEP-P) Focuses on level of physical functioning, activity, and energy, including disturbance in sleep pattern and changes in appetite and/or weight loss.

Mania

Activity Level (MAN-A) Focuses on overinvolvement in a wide variety of activities in a somewhat disorganized manner and the experience of accelerated thought processes and behavior

Grandiosity (MAN-G) Focuses on inflated self-esteem, expansiveness, and the belief that one has special and unique skills or talents.

Irritability (MAN-I) Focuses on the presence of strained relationships due to the respondent's frustration with the inability or unwillingness of others to keep up with their plans, demands, and possibly unrealistic ideas.

Paranoia

Hypervigilance (PAR-H) Focuses on suspiciousness and the tendency to monitor the environment for real or imagined slights by others.

Persecution (PAR-P) Focuses on the belief that one has been treated inequitably and that there is a concerted effort among others to undermine ones interests

Resentment (PAR-R) Focuses on a bitterness and cynicism in interpersonal relationships, and a tendency to hold grudges and externalized blame for any misfortunes.

Schizophrenia

Psychotic Experiences (SCZ-P) Focuses on the experience of unusual perceptions and sensations, magical thinking, and/or other unusual ideas that may involve delusional beliefs.

Social Detachment (SCZ-S) Focuses on social isolation, discomfort and awkwardness in social interactions.

Thought Disorder (SCZ-T) Focuses on confusion, concentration problems, and disorganization of thought processes.

Table 2. (continued)

Borderline Features

Affective Instability (BOR-A)	Focuses upon emotional responsiveness, rapid mood changes, and poor emotional control.
Identity Problems (BOR-I)	Focuses upon uncertainty about major life issues and feelings of emptiness, unfulfillment, and an absence of purpose.
Negative Relationships (BOR-N)	Focuses upon a history of ambivalent, intense relationships in which one has felt exploited and betrayed.
Self-Harm (BOR-S)	Focuses upon impulsivity in areas that have high potential for negative consequences.

Antisocial Features

Antisocial Behaviors (ANT-S)	Focuses on a history of antisocial acts and involvement in illegal activities.
Egocentricity (ANT-E)	Focuses on a lack of empathy or remorse and a generally exploitive approach to interpersonal relationships.
Stimulus-Seeking (ANT-S)	Focuses on a craving for excitement and sensation, a low tolerance for boredom, and a tendency to be reckless and risk-taking.

Aggression

Aggressive Attitude (AGG-A)	Focuses on hostility, poor control over anger expression, and a belief in the instrumental utility of aggression.
Verbal Aggression (AGG-V)	Focuses on verbal expressions of anger ranging from assertiveness to abusiveness, and a readiness to express anger to others.
Physical Aggression (AGG-P)	Focuses on a tendency to physical displays of anger, including damage to property, physical fights, and threats of violence.

Validation

The second part of the construct validation picture is the *validation*. Once a construct has been identified and the major elements of the construct delineated, the putative indicators of the construct need to be examined for validity. While this sounds simple enough, it is critical to understand that the validation of an indicator is a complex process, and the validity of an indicator cannot be reduced to a single coefficient. The importance of validation has been understood since the beginnings of psychometrics, but the multifaceted nature of validity has not been clearly recognized until relatively recently. In particular, the literature on test development and validation is replete with studies documenting *convergent validity*, or the association between indicators that supposedly measure the same construct. However, two other important aspects of validation often receive short shrift in the test construction literature, and the construct validation approach has been central in highlighting the importance of these overlooked aspects. The following sections examine two of these areas, namely *content validity* and *discriminant validity*.

Content Validity

The content validity of a measure involves the adequacy of sampling of content across the construct being measured. Often, this characteristic of a test is confused with "face validity," referring to whether the instrument appears to be measuring what it is intended to measure, particularly as it appears to a lay audience. These are not synonymous terms; a test for depression that consists of a single item such as "I am unhappy" may appear to be highly related to depression (i.e., high face validity) but provides a very narrow sampling of the content domain of depression (i.e., low content validity). The construction of the PAI sought to develop scales that provided a balanced sampling of the most important elements of the constructs being measured. This content coverage was designed to include both a consideration of *breadth* as well as *depth* of the construct. The *breadth* of content coverage refers to the diversity of elements subsumed within a construct. For example, as described earlier, in measuring depression it is important to inquire about physiological and cognitive signs of depression as well as features of affect. Any depression scale that focuses exclusively on one of these elements at the expense of the others will have limited content validity, with limited coverage of the breadth of the depression construct. The PAI sought to insure breadth of content coverage through the use of subscales representing the major elements of the measured constructs, as indicated by the theoretical and empirical literature on the construct.

The issue of construct breadth brings up one illustration of where two supposedly desirable aspects of a measure can actually be inversely related. Coefficient alpha (Cronbach, 1951) and its dichotomous version, KR-20, are measures of internal consistency that provide an estimate of a generalized split-half reliability. Many texts (e.g., Hammill, Brown, & Bryant, 1993) state that a high coefficient alpha (e.g., one above .80) is a desirable property of a test, and test construction procedures that use part-whole correlations or factor-analytic structures essentially attempt to maximize this psychometric property. However, sometimes internal consistency can be *too* high, an issue described as the "attenuation paradox" by Loevinger (1954) over 40 years ago. High internal consistency indicates that all test items are measuring the same thing, which at its extreme can result in highly redundant items that address a very narrow portion of a complex construct. As an example, a depression test which consists of 10 questions that all ask about difficulties in falling asleep might be highly internally consistent, but such a test would miss a considerable portion of the breadth of the depression construct, including mood and relevant cognitions.

The construction of the PAI sought to assure breadth of content validity in two ways. First, a subscale structure was specified (shown in Table 2) that represented the major facets of the constructs being measured. For example, the best way to insure that depressive cognitions were not underrepresented on the Depression scale was to include a subscale targeting these cognitions. Second, the item selection strategy sought to identify those items that did not contribute independent variance to scale scores. As an item selection criterion, the squared multiple correlation between each item and all other items from the same scale was calculated. These values were useful in identifying highly redundant items, since the response to a redundant item should be easily predicted from the other items in the scale.

The *depth* of content coverage refers to the need to sample across the full range of severity of a particular element of a construct. To assure adequate depth of coverage, the scales were designed to include items that addressed the full range of severity of the construct, including both its milder as well as most severe forms. One aspect of the PAI that resulted from this consideration was the item response scaling; the test items are answered on a four-alternative scale, with the anchors "Totally False," "Slightly True," "Mainly True," and "Very True." Each response is weighted according to the intensity of the feature that the different alternatives represent; thus, a client who answers "Very True" to the question "Sometimes I think I'm worthless" adds three points to his or her raw score on the Depression scale, while a client who responds "Slightly True" to the same item adds only one point. As a result, each item can capture differences in the severity of the manifestation of a feature of a particular disorder. The use of this four-alternative scaling is further justified psychometrically in that it allows a scale to capture more true variance per item, meaning that even scales of modest length can achieve satisfactory reliability. In addition, the use of four response options eliminates the central alternative that would be available if an odd number of response options were to be used. The use of an even number of response options is desirable from a psychometric perspective as reliable differences exist among individuals who make use of the central option (Nunnally, 1979). The use of four alternatives is also justified clinically, because sometimes even a "slightly true" response to some constructs (such as suicidal ideation) may merit clinical attention. Furthermore, clients themselves often express dissatisfaction with being forced to choose from dichotomous alternatives, expressing the belief that the true state of affairs lies somewhere "in the middle" of the two extremes presented.

In addition to differences in depth of severity of problems reflected in the response options, the items themselves were constructed to tap different levels of severity in the manifestation of a problem. Underlying all of the PAI scales is the assumption that members of the same diagnostic category can differ in degree in meaningful ways, with the severity of the problems reflecting this quantitative difference. For example, cognitive elements of depression can vary in severity from mild pessimism to severe feelings of hopelessness, helplessness, and despair. One statistical model that holds some promise for representing this dimensionality is item response theory (Hulin, Drasgow, & Parsons, 1983; Lord, 1980). Item response theory attempts to estimate the value of an individual on some latent trait using information contained in the responses of specific items. Tests developed from an item response approach attempt to provide items that sample information across the entire relevant range of the construct, rather than including items that optimally make a given discrimination. Scales that are developed with reference to an external criterion, such as those on the MMPI, are examples of the latter approach; if items are selected with respect to a particular discrimination (such as schizophrenic vs. normal), they will only provide information that is optimal for that particular distinction.

As an example, consider the hypothetical distributions of three groups on the construct of "thought disorder" shown in Figure 1. If items are selected on the basis of their ability to make a discrimination between two particular groups (e.g., schizophrenics vs. controls), those items that provide information at the point of rarity between the distributions of the two groups on the severity continuum will be seen as most useful. For the example in Figure 1, in differentiating schizophrenia from normality, items calibrated around point A will provide the most information for making this distinction. However, in differentiating schizophrenia from affective disorder, item information should be maximized around point B. If a scale is intended to be useful in making a variety of such distinctions, one would prefer a scale to be comprised of items that contain information relevant to discriminations across the entire relevant range – or the full depth – of the construct. In other words, a scale should be comprised of items sampling inform-

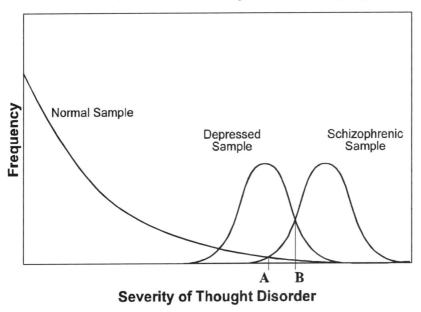

Figure 1. An example of the relationship between the severity of psychopathology represented by an item and its utility in making different diagnostic distinctions.

ation across the full spectrum of the concept if it is to be able to make a variety of different diagnostic distinctions.

In selecting items for the final version of the PAI, the item response model was used as a conceptual guide in an attempt to select items that provided information across the full spectrum of the diagnostic concept. Through examining the item characteristic curves of potential items, the final items were selected to provide information across the full range of construct severity. The nature of the severity continuum varies across the constructs. For example, for the Suicidal Ideation (SUI) scale, this continuum involves the imminence of the suicidal threat. Thus, items on this scale vary from vague and ill-articulated thoughts about suicide to immediate plans for self-harm.

Discriminant Validity

A test is said to have *discriminant validity* if it provides a measure of a construct that is specific to that construct; in other words, the measurement is free from the influence of other constructs. Although discriminant validity has been long recognized as an important facet of construct validity, it traditionally has not played a major role in the construction of psychological tests. This is unfortunate, since discriminant validity represents one of the largest challenges in the assessment of psychological constructs.

There are a variety of threats to validity where discriminability plays a vital role. Three of the major areas include *discrimination among psychopathologic constructs*, the influence of *response sets and response styles*, and the operation of *test bias*. The following paragraphs review these discriminant validity issues and discuss their handling in the development of the PAI.

Discrimination among constructs. This aspect of discriminant validity is a major challenge to instruments in the realm of psychopathology. Psychiatric diagnoses tend to be highly "comorbid" (e.g., Maser & Cloninger, 1990), which in essence means that an individual manifesting any type of mental health problem is at greatly increased risk to simultaneously manifest another such problem. This means that clinical problems are positively correlated in the population at large, and some (e.g., depression and anxiety, or the different personality disorders) are quite highly correlated. This poses an obvious challenge to the discriminant validity of any instrument that seeks to measure such constructs.

Throughout the development of the PAI, a number of procedures were implemented in an attempt to maximize discriminant validity. Items were written with particular attention to specificity concerns. Before any data were collected, expert diagnosticians provided a blind sorting of items into scale constructs to determine if they could accurately relate items to the appropriate constructs. The contrast sets for these discriminations were constructed to examine a number of particularly difficult phenomenological discriminations, such as between mania, aggressiveness, and paranoia, or between schizophrenia and social phobia. Also, at two different stages of data analysis items were examined to insure that they were more highly associated with their "parent" constructs than with any other constructs measured by the test, a critical step in the sequential strategy outlined by Douglas Jackson (e.g., Jackson, 1970, 1971).

Another practice that compromised the discriminant validity of many previous multi-scale inventories was the use of overlapping items, i.e., items that are scored on more than one scale. Overlapping items force a certain correspondence in the measurement of presumably distinct constructs; as such, the relationship between scales can be entirely artifactual rather than represent a true association between distinct disorders. Given that such constructs are inherently challenging to distinguish, a methodological handicap such as item overlap is indeed ill-advised. Many of the other instruments of this type contain large amounts of item overlap that lead to considerable discriminant validity problems (e.g., Welsh, 1952; Retzlaff & Gilbertini, 1987). The PAI contains no item overlap to reduce this potential source of discrimination problems; each scale is comprised of items loading only on that scale.

Response styles. Over the past thirty years, the issue of response styles has been a hotly debated topic in the field of objective psychopathology assessment. A classic review of this area by Wiggins (1962) distinguished between three components of variance in responding to self-report questionnaire items: *strategic, method,* and *stylistic* variance. Strategic variance is directly related to the discriminative purpose of the test and is determined by the subject's "true" positioning on the construct of interest. Method variance is affected by structural aspects of the instrument, such as phrasings of statements, format of response options, and directionality of item keying. Finally, stylistic variation consists of response consistencies that exist independent of the test itself, and notions of such as an "acquiesence set" or a "social desirability" set have been proposed as examples. However, there have been many debates over the nature of various constructs as to whether they represent strategic or stylistic variance in the measurement of personality (Helmes, this volume). For example, the construct of "social desirability" has been alternatively interpreted as a tendency for individuals to endorse unrealistically positive statements when describing themselves (e.g., Edwards, 1957), or as an indicator of a personality style related to autonomy, extroversion, optimism and ego strength (Block, 1965; McCrae & Costa, 1983).

The approach taken to the development of the PAI involved a careful consideration of the possible influence of response styles by considering the issue as one of discriminant validation. In other words, response styles were not viewed either as totally artifactual contributions to variance to be eliminated, nor as unimportant features to be ignored. Rather, the influence of response styles was examined at the level of the individual items, with the aim of eliminating items that seemed to measure stylistic or method variance to a greater extent than strategic variance. Response styles (either method or stylistic) were thus treated as independent constructs from which measured constructs should be distinguishable. The idea of eliminating all stylistic variance from the test was neither desirable nor practical, since there is no reason to suspect that certain response styles will be orthogonal to certain syndromes of mental disorder or to certain personality traits. The psychological phenomena experienced by the schizophrenic will never be seen as socially desirable, while the depressed individual usually manages to see the black cloud surrounding every silver lining. While orthogonality was not the aim, discriminant validity was the aim. Consistent with the Jackson approach to construct validation, items were selected only if they were better measures of their "parent" construct than they were of other constructs, including measures representing method and stylistic variance. To achieve this aim, a number of investigations were carried out using traditional approaches to studying the influence of response styles, such as the examination of measures of social desirability and acquiesence sets, and the use of experimental instructional sets simulating malingering and positive impression response patterns. If such analyses suggested that these response sets contributed more to variation in item responses than did variability in the target constructs, the item was not included in the final version of the instrument.

Test bias.   One implication of discriminant validity is that a test that is intended to measure a psychological construct should not be measuring a demographic variable, such as gender, age, or race. This does not mean that psychological tests should never be correlated with age, or gender, or race. However, the magnitude of any such correlations should not exceed the theoretical overlap of the demographic feature with the construct. For example, nearly every indicator of antisocial behavior suggests that it is more common in men than in women; thus, it would be expected that an assessment of antisocial behavior would yield average scores for men that are higher than those for women. However, the instrument should demonstrate a considerably greater correlation with other indicators of antisocial behavior than it does with gender; otherwise, it may be measuring gender rather than measuring the construct it was designed to assess.

In constructing the PAI, a number of different steps were taken to minimize the likelihood of test bias. First, every item on the instrument was reviewed by a bias panel (consisting of lay and professional individuals, both men and women, of diverse racial and ethnic backgrounds) to identify items that, although written to identify emotional and/or behavioral problems, might instead reflect other factors, such as sociocultural background. This panel represented a conceptually based approach to this particular aspect of discriminant validity. A second, empirical strategy for eliminating test bias involved the examination of item psychometric properties as a function of demography. In particular, associations between a given item and its corresponding full scale were evaluated using regression models, and items were chosen to display minimal variation in slope or intercept parameters as a function of demographic variables (Cleary, 1968). The intent of this approach was to eliminate items that had different meanings for different demographic groups; for example, if an item inquiring about "crying easily" seemed to be related to other indicators of depression in women but not in men, then that item was eliminated because interpretation of the item would vary as a function of gender. Note that this strategy will not eliminate mean demographic differences in scale scores. For example, an item inquiring about stealing may have a similar meaning for identifying antisocial personality for both men and women, yet still be more common among men. In this example, the resulting gender difference is not a function of test *bias;* rather, it is an accurate reflection of gender differences in the disorder. Although the PAI scales demonstrate relatively few demographic differences, it is important to recognize that such differences are *not* necessarily a sign of bias, and that a test with no such differences can in fact be quite biased.

THE PAI'S TEST CONSTRUCTION

Once the constructs to be measured by the PAI had been selected and the major facets of each construct delineated, items were written to tap these constructs. In generating and revising test items, it was always assumed that the content of a self-report item is critical to its utility as a measure of some phenomenon. Thus, items were written to reflect the phenomenology of various disorders and traits. The main attempt in writing items was to capture the experience of the person in order to determine if this experience is consistent with various phenomena relevant to mental health. For example, the experience of the paranoid individual is not one of being unreasonably suspicious, even though this feature is readily apparent to outside observers and is what is clinicians consider to be the core of the disorder. Rather, the paranoid individual feels surrounded by obstacles and barriers, created by others who may be envious of his or her potential. In writing items, care was taken not to confuse the experience of the clinician with that of the examinee.

   The items were written so that the content would be directly relevant to the different constructs measured by the test. Empirically derived tests may include items on a scale that have no apparent relation to the construct in question. However, research over the years (e.g., Holden, 1989; Holden & Fekken, 1990; Peterson, Clark, & Bennett, 1989) has continually indicated that such items add little or no validity to self-report tests. The available empirical evidence is entirely consistent with the assumption that the content of a self-report item is critical in determining its utility in measurement. This assumption does not preclude the potential utility of items that are truly "subtle" in the sense that a lay audience cannot readily identify the relationship of the item to mental health status. However, the assumption does suggest that the implications of such items for mental health status should be apparent to expert diagnosticians if the item is to prove useful.

Thus, the process of item development was done with a careful eye cast toward the content validity of the resultant scale, with respect to both breadth and depth of the construct as described above. A research team (which included assessment researchers, faculty, clinical practitioners, post-doctoral fellows, and graduate students in clinical psychology) independently generated items using the constructs described earlier as a guide. These item writers used the research literature, classic texts, the DSM and ICD manuals, and their own clinical experience as sources for item content. To insure that the PAI would represent a fresh approach to self-report assessment, items were generated completely independent of any other personality tests; many earlier clinical tests were developed from the same pool of items and hence shared many difficulties. Collectively, the research group produced a pool of over 2200 items; for each proposed scale, the pool included at least three times as many items as were planned for the final version of the test. These items were reduced to a final set of 344 through a number of procedures, both conceptual and empirical. The following paragraphs describe some of these procedures.

Conceptual Evaluation

As mentioned previously, the development of PAI items was based on the assumption that the content of a self-report item is critical to its utility as a measure of a clinical phenomenon. Thus, items were written so that the content would be directly relevant to the different constructs measured by the test, and it was assumed that the clinical implications of these items should be apparent to expert diagnosticians. Thus, the first stage of evaluation of the initial PAI item pool consisted of studies of the conceptual meaning of item content.

One study involved a rating task, in which members of a diagnostic research team independently evaluated the adequacy of item content for the construct in question. Each item in the pool was rated by at least four members of a research team that was diverse with respect to clinical experience, as well as gender, race, and religious background. The rating task had two components: (a) an assessment of the quality of the item; and (b) an assessment of the appropriateness of the subscale assignment for the item. In evaluating the quality of items, raters were given five guidelines to assist in decision-making:

1. The item should not be offensive to any gender, ethnic, economic, religious, or other group, nor potentially biased with respect to these groups.

2. The item should be worded unambiguously, at a 4th to 6th grade level. Items should have no more than 10 words if possible. No double negations should be used and single negations should be avoided if possible.

3. Colloquialisms or slang should be avoided, to avoid test items that would become dated within a few years or be difficult to translate into other languages.

4. Items should be reasonably specific to the syndrome under consideration, although they should not reflect only the most severe manifestations of the disorder.

5. No "damned if you do, damned if you don't" items were allowed. The meaning of endorsing an item as being true or false should be readily apparent.

In conjunction with the rating task described above, research team members were also asked to assign clinical scale items to the conceptual subscales that had emerged from reviewing the literature. Target agreement among the raters for the subscale assignment task was 75%; items that did not reach this level of agreement were rewritten or dropped from further consideration.

A second conceptual study of potential items involved the use of the bias review panel described earlier. This panel included professionals and citizens from varying backgrounds. These individuals were given a listing of the preliminary PAI items and were instructed to determine whether any of these items could be perceived as offensive on the basis of sex, race, religion, or ethnic group membership. Members of the panel were asked to mark any such items and indicate the reason for their determination as a guide to revising the item. The panel identified a number of items that could be endorsed in a pathological direction because of beliefs that were normative within a particular subculture. Also, panel members identified a few items as being potentially offensive and/or confusing. All such items were deleted or revised before the creation of the Alpha version of the PAI.

A third conceptual item evaluation involved a sorting study of item content using external experts in specific fields. Because all PAI items were written from the assumption that item content appropriate to the phenomenology of the mental disorder is crucial in determining the ultimate success or failure of a scale, an expert sorting task was developed to assess the appropriateness of item content as assessed by a panel of experts in psychopathology. The cooperation of eight experts was solicited in this project; each of these experts was internationally recognized in the assessment of constructs relevant to those measured by the PAI. The preliminary items were divided into four roughly equivalent groups within which sorting contrasts were made, with each contrast group comprised of items from five PAI scales. The assignment of PAI scales to these contrast groups was not random, in that certain discriminations were of particular interest. For example, the Schizophrenia and Anxiety-Related Disorders were placed within the same contrast group to determine if the experts could distinguish items tapping schizophrenic social detachment from those tapping heightened social anxiety and phobic avoidance. Similarly, Schizophrenia and Negative Impression items were placed into the same contrast group to determine if experts could distinguish items tapping psychotic aspects of schizophrenia from items written to represent a malingered psychosis.

The results of the sorting task indicated 89.8% agreement across all judgments of the preliminary items. For every scale, agreement values were substantially higher than the 20% agreement that would be expected from a chance assignment of items to the five scales in the contrast group. Items that did not achieve satisfactory agreement were dropped, and thus overall agreement for the items included on the Alpha version of the PAI was 94.3%. The results of the expert item sorting task therefore supported the conclusion that the content of PAI items could be reliably related to the relevant constructs by leading experts in the field.

Empirical Evaluation

After eliminating items on the basis of the rating task, bias panel review and expert judge sortings, a pool of 776 items remained. From these items, the final total of 344 items were selected on the basis of a two-tiered empirical evaluation strategy using an alpha and a beta version of the test. These studies examined a number of the psychometric properties of each item in a variety of different samples. The goal was to include items that struck a balance between different desirable item parameters, including content coverage as well as empirical characteristics, so that the scales could be useful across a number of different applications. Of paramount importance in this stage of item selection was the assumption that *no single quantitative item parameter should be used as the sole criterion* for item selection. An overreliance on a single parameter in item selection typically leads to a scale with one desirable psychometric property and numerous undesirable ones. In doing so, the construct validation approach can avoid the many pitfalls associated with "naive empiricism" in test construction.

The following psychometric parameters were considered in item selection:

Item means and standard deviations. In selecting items, item means and standard deviations were examined for normal subjects, patients in general, and patients who carried a diagnosis relevant to the scale from which the item had been selected. Such differences, while informative, by no means served as the sole or even primary criterion for empirical item selection. Nonetheless, there were many scales in which pronounced clinical/normal differences should be expected (e.g., Depression) while for others no differences were desired (e.g., Infrequency). Thus, these comparisons served as a basis for item selection on these scales.

Item-total correlations. This commonly-used parameter involved the corrected part-whole correlation of the item, reflected the correlation of the item with the sum of other items from the same scale. Items with negative values or values near zero were deleted if obtained in samples with reasonable variability in the construct in question.

Squared multiple correlations. As an adjunct to the part-whole correlation, the squared multiple correlation between each item and all other items from the same scale was calculated. These values were useful in identifying highly redundant items, since the response to a redundant item should be easily predicted from other items in the scale. Thus, with respect to this parameter, the ideal item should be consistent but not redundant with other items from the same scale in order to maximize the efficiency of the test. Where these values were very large (e.g., above .70), individual item intercorrelations were examined to isolate redundancies and the better of the two items (on other parameters) was retained.

Item "difficulty". This item parameter was derived from a one-parameter or Rasch modeling of item information curves. Items were selected such that this parameter would be reasonably variable across items, with the aim of providing items that sampled across the severity dimension of the construct in question. The other item parameters (e.g. slope and "guessing" parameters) were viewed as either irrelevant to a clinical instrument or rendered less important by the four-response option.

Item transparency. This item characteristic was operationalized as the F-value of the analysis of variance between subjects in standard, positive impression, and malingering instructional conditions. Larger F-values indicated more transparent items, suggesting that responses to the item could be affected by an examinee attempting to distort their profile in either a positive or negative direction. Since many key symptoms of mental disorder (such as hallucinations) are easily identified by a naive subject as pathological, transparency alone was not grounds for deletion of an item. However, items were selected to insure a range of transparency (i.e., including both obvious and more subtle indicators of a syndrome). Furthermore, where items were equivalent in other respects, less transparent items were selected over more transparent ones.

Response styles. This item characteristic also attempted to identify potential stylistic sources of variance in responses to an item. Here, the correlation of each item with the Marlowe-Crowne Social Desirability scale and the Positive Impression and Negative Impression scales were calculated. Items were candidates for deletion if the correlation with any of these scales approached or was higher than its corrected part-whole correlation with the parent construct.

Response sets. These analyses involved an investigation of a potential response set in utilizing the four-point answer scale of the PAI. This analysis sought, for example, to determine the influence of a tendency to use the left (i.e., "False", "Slightly True") or the right (i.e., "Very True", "Mainly True") on the response to individual questions, regardless of the content of the question. Although item content is generally found to be a much more powerful determinant of test results than such response sets (Koss, 1979), it was possible that the predominantly "true" response keying of PAI items could lead to problems in distinguishing stylistic from substantive variance. To address this issue, a score was calculated for each subject that was based upon the frequency of use of different response alternatives. These scores were then considered as discriminant validity indicators; items were expected to demonstrate higher correlations with other items from their scale than with any such indicators of response set tendencies.

Cross-scale correlations. This parameter sought to insure that items were related to their parent construct to a greater extent than to any other construct. It was assumed that an item that demonstrated sizable correlations with other scales from the test would have discrimination problems. Thus, items were candidates for deletion if they demonstrated greater correlation with other scales than with their own scale, or if they were highly correlated with a number of other scales in addition to their own.

Demographic differences. This parameter involved demographic differences in item endorsement. Mean values for items were examined to determine if large disparities existed as a function of gender, race, or age. It is important to point out that different endorsement rates are neither sufficient nor necessary evidence of item bias. Items can be biased with equivalent endorsement rates between groups, and they can also be unbiased where observed item differences are indicative of actual group differences on the construct. No attempt was made to equate mean values across these demographic features, since certain mental disorders are in fact associated with such variables. For example, it is well established that antisocial personality is more frequently observed in men than women, and also more common in younger as opposed to older patients – as a result, attempting to equate mean scores of these groups would not yield results reflecting the true nature of the disorder. Rather, the effort was made to insure that items were equally useful indicators of disorder across the different demographic groups using the regression-based procedure described below. However, where equivalent in other respects, items with no demographic differences were selected over those with discernible differences.

Item bias analyses. These analyses involved regression-based examinations of the relationship between each item and its parent scale, as a function of gender, race, or age, in an effort to identify and eliminate items that were biased demographically. Separate regressions were performed for men and women, whites and non-whites, and people under 40 years and those 40 and older, and differences in slope and intercept parameters of these regressions were noted. Items that yielded parameters that were significantly different across demographic groups were targets for deletion.

THE PAI: VALIDATION AND EXTENSION

The final step in the construct validation strategy involves the gathering of evidence of convergent and discriminant validity as gauged against other indicators of relevant constructs.   As such, the validation is never complete, but rather it is an ongoing process that provides feedback that is important in refining the use and interpretation of the test.

A full description of the validity studies of the PAI that have been conducted is beyond the scope of this chapter. The PAI manual alone contains information about correlations of individual scales with over 50 concurrent indices of psychopathology (Morey, 1991a), and numerous validity studies have been conducted since the publication of the test, many of which are summarized in the *Interpretive Guide* (Morey, 1996). The following sections touch on a few issues as example of the final stages of the construct validation process.

Reliability of the PAI

In classical test theory, reliability was considered to be a critical aspect of an instrument as it was interpreted as "freedom from random measurement error" and thus a constraining factor on validity. More modern conceptualizations, such as generalizability theory (Cronbach & Gleser, 1964) and item response theory (Hulin, Drasgow, & Parsons, 1983), make it apparent that such properties as internal consistency and temporal stability themselves must be understood as part of the nomological network. For example, assumptions about temporal stability in the measurement of mood state may be quite different from those in measuring intelligence. Thus, while these properties remain informative characteristics of any measures, it is important to place even these properties in the context of the construct.

The reliability of the PAI has been examined in a number of different studies that have examined the internal consistency, test-retest reliability, and configural stability of the instrument. Internal consistency has been examined in a number of different populations (Morey, 1991a: Boyle & Lennon, 1994; Alterman et al., 1995; Schinka, 1995; Rogers, Flores, Ustad, & Sewell, 1995b), ranging from a median alpha across scales of .78 in a sample of methadone maintenance patients (Alterman et al., 1995) to a median alpha of .86 in an alcoholic sample (Schinka, 1995). These medians include internal consistency estimates for the Inconsistency (ICN) and Infrequency (INF) scales, which are consistently lower than those for other scales since these scales do not measure theoretical constructs but rather the care with which the respondent completed the test. Lower alphas for such scales would be anticipated since carelessness might vary within an administration; for example, a subject might complete the first half of the test accurately but complete the last half haphazardly.

The lowest internal consistency estimates for the PAI reported in the literature were obtained using the Spanish version of the instrument (Rogers et al., 1995a), where an average alpha of .63 was obtained. Rogers and colleagues concluded that the internal consistency of the treatment consideration scales seemed to be most affected by the translation of the test. A subsequent study by this group indicated that the translated PAI demonstrated moderate convergent validity that was at least equal, and superior in some respects, to a Spanish translation of the MMPI-2 (Fantoni-Salvador & Rogers, 1997). Examination of internal consistency estimates for the PAI full scales for groups defined by various demographic characteristics (Morey, 1991a) does suggest that there is little variability in internal consistency as a function of race (median scale alpha for whites = .77, nonwhites = .78), gender (men = .79, women = .75), or age (under 40 = .79, 40 and over = .75). The Fantoni-Salvador and Rogers study also found no effect of ethnicity after controlling for symptom status.

The temporal stability of PAI scales has been examined by administering the test to subjects on two different occasions (Morey, 1991a; Boyle & Lennon, 1994; Rogers et al., 1995b). For the standardization studies, median test-retest reliability values, over a four-week interval, for the eleven full clinical scales was .86 (Morey, 1991a), leading to standard error of measurement estimates for these scales on the order of three to four T score points. Boyle and Lennon (1994) reported a median test-retest reliability of .73 in their normal sample over 28 days. Rogers et al. (1995b) found an average stability of .71 for the Spanish version of the PAI, administered over a two-week interval.

Since multiple-scale inventories are often interpreted configurally, additional questions should be asked concerning the stability of configurations on the eleven PAI clinical scales. One such analysis involved determining the inverse (or Q-type) correlation between each subject's profile at time one and the profile at time two. Correlations were obtained for each of the 155 subjects in the full retest sample, and a distribution of these within-subject profile correlations was obtained. Conducted in this manner, the median correlation over time of the clinical scale configuration was .83, indicating a substantial degree of stability in profile configurations over time (Morey, 1991a).

Validity Evidence

Considerable research on the convergent and discriminant validity has begun to accumulate. Much of this research has focused upon the "validity scales" and upon the scales targeting clinical constructs. The following sections provide examples of some of the research that has begun to elaborate the construct validation network for the PAI scales.

Validity scales and indices

One constant concern in psychological assessment involves the accuracy of self reported information as an indication of psychological status. The reasons offered as to why self-report may be distorted are myriad. One source of distortion may arise from an intention to deceive the recipient of the information. Such examinees may attempt to distort their responses to appear either better adjusted or more poorly adjusted than is actually the case. A second source of distortion may arise from limited insight or self-deception. These examinees may genuinely believe that they are doing quite well or quite poorly, but this belief might be at odds with the impression of objective observers. A third source of distortion can also arise from carelessness or indifference in taking a test; examinees who answer questions with little reflection (or even randomly) may yield results that do not accurately mirror their experiences. Fortunately, there are a variety of ways to detect such distortion with the PAI.

The first step in establishing profile validity involves using the PAI scales designed for this purpose. The PAI offers four scales that are designed to provide an assessment of factors which could distort the results of a self-report questionnaire. Two of these scales, Inconsistency (ICN) and Infrequency (INF) were developed to assess inconsistent or idiosyncratic responding, while the other two validity scales, Negative Impression (NIM) and Positive Impression (PIM) were developed to provide an assessment of efforts at impression management by the respondent.

There have been a number of correlational and simulation studies of these validity scales. For ICN and INF, the simulations have involved generation of random responses to the PAI, and the manual describes cutoff scores that will successfully identify the vast majority of such profiles as invalid (Morey, 1991a). For the NIM and PIM scales, a number of studies have been performed in which subjects were instructed to manage their impressions in either a positive or negative direction. Comparison of profiles for actual respondents (normal subjects or clinical subjects) and the response style simulation groups generally demonstrates a clear separation between scores of the actual respondents and the simulated responses (Morey, 1991a, Rogers, Ornduff, & Sewell, 1993; Cashel, Rogers, Sewell, & Martin-Cannici, 1995; Fals-Stewart, 1996). However, these simulation studies often indicate that the recommended cutoffs for NIM and PIM (92T and 68T, respectively) may be somewhat conservative when the base rate of distortion is relatively high. Under such conditions, Morey (1991) identified an optimal cutoff of 84T for NIM and 57T for PIM.

Table 3. A sample of instruments used in the validation of the PAI to date.

Beck Depression Inventory (Beck & Steer, 1987)
Beck Anxiety Inventory (Beck & Steer, 1990)
Beck Hopelessness Scale (Beck & Steer, 1988)
Bell Object Relations Inventory (Bell Inventory; Bell, Billington, & Becker, 1985)
Brief Psychiatric Rating Scale (Overall & Gorham, 1962)
Drug Abuse Screening Test (Skinner, 1982)
Fear Survey Schedule (Wolpe & Lang, 1964);
Hamilton Rating Scale for Depression (Hamilton, 1960)
Interpersonal Adjective Scale (IAS-R; Trapnell & Wiggins, 1990)
Maudsley Obsessive-Compulsive Inventory (Rachman & Hodgson, 1980)
Michigan Alcoholism Screening Test (Selzer, 1971)
Mississippi Scale for Combat-Related Posttraumatic Stress Disorder (Keane, Caddell, & Taylor, 1988)
MMPI-2 (Butcher et al., 1989)
MMPI clinical and research scales (Hathaway & McKinley, 1967; Morey, Waugh, & Blashfield, 1985; Wiggins, 1966)
NEO-PI (Costa & McCrae, 1985)
Perceived Social Support scales (Procidano & Heller, 1983)
Personality Disorder Examination (Loranger et al., 1987)
Psychopathy Checklist-Revised (Hare et al, 1990)
Referral Decision Scale (Teplin & Schwartz, 1989)
Schedule of Recent Events (Holmes & Rahe, 1967)
Schedule of Affective Disorders and Schizophrenia (Spitzer et al., 1979)
Self-Report Psychopathy test (Hare, 1985)
Suicide Probability Scale (Cull & Gill, 1982)
State-Trait Anger Expression Inventory (Spielberger, 1988)
State-Trait Anxiety Inventory (Spielberger, 1983)
Structured Clinical Interview of DSM-III-R Disorders (Spitzer et al., 1990)
Structured Interview of Reported Symptoms (Rogers, Bagby, & Dickens, 1992)
Wahler Physical Symptoms Inventory (Wahler, 1983)

A second strategy for the evaluation of profile validity is based upon the consideration of various configural elements of the PAI profile. For example, the Defensiveness and Malingering Indices (Morey, 1996) consist of features that tend to be observed only in distorted profiles. Use of discriminant function analysis to identify defensive (Cashel et al., 1995) and malingered (Rogers et al., 1996) responding has also been found to yield good identification rates that cross validate across different studies (Morey, 1996; Morey & Lanier, 1998). Finally, the specific issue of defensiveness about alcohol and/or drug use has been addressed with a regression-based strategy that seeks to identify underreporting of substance use based upon various configural predictors (Morey, 1996). Each of these strategies should be used to supplement the validity scales to insure that the PAI profile can be interpreted in a straightforward manner.

Clinical scales

The clinical scales of the PAI were assembled to provide information about critical diagnostic features of important clinical constructs. A large number of different indicators have been used to provide information on the convergent and discriminant validity of the PAI clinical scales. The manual alone (Morey, 1991a) provides validity coefficients on over 50 commonly used measures of clinical and personality status, and a number of subsequent investigations have greatly expanded this literature (e.g., Montag & Levin, 1994; Osborne, 1994; Greenstein, 1993; Cherepon & Prinzhorn, 1994; Costa & McCrae, 1992; Ban et al., 1993; Boyle & Lennon, 1994; Fantoni-Salvador & Rogers, 1997; Kurtz, Morey, & Tomarken, 1992; Alterman, Zabarello, Lin, Siddiqui, Brown, Rutherford, & McDermott, 1995; Bell-Pringle, 1994; Rogers et al., 1995b; Rogers, Ustad & Salekin, 1998; Trull, 1995; Trull, Useda, Conforti, & Doan, 1997; Wang et al., 1997). Markers used as validation indicators, some of which are shown in Table 3, have included many of the most commonly used clinical measures. Although a full review of this literature is beyond the scope of the chapter, the scales of the PAI have been found to associate with most major instruments for the assessment of diagnosis and treatment efficacy in theoretically concordant ways, indicating that the process of construct validation for the instrument continues to evolve.

CONCLUSION

The construct validation approach to psychological assessment appears deceptively simple, yet the subtleties become much more apparent in the process of developing and validating a multiscale instrument. It was really only after performing such an exercise that I really began to appreciate Douglas Jackson's contributions to this field. I also believe that, through his efforts and the efforts of the other contributors to this volume, psychological assessment has more to offer the researcher and clinician today than it did four decades ago. The construct validation approach yields instruments that are straightforward in terms of meaning and interpretation; because the measures are tied explicitly to constructs, the interpretation of a scale score generally corresponds directly to the name of the scale, which remarkably has often not been the case in the history of assessment. For example, on the PAI, if a person obtains an elevated score on DEP it is safe to conclude that the person is reporting experiencing signs and symptoms of depression. However, this parsimony of interpretation should not be viewed as a limit, but rather as a solid beginning point for the new user. Because of the relatively recent introduction of the PAI, the configural power of the instrument is only beginning to be understood and tapped. In recent years, actuarial checklists have being introduced that are useful identifying individuals who are attempting to distort their self-presentation, those who deny substance misuse, those at risk for suicide or violence, and those who may be particularly difficult to engage in therapy. As these indices gather cross-validation support, they may provide a valuable supplement to the standard PAI scales, in many cases providing alternative means of answering some of the most challenging issues in assessment.

Ultimately, the goal for an assessment instrument is the same as the goal for a more general science of psychology, this being a thorough elaboration of the nomological network relating important constructs and their various indicators. Because of the efforts of assessment pioneers such as Douglas Jackson, the field has a more clear sense of the steps needed to achieve this goal. I have little doubt that these efforts will continue to serve as the foundation for the development of psychological theory and measurement well into the coming century.

REFERENCES

Alterman, A.I., Zaballero, A.R., Lin, M.M., Siddiqui, N., Brown, L.S., Rutherford, M.J., & McDermott, P.A. (1995). Personality Assessment Inventory (PAI) scores of lower socioeconomic African American and Latino methadone maintenance patients. *Assessment*, **2**, 91-100.

Ban, T.A., Fjetland, O.K., Kutcher, M., & Morey, L.C. (1995). CODE-DD: Development of a diagnostic scale for depressive disorders. In I. Hindmarch & P. Stonier (eds.), *Human psychopharmacology: Measures and Methods. Volume 4.*

Beck, A.T. (1967). *Depression: Clinical, experimental, and theoretical aspects.* New York: Harper & Row.

Beck, A.T., & Emery, G. (1979). *Cognitive therapy of anxiety and phobic disorders.* New York: Guilford.

Beck, A.T., & Steer, R.A. (1987). *Beck Depression Inventory manual.* San Antonio: The Psychological Corporation.

Beck, A.T., & Steer, R.A. (1988). *Beck Hopelessness Scale manual.* San Antonio: The Psychological Corporation.

Beck, A.T., & Steer, R.A. (1990). *Beck Anxiety Inventory manual.* San Antonio: The Psychological Corporation.

Bell, M.J., Billington, R., & Becker, B. (1985). A scale for the assessment of object relations: Reliability, validity, and factorial invariance. *Journal of Clinical Psychology*, **42**, 733-741.

Bell-Pringle, V.J. (1994). *Assessment of borderline personality disorder using the MMPI-2 and the Personality Assessment Inventory.* Doctoral Dissertation, Georgia State University, Atlanta, GA.

Blashfield, R.K., & McElroy, R.A. (1987). The 1985 journal literature on the personality disorders. *Comprehensive Psychiatry*, **28**, 536-546.

Block, J. (1965). *The challenge of response sets: Unconfounding meaning, acquiescence, and social desirability in the MMPI.* New York: Appleton-Century-Crofts.

Boyle, G. J., & Lennon, T.J. (1994) Examination of the reliability and validity of the Personality Assessment Inventory. *Journal of Psychopathology and Behavior Assessment*, **16**, 173-188.

Butcher, J.N., Dahlstrom, W.G., Graham, J.R., Tellegen, A., & Kaemmer, B. (1989). *Minnesota Multiphasic Personality Inventory-2: Manual for Adminstration and Scoring.* Minneapolis: University of Minnesota Press.

Campbell, D.T., & Fiske, D.W. (1959). Convergent and discriminant validation by the multitrait-multimethod matrix. *Psychological Bulletin*, **56**, 81-105.

Cashel, M.L., Rogers, R., Sewell, K., & Martin-Cannici, C. (1995). The Personality Assessment Inventory and the detection of defensiveness. *Assessment*, **2**, 333-342.

Cherepon, J.A., & Prinzhorn, B. (1994). The Personality Assessment Inventory profiles of adult female abuse survivors. *Assessment, 1,* 393-400.

Costa, P.T., & McCrae, R.R. (1985). *The NEO Personality Inventory manual.* Odessa, FL: Psychological Assessment Resources.

Costa, P.T., & McCrae, R.R. (1989). *The NEO-PI/FFI manual supplement.* Odessa, FL: Psychological Assessment Resources.

Costa, P.T., & McCrae, R.R. (1992). Normal personality in clinical practice: The NEO Personality Inventory. *Psychological Assessment, 4,* 5-13.

Cleary, T.A. (1968). Test bias: Prediction of grades of Negro and white students in integrated colleges. *Journal of Educational Measurement, 5,* 115-124.

Cronbach, L.J. (1951). Coefficient alpha and the internal structure of tests. *Psychometrika, 16,* 297-334.

Cronbach, L.J., & Gleser, G.C. (1964). The signal-noise ratio in the comparison of reliability coefficients. *Educational and Psychological Measurement, 24,* 467-480.

Cronbach, L. J & Meehl, P. E. (1955). Construct validity in psychological tests. *Psychological Bulletin, 52,* 281-302.

Cull, J.G., & Gill, W.S. (1982). *Suicide Probability Scale manual.* Los Angeles, CA: Western Psychological Services.

Cronbach, L.J., & Meehl, P.E. (1955). Construct validity in psychological tests. *Psychological Bulletin, 52,* 281-302.

Edwards, A. L. (1957). *The social desirability variable in personality assessment and research.* New York: Dryden.

Fals-Stewart, W. (1996). The ability of individuals with psychoactive substance use disorders to escape detection by the Personality Assessment Inventory. *Psychological Assessment, 8,* 60-68.

Fantoni-Salvador P., & Rogers, R. (1997). Spanish versions of the MMPI-2 and PAI: An investigation of concurrent validity with Hispanic patients. *Assessment, 4,* 29-39.

Faravelli, C., Albanesi, G., & Poli, E. (1986). Assessment of depression: a comparison of rating scales. *Journal of Affective Disorders, 11,* 245-253.

Faust, D., & Miner, R.A. (1986). The empiricist and his new clothes: DSM-III in perspective. *American Journal of Psychiatry, 143,* 962-967.

Greenstein, D.S. (1993). *Relationship between frequent nightmares, psychopathology, and boundaries among incarcerated male inmates.* Doctoral dissertation, Adler School of Professional Psychology, Chicago, IL.

Hamilton, M. (1960). A rating scale for depression. *Journal of Neurology, Neurosurgery, and Psychiatry, 23,* 56-62.

Hammill, D.D., Brown, L., & Bryant, B.R. (1993). *A consumer's guide to tests in print.* Austin, TX: Pro-Ed.

Hare, R. D. (1985). Comparison of procedures for the assessment of psychopathy. *Journal of Consulting and Clinical Psychology, 53,* 7-16.

Hare, R.D., Harpur, T.J., Hakstian, A.R., et al. (1990). The revised Psychopathy Checklist: Reliability and factor structure. *Psychological Assessment, 2,* 338-341.

Hathaway, S.R., & McKinley, J.C. (1967). *MMPI manual (revised edition).* New York: Psychological Corporation.

Helmes, E. (1999). The role of social desirability in the assessment of personality constructs. In R.D. Goffin and E. Helmes (Eds.) *Problems and Solutions in Human Assessment.* Norwell, MA: Kluwer Academic Publishers.

Holden, R.R. (1989). Disguise and the structured self-report assessment of psychopathology: II. A clinical replication. *Journal of Clinical Psychology, 45,* 583-586.

Holden, R. R.. (1999). Application of the construct heuristic to the screening of psychopathology: The Holden Psychological Screening Inventory (HPSI). In R.D. Goffin and E. Helmes (Eds.) *Problems and Solutions in Human Assessment.* Norwell, MA: Kluwer Academic Publishers.

Holden, R.R., & Fekken, G.C. (1990). Structured psychopathological test item characteristics and validity. *Psychological Assessment, 2,* 35-40.

Holmes, T.H., & Rahe, R.H. (1967). The social readjustment rating scale. *Journal of Psychosomatic Research, 11,* 213-218.

Hulin, C.L., Drasgow, F., & Parsons, C.K. (1983). *Item response theory: Application to psychological measurement.* Homewood, IL: Irwin.

Jackson, D. N. (1967). *Personality Research Form manual.* Goshen, NY: Research Psychologists Press.

Jackson, D.N. (1970). A sequential system for personality scale development. In C.D. Spielberger (Ed.), *Current topics in clinical and community psychology, volume 2*, pp.62-97. New York: Academic Press.

Jackson, D.N. (1971). The dynamics of structured personality tests. *Psychological Review, 78*, 229-248.

Keane, T.M., Caddell, J.M., & Taylor, K.L. (1988). Mississippi scale for combat-related posttraumatic stress disorder: Three studies in reliability and validity. *Journal of Consulting and Clinical Psychology, 56*, 85-90.

Koss, M.P. (1979). MMPI item content: recurring issues. In J.N. Butcher (Ed.), *New developments in the use of the MMPI*, pp. 3-38. Minneapolis: University of Minnesota Press.

Kurtz, J.E., Morey, L.C., & Tomarken, A.J. (1993) The concurrent validity of three self-report measures of borderline personality. *Journal of Psychopathology and Behavioral Assessment, 15*, 255-266.

Loevinger, J. (1954). The attenuation paradox in test theory. *Psychological Bulletin, 51*, 493-504.

Loevinger, J. (1957). Objective tests as instruments of psychological theory. *Psychological Reports, 3*, 635-694.

Loranger, A.W., Susman, V.L., Oldham, J.M., & Russakoff, L.M. (1987). The Personality Disorder Examination: A preliminary report. *Journal of Personality Disorders, 1*, 1- 13.

Lord, F.M. (1980). *Applications of item response theory to practical testing problems.* Hillsdale, NJ: Erlbaum.

Louks, J., Hayne, C., & Smith, J. (1989). Replicated factor structure of the BeckDepression Inventory. *Journal of Nervous and Mental Disease, 177* , 473-479.

Maser, J.D., & Cloninger, C.R. (1990). *Comorbidity of mood and anxiety disorders.* Washington DC: American Psychiatric Press.

McCrae, R. R., & Costa, P. T. (1983). Social desirability scales: More substance than style. *Journal of Consulting and Clinical Psychology, 31*, 882-888.

Meehl, P.E. (1977). Specific etiology and other forms of strong influence: Some quantitative meanings. *Journal of Medicine and Philosophy, 2*, 33-53.

Montag, I., & Levin, J. (1994). The five factor model and psychopathology in nonclinical samples. *Personality and Individual Differences, 17*, 1-7.

Morey, L.C. (1988). Personality disorders under DSM-III and DSM-III-R: An examination of convergence, coverage, and internal consistency. *American Journal of Psychiatry, 145*, 573-577.

Morey, L.C. (1991a). *The Personality Assessment Inventory Professional Manual.* Odessa, FL: Psychological Assessment Resources, Inc.

Morey, L.C. (1991b). The classification of mental disorder as a collection of hypothetical constructs. *Journal of Abnormal Psychology, 100*, 289-293.

Morey, L.C. (1996). *An interpretive guide to the Personality Assessment Inventory.* Odessa, FL: Psychological Assessment Resources, Inc.

Morey, L.C., & Lanier, V.W. (1998). Operating characteristics for six response distortion indicators for the Personality Assessment Inventory. *Assessment, 5*, 203-214.

Morey, L.C., Waugh, M.H., & Blashfield, R.K. (1985). MMPI scales for DSM-III personality disorders: Their derivation and correlates. *Journal of Personality Assessment, 49*, 245-251.

Nunnally, J.C. (1979). *Psychometric theory (second edition).* New York: McGraw- Hill.

Osborne, D. (1994). *Use of the Personality Assessment Inventory with a medical population.* Paper presented at the meetings of the Rocky Mountain Psychological Association, Denver, CO, April, 1994.

Overall, J.E., & Gorham, D.R. (1962). The Brief Psychiatric Rating Scale. *Psychological Reports, 10*, 799-812.

Peterson, G.W., Clark, D.A., & Bennett, B. (1989). The utility of MMPI subtle, obvious scales for detecting fake good and fake bad response sets. *Journal of Clinical Psychology, 45*, 575-583.

Procidano, M.E., & Heller, K. (1983). Measures of perceived social support from friends and from family: Three validation studies., *American Journal of Community Psychology, 11*, 1-24.

Rachman, S.J., & Hodgson, R.J. (1980). *Obsessions and compulsions.* Englewood Cliffs, NJ: Prentice-Hall.

Retzlaff, P., & Gilbertini, M. (1987). Factor structure of the MCMI basic personality scales and common-item artifact. *Journal of Personality Assessment, 51*, 588-594.

Rogers, R., Bagby, R.M., & Dickens, S.E. (1992*). Structured Interview for Reported Symptoms (SIRS) and professional manual.* Odessa, FL: Psychological Assessment Resources.

Rogers, R., Flores, J., Ustad, K., & Sewell, K.W. (1995a). Initial validation of the Personality Assessment Inventory-Spanish Version with clients from Mexican American communities. *Journal of Personality Assessment, 64*, 340-348.

Rogers, R., Ornduff, S.R., & Sewell, K. (1993). Feigning specific disorders: A study of the Personality Assessment Inventory (PAI). *Journal of Personality Assessment*, **60**, 554-560.

Rogers, R, Sewell, K.W., Ustad, K, Reinhardt, V., & Edwards, W. (1995b). The referral decision scale with mentally disordered inmates - a preliminary-study of convergent and discriminant validity. *Law and Human Behavior*, **19**, 481-492.

Rogers, R., Sewell, K.W., Morey, L.C., & Ustad, K.L. (1996). Deterction of feigned mental disorders on the Personality Assessment Inventory: A discriminant analysis. *Journal of Personality Assessment*. **67**, 629-640.

Rogers, R., Ustad, K.L., & Salekin, R.T. (1998). Convergent validity of the personality assessment inventory: A study of emergency referrals in a correctional setting. *Assessment*, **5**, 3-12.

Schinka, J.A. (1995). Personality Assessment Inventory scale characteristics and factor structure in the assessment of alcohol dependency. *Journal of Personality Assessment*, **64**, 101-111.

Schinka, J.A. & Borum, R. (1993). Readability of adult psychopathology inventories. *Psychological Assessment*, **5**, 384-386.

Schwartz, M.A., & Wiggins, O.P. (1987). Empiricism and DSM-III. *American Journal of Psychiatry*, **144**, 837-838.

Selzer, M. L. (1971). The Michigan Alcoholism Screening Test: The quest for a new diagnostic instrument. *American Journal of Psychiatry*, **127**, 1653-1658.

Skinner, H.A. (1981). Toward the integration of classification theory and methods. *Journal of Abnormal Psychology*, **90**, 68-87.

Skinner, H.A. (1982). The drug abuse screening test. *Addictive Behaviors*, 7, 363-371.

Skinner, H.A. (1986). Construct validation approach to psychiatric classification. In T. Millon & G.L. Klerman (eds.), *Contemporary directions in psychopathology*, pp. 307-330. Yew York: Guilford Press.

Spielberger, C.D. (1983). *Manual for the State-Trait Anxiety Inventory*. Palo Alto, CA: Consulting Psychologists Press.

Spielberger, C.D. (1988). *State-Trait Anger Expression Inventory.* Odessa, FL: Psychological Assessment Resources.

Spitzer, R.L., Williams, J.B., Gibbon, M., & First, M. (1990). *Structured clinical interview for DSM-III-R*. Washington, DC: American Psychiatric Press.

Spitzer, R.L., & Endicott, J. (1979). *Schedule for Affective Disorders and Schizophrenia*. New York: New York State Psychiatric Institute, Biometrics Research.

Steer, R, A., Ball, R., Ranieri, W.F., & Beck, A. T., (1999). Dimensions of the Beck Depression Inventory-II in clinically depressed outpatients. *Journal of Clinical Psychology*. **55**, 117-128.

Teplin, L.A., & Swartz, J. (1989). Screening for severe mental disorder in jails - the development of the Referral Decision Scale. *Law and Human Behavior*, **13**, 1-18.

Trapnell, P.D., & Wiggins, J.S. (1990). Extension of the Interpersonal Adjective Scale to include the big five dimensions of personality. *Journal of Personality and Social Psychology*, **59**, 781-790.

Trull, T.J. (1995). Borderline personality disorder features in nonclinical young adults: 1. Identification and validation. *Psychological Assessment*, 7, 33-41.

Trull, T.J., Useda, J.D., Conforti, K., & Doan, B.T. (1997). Borderline personality disorder features in nonclinical young adults .2. Two-year outcome. *Journal of Abnormal Psychology*, **106**, 307-314.

Wahler, H.J. (1983). *Wahler Physical Symptoms Inventory, 1983 edition*. Los Angeles: Western Psychological Services.

Wang, E.W., Rogers, R., Giles, C.L.,, Diamond, P.M., Herrington-Wang, L.E., & Taylor, E.R. (1997). A pilot study of the Personality Assessment Inventory (PAI) in corrections: Assessment of malingering, suicide risk, and aggression in male inmates *Behavioral Sciences & The Law* , **15**, 469-482.

Welsh, G. S. (1952). A factor study of the MMPI using scales with item overlap eliminated. *American Psychologist*, 7, 341.

Wiggins, J.S. (1962). Strategic, method, and stylistic variance in the MMPI. *Psychological Bulletin*, **59**, 224-242.

Wiggins, J.S. (1966). Substantive dimensions of self-report in the MMPI item pool. *Psychological Monographs, 80*, **22** (whole No. 630).

Wolpe, J., & Lang, P. (1964). A fear survey schedule for use in behavior therapy. *Behavior Research and Therapy*, **2**, 27-30.

8 INDIVIDUAL DIFFERENCES AND SCIENTIFIC PRODUCTIVITY

J. Philippe Rushton

OVERVIEW

This chapter features Jackson's and my (independent) work on the personality traits, values, and motives of productive scientists. It shows that the distribution of scientific achievement is J-shaped, implying that the underlying causes combine multiplicatively rather than additively. It reviews my own research using peer- and self-ratings on 29 traits, including those from Jackson's *Personality Research Form*, in which impactful scientists were found to be ambitious, enduring, seeking definiteness, dominant, showing leadership, intelligent, aggressive, independent, not meek, and non-supportive. It reviews Jackson's research finding that strong theoretical interests, curiosity, an autonomous personality, and achievement motivation are salient in successful scientists. It also reviews his suggestions that administrators need to take the unique attributes of scientists into account to create the conditions maximally conducive to productivity. These include freedom from bureaucratic interference, good financial rewards, and incentives for career advancement. It concludes by touching on the important role Doug Jackson played defending academic freedom in Canada.

A PERSONAL NOTE

Back in 1977 when I began my career at the University of Western Ontario, Doug Jackson (to whom I largely owed my appointment) was one of the most prolific and cited psychologists in North America. Year after year, he routinely published about 10 articles, book chapters, research bulletins, and psychology test manuals. I was keen to find out how he generated the quality and quantity of his output as I had developed a research program on productivity and impact (Rushton & Endler, 1977). I was also delighted to learn Doug shared my interest in the causes of high productivity.

Regular lunch partners, Doug and I have frequently discussed progress in science. By 1985 this mutual interest led us to co-host a conference on scientific excellence at the University of Western Ontario. Supported by grants from the Academic Development Fund at the university and the Social Sciences and Humanities Research Council of Canada, the conference resulted in an edited book, *Scientific Excellence: Origins and Assessment* (Jackson & Rushton, 1987).

STUDIES OF SCIENTIFIC ACHIEVEMENT

One of the most salient features of scientific achievement is its unequal distribution. Whereas personality and intelligence are normally distributed, scientific achievement is not. A very few scientists are responsible for the great majority of creative works. Across scientific disciplines, the most productive 10% of scientists typically account for 50% of the publications (Dennis, 1955; Shockley, 1957). Studies of academic psychologists show a similar distribution (Endler, Rushton & Roediger, 1978; Rushton & Endler, 1977; Rushton, 1989). Consider, for example, the citation and publication counts reported in Table 1. These cumulative percentage frequencies are based on 4,070 faculty members studied by Endler et al. (1978) in an analysis of the top 100 departments of psychology in the United States, Canada, and the United Kingdom. Over half (52%) of the sample did not publish an article in 1975 in any of the journals reviewed by the *Social Sciences Citation Index*. The picture is similar for citations, the great majority of academic psychologists having relatively few. For example, only about 25% of psychologists had more than 15 citations in 1975 and only 1% had more than 100 citations.

"Ageist," "sexist," and "elitist" factors contribute to the positive skew shown in these distributions. Productivity increases with age up to around 40-45 years, then gradually diminishes. Women are not only under-represented in science but, on a per capita basis, produce less than their male counterparts (Cole, 1981). Individuals who received doctorates from more prestigious institutions and/or who obtained their first academic positions at high prestige universities are more productive than those who graduated from or were appointed to less esteemed institutions (Gaston, 1978).

Why? As Walberg, Strykowski, Rovai, and Hung (1984) explain, the normal distribution does not apply to exceptional performance. Instead, J-shaped distributions such as those shown in Table 1, are characteristic. J-shaped distributions – monotonically decreasing at a decelerating rate – typically occur when the underlying causes combine multiplicatively rather than additively. (Additive causes typically produce normal distributions). Walberg et al. (1984) show that learning is a multiplicative, diminishing-returns function of student ability, time, motivation, and amount and quality of instruction. (Those instances in which no learning at all takes place occur because any zero score in the equation yields a product of zero.)

Table 1. Frequencies and Cumulative Percentage for the Distribution of Citations of and Publications by Faculty Members at the Top 100 British, Canadian, and American Graduate Department of Psychology

Number of Citations or Publications	Citations		Publications	
	Cumulative Frequency	Percentage	Cumulative Frequency	Percentage
>100	134	100	-	-
26-99	556	97	-	-
21-25	164	83	1	100
16-20	223	79	1	99
11-15	338	74	1	99
10	97	65	3	99
9	82	63	4	99
8	102	61	12	99
7	105	58	18	99
6	125	56	37	99
5	187	53	54	98
4	187	48	147	97
3	207	44	259	93
2	302	38	468	87
1	365	31	971	75
0	896	22	2094	52
Total	4070		4070	

Note. From the 1975 *Social Sciences Citation Index.* (From Endler, Rushton, and Roediger, 1978, p. 1079, Table 5). Copyright 1978 by the American Psychological Association. Reprinted by permission.

Creative achievement is a multiplicative function of cognitive, personality, and environmental variables. *Cognitive* abilities (such as intelligence, acquired knowledge, technical skills, and special talents) combine with *personality* traits (such as internal motivation, confidence, non-conformity, persistence and originality) and *environmental* variables (such as political-religious, socioeconomic, and educational factors) in producing truly creative achievements. Many of these variables are likely to act in a multiplicative (synergistic) rather than an additive manner. Assuming independence of each of these traits, a scientist who is at the 90th percentile on intelligence, internal motivation, independence, and endurance is a person who is one in ten thousand.

THE SCIENTIFIC PERSONALITY

The portrayal of the "scientific personality" in some biographies leaves little doubt as to the characteristics of the ideal scientist: objectivity, emotional neutrality, rationality, open-mindedness, superior intelligence, integrity, and a communal, open, and cooperative attitude toward sharing knowledge. Indeed, the history of science is sometimes "as inspiring in its human values as are the legends of the saints" (Knickerbocker, 1927, p. 305).

Biographies also show the gap between reality and this idealized portrait (Eysenck, 1995). Scientists often engage in emotionally charged ideological battles, where personal success and the destruction of opponents override objectivity, where selective perceptions and distortion of facts diminish rationality, and where personal biases lead to editorial rejection of contrary ideas. At times, outright deception and fraud undermine the ideal of honest integrity, and secrecy, suspicion, and aggressive competition in the race to be "number one" displace any altruistic desire to share knowledge and cooperate. Nonetheless, inspirational cases are there to be found, as in Eysenck's (1995) example of "unconquerable will" and achievement exemplified by George Washington Carver who was born a slave but rose against the odds to considerable heights of scientific achievement.

The scientific investigation into the psychological characteristics of eminent scientists began with Francis Galton (1869, 1874). His pioneering work was expanded by J. M. Cattell (1903, 1910), Havelock Ellis (1904), Cox (1926), Roe (1952), R. B. Cattell and Drevdahl (1955), Terman (1955), and by Taylor and Barron (1962), and others (see Jackson & Rushton, 1987; Eysenck, 1995; Sulloway, 1996; Vernon, 1987; for reviews). From this growing body of research it became clear that successful scientists are hardly "saints," either in their personality or work style. More often they display reclusive personalities, arrogant work styles, hostility to frustration, and intrinsic motivations bordering on the autistic.

One early investigation of the scientific personality is Terman's (1955) longitudinal study of 800 high-IQ men, which found that those who took science degrees at college differed from non-scientists. The scientists showed greater intellectual curiosity from an early age and were lower than average in sociability. Terman concluded that "the bulk of scientific research is carried on by devotees of science for whom research is their life and social relations are comparatively unimportant" (p. 7). Earlier, Roe had found that scientists had difficulty in interpersonal situations and often tried to avoid them. Terman described Roe's sample of scientists as tending "to be shy, lonely, slow in social development, and indifferent to close personal relationships, group activities, or politics" (p. 7). However, Terman pointed out that these traits were not necessarily defects of personality since emotional breakdowns were no more common than among nonscientists. Instead, he suggested that a below-average interest in social relations and a heavy concentration of interest in the objective world was a statistical, but non-clinical departure from average, decidedly favorable for the professional development of a scientist.

Raymond Cattell's (1962, 1965; Cattell & Drevdahl, 1955) profile of the prototypic scientist emerges from both the qualitative study of biographies and from quantitative psychometric studies of leading physicists, biologists, and psychologists. Cattell found successful scientists to be reserved and introverted, intelligent, emotionally stable, dominant, serious-minded, expedient, venturesome, sensitive, radical thinking, self-sufficient, and having a strong and exacting self-concept. He noted that the physicists, biologists, and psychologists were similar in personality except that psychologists were less serious-minded and more "surgent" and talkative than non-psychologists. Creative scientists differed most from normals on his schizothymia-cyclothymia factor, with scientific researchers being toward the schizothymic end. Cattell thus describes scientists as being sceptical, internally preoccupied, precise, and critical individuals who are exacting and reliable.

Several studies were carried out by Barron and his colleagues (Barron, 1962; Taylor & Barron, 1962). Barron (1962), for example, found creative people generally to be cognitively complex (preferring complexity and imbalance in phenomena), to have a more differentiated personality structure, to be independent in their judgment and less conformist in social contexts (e.g., Asch group pressure situation), to be self-assertive and dominant, and to be low in using suppression as a mechanism for the control of impulses and thoughts (that is, they forbade themselves fewer thoughts). Chambers (1964) compared eminent researchers with those less eminent but matched on other relevant variables. Results indicated that the more creative scientists were also more dominant, had more initiative, were more self-sufficient, and were more motivated toward intellectual success. McClelland (1962) found successful scientists to be not only higher in need for achievement but also to be calculating risk-takers in the same way as are successful business entrepreneurs. Their risk-taking, however, involved dealing with nature or physical situations rather than social situations, for McClelland, too, found scientists to be decidedly avoidant of interpersonal relationships. Scientists, for instance, indicated a much higher preference for being a lighthouse keeper than a headwaiter (Item # 324 on the Strong Vocational Interest Blank). McClelland also argued that the need for scientific achievement was a strong aggressive drive "which is normally kept carefully in check and diverted into taking nature apart" (1962, p. 162). In short, the scientist is "introverted and bold" (Drevdahl & Cattell, 1958).

Publication and citation counts of psychologists can be predicted by those components of achievement motivation that concern the enjoyment of challenging tasks and hard work, but not by those components concerned with interpersonal competition or bettering others (Helmreich et al., 1978, 1980). Type A "workaholic" behavior (aggressive, incessantly struggling, time-oriented, hostile when frustrated) predicts the number of citations a psychologist's work earned from others (Matthews et al., 1980). Using structural equation modeling, Feist's (1993) model produced a good fit leading from hostile personality, internal motivation, and arrogant working style to objectively measured eminence in 100 physicists, chemists, and biologists at major research universities in California.

PERSONALITY, RESEARCH CREATIVITY, AND TEACHING EFFECTIVENESS

My own research includes two separate studies conducted with Harry Murray and Sampo Paunonen on the personality correlates of research and teaching effectiveness (Rushton, Murray & Paunonen, 1983; editor's note: Paunonen has contributed chapter 6 of this volume). We examined the importance of 29 personality traits, including 20 from Jackson's (1974) *Personality Research Form*. In the first study, 52 (46 male, 6 female) psychology professors at the University of Western Ontario were assessed by scale scores, self-ratings, student-ratings, and faculty peer-ratings. (Due to the small number of females, all analyses are collapsed across sex.)   Instructions emphasized that ratings were to be made relative to other professors rather than to people in general. Ratings were made on 9-point-scales, using the trait names and brief descriptions shown in Table 2 which also shows the split-half reliabilities for the faculty-peer and student judgments. The various assessments showed convergent validity (mean across methods = 0.48). Because we had complete data for the peer-ratings (n = 52; 12 ratings per faculty member) and not the other procedures, the analyses here will be limited to the former. In the second study we mailed a survey to 400 psychologists at other Canadian universities and asked them to rate their own personality in relation to other university professors and the importance to them of research and teaching. In Study 1, an index of research eminence was made from two measures: (1) total publications over the previous four years as listed in either the Social Science Cita-

Table 2. Split-half reliabilities of peer and student ratings of personality computed across professor targets for each of 29 personality traits (decimals omitted).

	Raters	
Personality trait and trait definition	Faculty (n=52)	Students (n=43)
1. Meek (mild mannered; subservient)	73	57
2. Ambitious (aspiring to accomplish difficult tasks; striving, competitive)	88	74
3. Sociable (friendly, outgoing, enjoys being with people)	74	63
4. Aggressive (argumentative, threatening; enjoys combat and argument)	84	62
5. Independent (avoids restraints; enjoys being unattached)	80	42
6. Changeable (flexible, restless; likes new and different experiences)	77	33
7. Seeks definiteness (dislikes ambiguity or uncertainty in information; wants all questions answered completely)	84	22
8. Defensive (suspicious, guarded, touchy)	72	56
9. Dominant (attempts to control environment; forceful, decisive)	87	60
10. Enduring (willing to work long hours; persevering, steadfast, unrelenting)	90	52
11. Attention seeking (enjoys being conspicuous, dramatic, colorful)	88	67
12. Harm avoiding (careful, cautious, pain-avoidant)	84	90
13. Impulsive (spontaneous, hasty, impetuous, and uninhibited)	89	31
14. Supporting (gives sympathy and comfort; helpful, indulgent)	84	36
15. Orderly (neat and organized; dislikes clutter, confusion, lack of organization)	77	56
16. Fun loving (playful, easygoing, light-hearted; does many things "just for fun")	88	75
17. Aesthetically sensitive (sensitive to sounds, sights, tastes, smells)	80	74

Table 2. (continued)

18. Approval seeking (desires to be held in high esteem; obliging, agreeable)	76	42
19. Seeks help and advice (desires and needs support, protection, love, advice)	80	86
20. Intellectually curious (seeks understanding; reflective, intellectual)	78	65
21. Anxious (tense, nervous, uneasy)	60	63
22. Intelligent (bright, quick, clever)	89	50
23. Liberal (progressive, seeks change, modern, adaptable)	81	29
24. Shows leadership (takes initiative and responsibility for getting things done)	86	54
25. Objective (just, fair, free of bias)	78	48
26. Compulsive (meticulous, perfectionistic, concerned with details)	69	50
27. Authoritarian (rigid, inflexible, dogmatic, opinionated)	70	52
28. Extraverted (has many friends; craves excitement; fond of practical jokes; is carefree, easygoing, optimistic)	90	71
29. Neurotic (a worrier; overly emotional; anxious, moody, and often depressed)	61	71
Mean	79	56

Note. Based on data from Rushton, Murray and Paunonen (1983).

tion Index or the Science Citation Index (whichever was larger for the particular individual and with credit assigned equally for senior and junior authorship), and (2) total citations for the previous three years in the same Citation Indices (with first authored self-citations excluded). Year-to-year stability was 0.60 for publications and 0.98 for citations. The two indices intercorrelated 0.28 ($p. < 0.05$) and were combined. A five-point rating of "overall effectiveness" as a teacher was determined from an average of five years of archival data based on end-of-course student evaluation of instructors.

In our follow-up of Study 1, we mailed a questionnaire to nine other psychology departments in Canada with 69 (68 male, 1 female) people responding. The same 29 personality traits and definitions were used. Respondents were instructed to rate themselves in percentiles, "relative to other Canadian university psychology professors." The distributions turned out to be roughly normal, with a mean percentile across traits of 55 and a standard deviation of 21. Socially desirable traits were rated higher than socially undesirable traits, with professors rating themselves at the 80th percentile on intelligence and at the 26th percentile on authoritarianism! Four items were aggregated to index research effectiveness: (1) total number of publications, (2) mean number of publications in last 5 years, (3) number of hours spent on research, and (4) rated enjoyment of research. Each of these was significantly associated with the others (mean correlation of 0.36; $p <$ 0.01).

Figure 1 plots the traits which loaded 0.30 or greater on either dimension in both studies. (The research and teaching effectiveness composites intercorrelated zero.) Coefficients of congruence across Studies 1 and 2 were 0.64 for the research factor and 0.74 for the teaching factor. Although low, these do show some consistency. Based on both studies combined, the ten main traits of productive researchers were: ambitious, enduring, seeking definiteness, dominant, showing leadership, aggressive, intelligent, independent, not meek, and non-supportive. The effective teacher, on the other hand, was described on eleven traits: liberal, sociable, showing leadership, extraverted, low in anxiety, objective, supporting, non-authoritarian, not defensive, intelligent, and aesthetically sensitive. The cluster of traits associated with being an effective researcher were essentially orthogonal to those characterizing the effective teacher, and were generally less socially desirable. The only variables loading positively on both the research and the teaching dimensions were intelligence and leadership, while meekness was associated with being poor in both.

JACKSON ON THE PERSONALITY CHARACTERISTICS AND VOCATIONAL INTERESTS OF SCIENTISTS

Jackson's work on the personality traits of scientists has grown out of his long-standing research program on vocational interests (Jackson, 1977, 1999). His 1987 chapter in *Scientific Excellence* well illustrates Jackson's ideas, style, and perceptiveness. Citing an important study by Eiduson (1962) contrasting research scientists and businessmen, he summarized three sets of differences pertaining to *cognitive processes, emotional variables*, and *motivational variables.*
Cognitively, scientists were rated significantly higher than businessmen on the following items:

- Seeks to depart radically from the usual, obvious, or hackneyed.
- Can loosen or relax controls without personality disorganization.
- Shows richness in symbolic and descriptive expression and association.
- Interests point to the theoretical and abstract rather than the practical and realistic.
- Has capacity for recombining, reorganizing visual conceptions.

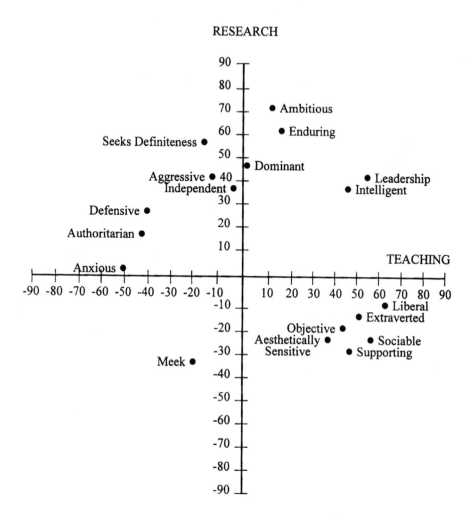

Figure 1. Plot of mean factor pattern coefficients of personality traits on dimensions of research productivity and teaching effectiveness, averaged across two studies. Only those traits with absolute values of >0.30 on either factor in both studies are shown (Based on data in Rushton, Murray & Paunonen, 1983).

In terms of emotional variables, the following were characteristics of scientists:
- Shows a tendency for sensuous gratification.
- Has strong emotional leanings for intellectual activity.
- Imitates and depends on others in thinking and action (reverse scored).
- Is challenged by frustration and anxiety-producing situations rather than being overwhelmed by them.

Motivationally, scientists were significantly higher on the following:
- Curiosity likely to be a prominent determinant of work.
- Uses parental ideals to set own goals (reverse scored).
- Seems to be strongly self-directed and self-disciplined.
- Strong ego involvement and conflict expressed in work.
- Motivated by a desire to master or interpret natural forces or reality.

Thus, the research scientist is seen as capable of relaxing controls and departing radically in expressions and thinking from the usual, shows a richness and novelty both in capacities and interest in ideational activity, seeks sensuous gratification, and is motivated to interpret the external world. It is particularly noteworthy that the scientist is motivated by a self-directed curiosity and is not particularly dependent upon others (or parents) in goal-setting or action.

A clear picture of the scientist emerges in Figure 2 which presents a factor plot involving personality measures from the Personality Research Form and occupational scales from the Strong Vocational Interest Blank (Siess & Jackson, 1970). Note that for the dimension defined by engineer and physical scientist, the personality scales for endurance, achievement, and understanding are positively salient, while the need for social recognition and succorance scales are negatively salient. This implies that the scientist is willing to work long hours to achieve a standard of excellence and intellectual mastery, while manifesting a singular disdain for fulfilling needs for social recognition and dependence.

Jackson (1977) has found that the vocational interests of scientists yield few surprises and are polar opposites of those of business managers. For example, a sample of 276 male chemists completing the Jackson Vocational Interest Survey (Jackson, 1977) indicated their strongest interests were in physical science, engineering, mathematics, and life science. They also showed marked interest in working in environments that required stamina, while showing limited interest in sales, social service, personal service, and performing arts (Figure 3).

It comes as no surprize that employment interviewers recognize the relevance of personality traits to scientific performance. In a series of studies, Jackson and his colleagues (Jackson, Peacock, & Smith, 1980; Rothstein & Jackson, 1980; see also Rothstein & Goffin's chapter in this volume) asked employment interviewers

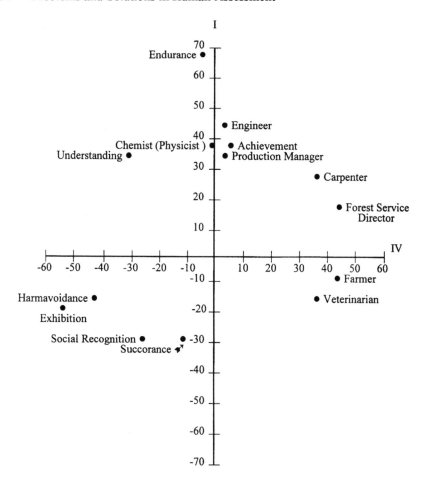

Figure 2. Factor plot of dimensions derived from multimethod factor analysis: Factor I – Technically-Oriented Achievement versus Social Recognition, and Factor IV – Practical (Based on data in Seiss & Jackson, 1970).

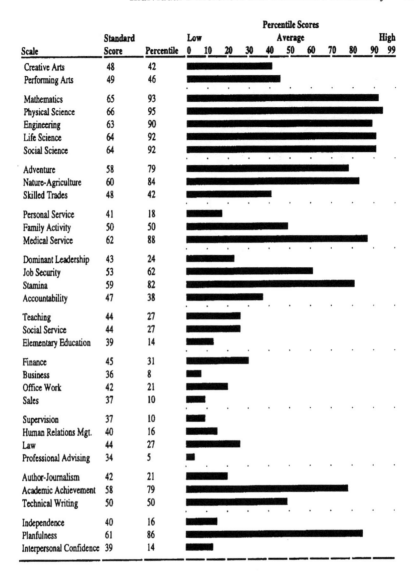

Scale	Standard Score	Percentile	Percentile Scores
Creative Arts	48	42	
Performing Arts	49	46	
Mathematics	65	93	
Physical Science	66	95	
Engineering	63	90	
Life Science	64	92	
Social Science	64	92	
Adventure	58	79	
Nature-Agriculture	60	84	
Skilled Trades	48	42	
Personal Service	41	18	
Family Activity	50	50	
Medical Service	62	88	
Dominant Leadership	43	24	
Job Security	53	62	
Stamina	59	82	
Accountability	47	38	
Teaching	44	27	
Social Service	44	27	
Elementary Education	39	14	
Finance	45	31	
Business	36	8	
Office Work	42	21	
Sales	37	10	
Supervision	37	10	
Human Relations Mgt.	40	16	
Law	44	27	
Professional Advising	34	5	
Author-Journalism	42	21	
Academic Achievement	58	79	
Technical Writing	50	50	
Independence	40	16	
Planfulness	61	86	
Interpersonal Confidence	39	14	

Figure 3. Jackson Vocational Interest Survey profile of 276 male chemists.

and others to judge the probable satisfaction, suitability, and hireability of interviewees. Among the characteristics valued by employment interviewers in hiring engineers (and identified independently in empirical studies of test scores), were high endurance, understanding, and achievement, and low social recognition and succorance. Different traits, namely high need for cognitive structure and order, and low impulsivity, autonomy, and need for change, were considered important in hiring decisions for the job of accountant.

THE VALUES OF SCIENTISTS

Jackson is fond of quoting Robert Oppenheimer's (1956) poetic phrase to the effect that their search for "elegant, virtuous, and beautiful solutions" sets scientists apart. Achieving these solutions requires long hours of arduous work mastering complex and sometimes recalcitrant problems. This view of research is unlikely that of the typical corporate financial officer or university administrator, who sees research as a means to the end of either profits or enhanced institutional prestige.

As Jackson (1987) noted, insufficient communication by scientists of their values and inadequate attempts by administrators to appreciate the unique motives of the scientist both contribute to the less than fully optimal environments in which researchers and development groups sometimes find themselves. Traditionally, scientists worked as individuals in universities or elsewhere. Conflicts based on values were few. With the emergence of organized science replete with research directors and vice presidents for research and development, however, the opportunities for conflict over values have greatly increased. Jackson (1987) has represented this conflict of values between scientists and non-scientists in terms of Max Weber's theory of domination. Table 3 distinguishes: (1) the characteristic beliefs that legitimize the exercise of power over individuals; (2) the characteristics of the followers; and (3) the administrative structure through which power is exercised. Conflict occurs when *the purposive-rational style* of leadership characteristic of managers comes head-to-head with the *value-rational style* more typical of scientists. Purposive-rational types are dominated by economic and political considerations, obey rules and formal authority, are flexible in regard to means and ends, see as a source of authority legal and bureaucratic rules, act for an organization or group, and prefer a hierarchical structure based on authority. Value-rational types, on the other hand, are dominated by ideas, obey ideology and norms rather than rules and law, seek an absolute goal – knowledge, and see legitimate authority as springing from expertise, with the goal of accumulating a body of knowledge. Value-rational types recognize individual authority and prefer a polycentric organizational structure, a company of equals, and decisions based on individual judgment.

Table 3. Weber's Types of Leadership Styles

Type Domination	Power Legitimation	Follower Characteristics	Administrative Structure
Charismatic	Unquestioning belief in potency of leader	Faith	Disciples
Traditional	Rightness of the past, and the inheritance of leadership	Loyalty	Feudal
Purposive-rational	Rightness of law	Law-abiding	Rules through Bureaucracy
Value-rational	Rightness of knowledge	Professionalism; intellectual elite	Collegial, polycentric

Although these are ideal types, Jackson suggests that they are strongly associated with management and science, respectively. Thus one challenge for productively organizing the activities of scientists is to reconcile the pragmatic, perhaps profit-oriented motivations of the traditional manager with the values implicit in the quest for truth by scientists. The manager operating within a purposive-rational culture is concerned with doing, with short-term goals, with mastery over nature and "the competition," and with achieving ends by persuasion and other interpersonal strategies. The value-rational culture, on the other hand, is concerned with knowing, with long-term rather than short-term goals (a book on the one-minute scientist has yet to appear), with goals of understanding and having a harmonious relation to nature, and favors individuality (Lane, 1977). A prototypical purposive-rational type, namely the financial manager with an accounting background, is comfortable in a predictable environment and is made uncomfortable by risk, whereas research and development involves inherent risks.

THE MOTIVATION OF THE SCIENTIST AND THE NATURE OF ACHIEVEMENT MOTIVATION

Much of the research on achievement motivation has been conducted not on university students, but on business people. The resulting theory of achievement motivation has frequently failed to distinguish the various facets of this construct and also failed to recognize how the motivation of the scientist differs from that of the entrepreneurial businessperson.

In a multitrait-multimethod matrix (Campbell & Fiske, 1959), using five methods of measurement, Jackson, Ahmed, and Heapy (1976) identified six dimensions of achievement: *concern for excellence, status with experts, status with peers, competitiveness, acquisitiveness,* and *achievement by independence.* Figure 4 shows the results from a second-order factor analysis and indicates the independence of concern for excellence and a dimension marked by competitiveness and acquisitiveness. Far from being co-linear with competitiveness and acquisitiveness, the concern for excellence may conflict with the rapid movement of products to the marketplace and represents another source of conflict between the R&D manager and the scientist. Of course, this conflict is not inevitable. Indeed, creative project planning seeks to identify achievable goals thereby providing a focus for the scientist's concern with excellence.

Jackson has also discussed how to reward achievement among scientists, noting that David McClelland (1951) made much of monetary remuneration as a method of "keeping score" for business people. McClelland argued that acquisitiveness is not a central part of achievement motivation but, rather, is a means of marking one's attainment. Jackson points out that comparable attention has not been given to a means for marking the scientists' progress.

It is true that some sociological accounts of academic prestige have suggested that a professor's annual salary taken together with the prestige of his or her university provides a basis for a status ranking, but it is recognized that salary is an imperfect index in that it tends to be substantially correlated with age and experience; tends to be influenced by extrinsic factors, such as market conditions within a specialty and for professors generally, budgetary exigencies, and local costs of living; and often represents reward for performance in other areas, such as administration and teaching. For the scientist, rewards are often, of necessity, intrinsic. As Heckhausen (1967) has pointed out, most people do not view achievement as having been realized unless there is *some* form of social recognition. For the scientist, this usually takes the form of publication, or at least this is a first step toward recognition. For the engineer, while some environments may encourage applications for patents and publication, many others do not.   An

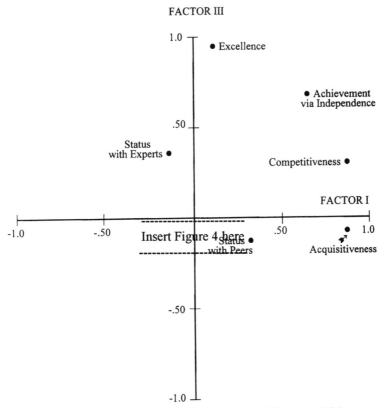

Figure 4. Second-order achievement factors: Competitive acquisitiveness and concern for excellence. (After Jackson, Ahmed, & Heapy, 1976)

indication of the importance placed upon the recognition stemming from publication is that in one study, more than 50% of scientists reported that they had experienced priority disputes of one kind or another. Programs involving intrinsic rewards for scientists and engineers should take account of a need on the part of the scientist to document and communicate findings and to achieve status among scientific peers.

Another aspect of the complexity of the relationships between achievement motivation and scientific attainment emerges from the work of Helmreich, Beane, Lucker, and Spence (1978). They identified three components of achievement motivation: intellectual mastery, orientation toward work, and competitiveness. Measures of these components did not singly correlate significantly with journal citations of scientists, but interactions between these dispositions did. The highest citation rate was found for those high on both work and mastery, and the lowest was for those low on work and high on mastery. They also found that when work motivation was high, *low* competitiveness was associated strongly and positively with citations, while among those with low work motivation, higher competitiveness was reflected in more citations. This implies that there are different achievement styles. Achievement profiles of scientists and their work environments warrant further study.

REINFORCEMENT PATTERNS OF SCIENTISTS AND ENGINEERS

If scientists value independence and the opportunity to engage in tasks requiring intellectual curiosity, one would expect scientists to express intrinsic rewards consistent with these values. This is indeed the case. In an early study by Riegal (1958), research personnel attached high importance to being challenged by projects assigned, to having freedom in managing their work, to seeing ideas put to use, and to associating with able professionals. These same characteristics were rated high in importance by engineers in product development, but in this sample the research engineers indicated that these intrinsic rewards were less frequently experienced than they were for the scientist.

How important is satisfaction for performance? The relationship between satisfaction and productivity is not a simple one, but in the area of scientific performance significant relationships have been reported between satisfaction and performance. For example, previous findings indicate that a positive performance-satisfaction relationship was facilitated by three individual characteristics: high motivation, internal rather than external control, and strong need for achievement; and four job characteristics: high organizational level, participation in decision making, high level of task difficulty, and low level of leader initiating structure.

Although several authors have commented on the importance of freedom in identifying problems and the importance of relieving a scientist of responsibilities in other areas (Eysenck, 1995), the classic study by Pelz (1967) of 1,300 scientists in 11 research and development laboratories adds some important perspective. He has argued persuasively that for creative work to flourish, certain tensions must exist. First, in regard to *science versus application*, Pelz found that highest levels of performance and productivity were not identified in individuals devoting 100% of their time to research. Rather, individuals devoting a portion of their efforts to development and invention, or technical services, were more effective. He argued that the challenges created by diversity provided impetus for combining elements in new ways and was therefore beneficial. Diversity was also effective in other regards. Persons who had two or three areas of specialization or who spent one-quarter of their time in teaching or administration also performed better as scientists.

Second, in regard to *independence versus interaction*, highly productive scientists were stimulated by previous work, by curiosity, and by the freedom to pursue their own ideas. They did not avoid people. The more creative conferred often, realizing a creative challenge by more frequent contacts, while acquiring information as well. (This information appears to contrast with some of the earlier descriptions of scientists as largely reclusive. Perhaps the reclusiveness of productive scientists applies mostly to social interaction for the sake of social interaction, whereas social interaction for the sake of potentially acquiring/sharing relevant information, may, in fact be highly rewarding.)

With regard to *age, specialization,* and *diversity,* there were distinct stages in the creative scientist's career. The young group was more concerned with security, technical performance, often spending a great deal of time on focused projects. After 40, creative scientist became more self-confident and were more willing to take risks. After 50, the typical pattern was for probing deeply or mapping broad areas.

With regard to their *relationship to the organization,* performance increased with greater autonomy up to a point. But when Ph.D. scientists had more than 30% of their time free to work on self-directed projects, their performance dropped. Scientists, like others, appear to be responsive to the need to be accountable. Pelz related this to the looseness versus tightness of the organization, arguing that the isolation from challenges stemming from too much autonomy was as injurious to productivity as was too rigid a control structure.

With regard to *sources of influence,* Pelz identified five: the scientist, peers, supervisors, management, and clients. Interestingly, performance was highest when all sources were active, a finding consistent with the idea that challenge for productive work originates in part from the social environment. Although creative scientists saw themselves as different in their responses to social influence, their work nevertheless benefited from constructive social interaction.

GUIDELINES FOR EFFECTIVE RESEARCH ADMINISTRATION

Managing the social world of science is a much neglected topic but obviously calls for another set of traits, especially in the increasingly complicated, high-tech, bureaucratized world of "Big Science." Even for the individual scientist, major innovations need to be "sold" through networking and social organisations to government bodies, the mass media, funding agencies, and scientific and professional groups. Perhaps the high autonomy and enduring personalities of some scientists make them less vulnerable to social blandishments and criticisms. But it would be a mistake to fixate on scientists as mavericks or Don Quixotes tilting at establishment windmills. Also, because a fairly clear personality profile of the innovative researcher emerges, it does not mean that individual differences do not exist! For example, although many scientists have historically been recognized as less sociable than average, Galileo, Leibnitz, and others were as fully at home in the social free-for-all of court circles as in the laboratory. Indeed, as Jackson has noted, far from believing that the optimal condition for scientific advance is absolute freedom to think in a far removed-from-it-all environment, evidence suggests that social constraints, and constructive social interaction are beneficial.

Both Jackson and I have reviewed a number of aspects of the personalities of scientists and Jackson has studied the characteristics of productive environments. The Jacksonian implications are clear. Environments that nurture the creative urges of the scientist, that offer recognition for inventive productivity, that harness a concern for excellence, that communicate organizational goals effectively, that combine autonomy with accountability, that avoid imposing the burdens of rigid bureaucratic organization and rules, that discourage nonscientist line administrators from close supervision of technical projects, and that offer monetary recognition and career paths for scientists parallel to advancement, have better prospects for success. Equally important, of course, is the careful selection of scientists and of technical managers with a flair for the unique kind of leadership needed for scientific and technical development.

JACKSON'S COMMITMENT TO ACADEMIC FREEDOM

Effective research administration depends upon, among other things, allowing the researcher sufficient autonomy and not imposing rigid rules on what gets researched, hence there must be academic freedom. Doug's beliefs in the value of unfettered enquiry led him to play a key role in defending academic freedom in Canada. When the U.S. based National Association of Scholars, an academic freedom society, intervened on behalf of Canadian researchers challenged by "Political Correctness" (Hunt, 1999), Doug lent his considerable prestige to founding a sister organization in Canada, the Society for Academic Freedom and Scholarship. As the founding Secretary-Treasurer of the nascent society, he drafted its Deed of Incorporation as an official charity and also its first constitution. He was active in many of its early cases, writing letters on its behalf, proferring expertise, and counseling injured parties. Since this took time from an already very busy schedule, Doug demonstrated his personal commitment to enduring personal liberty and freedom of enquiry for his colleagues.

REFERENCES

Barron, F. (1962). The needs for order and disorder as motives in creative activity. In C. W. Taylor, & F. Barron (Eds), *Scientific creativity: Its recognition and development*. (pp.139-152). New York: Wiley.

Campbell, D. T., & Fiske, D. W. (1959). Convergent and discriminant validation by the multitrait-multimethod matrix. *Psychological Bulletin*, 56, 81-105.

Cattell, J. M. (1903). A statistical study of eminent men. *Popular Science Monthly*, 32, 359-377.

Cattell, J. M. (1910). A further statistical study of American men of science. *Science*, 32, 633-648.

Cattell, R. B. (1962). The personality and motivation of the researcher from measurements of contemporaries and from biography. In C. W. Taylor & F. Barron (Eds), *Scientific creativity: Its recognition and development*. New York: Wiley.

Cattell, R. B. (1965). *The scientific study of personality*. Harmondsworth, England: Penguin.

Cattell, R. B., & Drevdahl, J. E. (1955). A comparison of the personality profile (16 PF) of eminent researchers with that of eminent teachers and administrators, and of the general population. *British Journal of Psychology*, 46, 248-261.

Chambers, J. A. (1964). Creative scientists of today. *Science*, 145, 1203-1205.

Cole, J. R. (1981). Women in science. *American Scientist*, 69, 385-391.

Cox, C. M. (1926). *The early mental traits of three hundred geniuses*. Stanford CA: Stanford University Press.

Dennis, W. (1955). Variation in productivity among creative workers. *Scientific Monthly*, 80, 277-278.

Drevdahl, J. E., & Cattell, R. B. (1958). Personality and creativity in artists and writers. *Journal of Clinical Psychology*, 14, 107-111.

Eiduson, B. T. (1962). *Scientists: Their psychological world*. New York: Basic Books.

Ellis, H. (1904). *A study of British genius*. Oxford: Hurst and Blackwell.

Endler, N. S., Rushton, J. P., & Roediger, H. L. (1978). Productivity and scholarly impact (citations) of British, Canadian, and U.S. departments of psychology. *American Psychologist*, 33, 1064-1083.

Eysenck, H. J. (1995). *Genius: The natural history of creativity*. Cambridge: Cambridge University Press.

Feist, G. J. (1993). A structural model of scientific eminence. *Psychological Science*, 4, 366-371.

Galton, F. (1869). *Hereditary genius: An inquiry into its laws and consequences*. London: Macmillan.

Galton, F. (1874). *English men of science*. London: Macmillian.

Gaston, J. (1978). *The reward system in British and American Science*. New York: John Wiley.

Heckhausen, H. (1967). *The anatomy of achievement motivation*. New York: Academic Press

Helmreich, R. L., Beane, W. E., Lucker, G. W., & Spence, J. T. (1978). Achievement motivation and scientific attainment. *Personality and Social Psychology Bulletin*, 4, 222-226.

Helmreich, R. L., Spence, J. T., Beane, W. E., Lucker, G. W., & Matthews, K. A. (1980). Making it in academic psychology: Demographic and personality correlates of attainment. *Journal of Personality and Social Psychology*, 39, 896-908.

Hunt, M. (1999). *The new know-nothings*. New Brunswick, NJ: Transaction.

Jackson, D. N. (1977). *Jackson Vocational Interest Survey manual*. Port Huron, MI: Sigma Assessment Systems.

Jackson, D. N. (1984). *Personality Research Form manual*. Port Huron, MI: Sigma Assessment Systems.

Jackson, D. N. (1987). Scientific and technological innovation: Its personological and motivational context. In D. N. Jackson and J. P. Rushton (Eds.), *Scientific excellence: Origins and assessment*. Beverly Hills, CA: Sage.

Jackson, D. N. (1999). *Jackson Vocational Interest Survey manual*. Port Huron, MI: Sigma Assessment Systems.

Jackson, D. N., Ahmed, S. A., & Heapy, N. A. (1976). Is achievement a unitary construct? *Journal of Research in Personality*, 10,1-21.

Jackson, D. N., Peacock, A. C., & Smith, J. P. (1980). Impressions of personality in the employment interview. *Journal of Personality and Social Psychology*, 39, 294-307.

Jackson, D. N., & Rushton, J. P. (Eds.). (1987). *Scientific excellence: Origins and assessment*. Beverly Hills, CA: Sage.

Knickerbocker, W. S. (1927). *Classics of modern science*. New York: Knopf.

Lane, H. W. (1977). *Managing innovation: A comparative analysis of program level research and development units*. Unpublished doctoral dissertation, Harvard University. (University Microfilms No. 77-16, 862).

McClelland, D. C. (1951). *Personality*. New York: Holt, Rinehart & Winston

McClelland, D. C. (1962). The calculated risk: An aspect of scientific performance. In C. W. Taylor & F.Barron (Eds.), *Scientific creativity: Its recognition and development*. New York: Wiley.

Matthews, K. A., Helmreich, R. L., Beane, W. E., & Lucker, G. W. (1980). Pattern A, achievement striving, and scientific merit: Does pattern A help or hinder? *Journal of Personality and Social Psychology*, 39, 962-967.

Oppenheimer, R. (1956). Analogy in science. *American Psychologist*, 11, 127-135.

Pelz, D. C. (1967). Creative tensions in the research and development climate. *Science*, 157, 160-165.

Roe, A. (1952). *The making of a scientist*. Westport, CT: Greenwood Press.

Riegal, J. W. (1958). *Administration of salaries and intangible rewards for engineers and scientists*. Michigan: Bureau of Industrial Relations. Ann Arbor, University of Michigan.

Rothstein, M., & Goffin, R. D. (1999). The assessment of personality constructs in industrial-organizational psychology. In R. D. Goffin & E. Helmes (Eds.), *Problems and solutions in human assessment: Honoring Douglas N. Jackson at seventy*. Norwell, MA: Kluwer Academic Publishers.

Rothstein, M., & Jackson, D. N. (1980). Decision making in the employment interview: An experimental approach. *Journal of Applied Psychology*, **65**, 271-283.

Rushton, J. P. (1989). A ten-year scientometric revisit of British psychology departments. *The Psychologist*, 64-68.

Rushton, J. P., & Endler, N. S. (1977). The scholarly impact and research productivity of Departments of Psychology in the United Kingdom. *Bulletin of the British Psychological Society*, **30**, 369-373.

Rushton, J. P., Murray, H. G., & Paunonen, S. V. (1983). Personality, research creativity, and teaching effectiveness in university professors. *Scientometrics*, **5**, 93-116. *Science Citation Index*. Philadelphia, PA: Institute for Scientific Information.

Shockley, W. (1957). On the statistics of individual variations of productivity in research laboratories.. *Proceedings of the Institute of Radio Engineers*, **45**, 279-290.

Siess, T. F., & Jackson, D. N. (1970). Vocational interests and personality: An empirical integration. *Journal of Counseling Psychology*, **17**, 27-35. *Social Science Citation Index*. Philadelphia, PA: Institute for Scientific Information.

Sulloway, F. J. (1996). *Born to rebel*. New York: Pantheon.

Taylor, C. W., & Barron, F. (1962).*Scientific creativity: Its recognition and development*. New York: Wiley.

Terman, L. M. (1955). Are scientists different? *Scientific American*, **192**, 25-29.

Vernon, P. E. (1987). Historical overview of research on scientific abilities. In D. N. Jackson & J. P. Rushton (Eds), *Scientific excellence: Origins and assessment* (pp. 40-66). Beverly Hills, CA: Sage.

Walberg, H., Strykowski, B. F., Rovai, E., & Hung, S. S. (1984). Exceptional performance. *Review of Educational Research*, **54**, 87-112.

9 RECENT STUDIES OF INTELLIGENCE AND PERSONALITY USING JACKSON'S MULTIDIMENSIONAL APTITUDE BATTERY AND PERSONALITY RESEARCH FORM

Philip A. Vernon

Since its publication in 1984, Jackson's *Multidimensional Aptitude Battery* (MAB) has been used quite extensively in a variety of programs of research. In this chapter, the MAB and its psychometric properties are first described, followed by sections illustrating different types of research that the MAB has been used in. As will be seen, the MAB has allowed considerable advances to be made in investigations of such topics as relationships between intelligence and speed of information-processing; behavioral genetic studies of cognitive abilities; the identification of biological correlates of human intelligence; a study of both the phenotypic and the genetic relationship between intelligence and dimensions of personality; and a study of environmental factors that contribute to the differential personality development of twins and non-twin siblings. It is not claimed that none of these investigations could have been conducted without the MAB, however the existence of the MAB has certainly contributed to the ability of researchers to obtain valid estimates of broad dimensions of intelligence from large samples of people much more quickly and easily than would be the case if they had had to employ an individually-administered IQ test such as the Wecshler or Binet.

THE MULTIDIMENSIONAL APTITUDE BATTERY

The Multidimensinal Aptitude Battery (MAB; Jackson, 1984) is a multiple-choice, group-administrable test of intelligence patterned quite closely after the Wechsler Adult Intelligence Scale-Revised (WAIS-R; Wechsler, 1981). Like the WAIS-R, the MAB consists of two subscales, Verbal and Performance, each comprising five subtests. The MAB is designed to be used with adolescents and adults between 16 and 74 years of age and is scored to provide Verbal, Performance, and Full-Scale IQs as well as subtest profiles.

In the Verbal Scale, subtests include *Information* (a 40-item test of general knowledge), *Comprehension* (a 28-item test measuring a person's understanding of various social situations or conventions); *Arithmetic* (26 items ranging in difficulty from simple arithmetic to complex numerical reasoning); *Similarities* (a 34-item test in which people must decide in what way two things are alike); and *Vocabulary* (46 items). Each of these subtests taps the same constructs as those in the WAIS-R, though all of the actual items are different. Note also that there is no MAB subtest comparable to the WAIS-R's Digit Span.

In the Performance Scale, the MAB subtests include *Digit Symbol* (a 35-item test in which the digits 1 to 9 are matched [or coded] with different symbols. Subjects are presented with strings of from 1 to 9 symbols and must identify which of five accompanying strings of digits correctly matches the symbols); *Picture Completion* (35 items in which pictures of objects with one missing part are presented. Accompanying each picture are the first letters of five possible missing parts. Subjects must first identify the correct missing part in each picture and then choose its first letter correctly from among the distractors); *Spatial* (a 50-item test in which subjects must spatially rotate a figure and match the rotation to one of five possible answers. This is the only MAB subtest that does not have a precise counterpart in the WAIS-R; it is the MAB's alternative to the WAIS-R's Block Design); *Picture Arrangement* (21 items in which subjects must mentally rearrange between 3 and 6 cartoon panels to tell a sensible story); and *Object Assembly* (a 20-item test in which between 3 and 6 numbered silhouetted parts of common objects are presented in the wrong order. Subjects must first identify the objects and then mentally rearrange their parts into the correct order).

Internal consistency reliability coefficients are reported in the MAB Manual (Jackson, 1984) for each of its subtests and for Verbal, Performance, and Full-Scale IQ scores. Subtest reliabilities range from .70 to .96 and VIQ, PIQ, and FSIQ reliabilities range from .94 to .98 in different age groups. Test-retest stability and split-half reliability coefficients are also reported in the MAB Manual: subtest stability coefficients range from .83 to .97, VIQ, PIQ, and FSIQ stability coefficients are .95, .96, and .97, respectively; subtest split-half reliabilities (Spearman-Brown corrected) range from .55 to .87, VIQ, PIQ, and FSIQ corrected reliabilities are .92, .94, and .95. Clearly, the MAB Scale scores are highly reliable and the reliabilities of its individual subtests are at least satisfactory.

A number of studies have investigated the construct validity of the MAB. In the MAB Manual, intercorrelations between the subtests and the results of a principal components analysis of these correlations are presented, based on data collected from over 3000 male and female high school students. All subtest intercorrelations are positive (ranging from .24 to .73) and the factor analysis yields a strong general factor (with all subtests loading between .53 to .82) and two rotated orthogonal factors clearly identifiable as Verbal and Performance factors, although the arithmetic and picture completion subtests have quite high loadings on both factors. In fact, there is a tendency for several of the Performance subtests to have low to moderate loadings on the Verbal factor (notably, *Picture Completion*, *Picture Arrangement*, and *Object Assembly*), reflecting the fact that these subtests require subjects to generate verbal responses. Kranzler (1991) also found that the MAB *Picture Completion* subtest loaded on a Verbal factor in a hierarchical factor analysis of data collected from high IQ University students. Kranzler (1991) also found a g factor accounting for the greatest amount of the variance in the MAB, as did Wallbrown, Carmin, and Barnett (1988, 1989) and Lee and Wallbrown (1990).

In addition to these factor analytic studies of the MAB, another source of information about its validity is its correlation with the WAIS-R. In the MAB Manual, a study of 145 subjects is reported in which the MAB and the WAIS-R were administered to 16- to 35-year-old university or high school students, psychiatric patients, or persons on probation from prison. Correlations between the tests' subtests range from .44 (MAB *Spatial* with WAIS-R *Block Design*) to .89 (for both *Arithmetic* and *Vocabulary*), with a median of .78. MAB and WAIS-R VIQ, PIQ, and FSIQ correlate .92, .79, and .91, respectively, which compares very favorably with the corresponding correlations between the WAIS-R and the WAIS (.82, .82, and .87 [averaged across two studies and reported in the MAB Manual]). These studies indicate that the MAB and the WAIS-R are highly related; insofar as the WAIS-R is accepted as a standard against which the validity of other tests of intelligence can be evaluated, the MAB performs very well.

In conclusion, like the WAIS-R the MAB measures a broad range of dimensions of mental ability and also defines a strong g factor. The MAB has excellent psychometric properties and can be used to provide reliable and valid measures of Verbal, Performance, and Full-Scale intelligence (bearing in mind that its Performance scores are also somewhat verbally saturated). Its relatively low cost, its ease and speed of administration, and its ability to be given to individuals or groups make it an attractive alternative to the WAIS-R, perhaps particularly in research applications. This having been established, attention will turn now to studies which have used the MAB in different researches.

INTELLIGENCE AND SPEED OF INFORMATION-PROCESSING

In the time that has elapsed since Charles Spearman (1904, 1927) first proposed a g or general intelligence factor to account for the positive correlations he observed among diverse tests of mental ability, a great deal of research has been conducted in an attempt to validate or invalidate this construct. Today, there is probably fairly widespread consensus that individual differences in performance on tests of reasoning, problem solving, and many other kinds of mental ability are in large part attributable to differences in general cognitive ability and, as described above, Jackson's MAB provides a good measure of g in addition to other broad and more specific ability factors. Of more concern during the past 20 years or so have been questions about the underlying cognitive and neuropsychological processes and mechanisms that contribute to individual differences in g itself. This section will provide a brief overview of one aspect of this more recent cognitive and biologically-oriented research: that which has focused on relationships between intelligence and speed of information-processing.

Much of the recent work in this area can be traced back to the pioneering research of Arthur Jensen, Earl Hunt, and others in the 1970's (e.g., Brand, 1979; Hunt, 1976; Jensen, 1979; Jensen & Munro, 1979; Keating & Bobbitt, 1978; Lally & Nettelbeck, 1977; Nettelbeck & Lally, 1976). Jensen, for example, conducted a number of early studies correlating people's simple and choice reaction times (RTs) to visual stimuli, presented on what he termed the *Hick apparatus*, with their IQ scores. In a 1987 chapter, Jensen summarized the results of 33 IQ/Hick RT studies, based on data collected from a total of almost 2000 subjects in 26 independent samples, reporting an average IQ/RT correlation of -.20 (or -.31 after correction for unreliability).

Reaction times on the Hick apparatus provide a measure of what might be called *general* speed of information-processing. Other researchers have focused on more specific cognitive processes, such as the speed with which persons can scan information in short-term memory (STM) (Dugas & Kellas, 1974; Keating & Bobbitt, 1978; Vernon, 1983); access and retrieve information from long-term-memory (LTM) (Hunt, 1976; Goldberg, Schwartz, & Stewart, 1977; Vernon, 1983); simultaneously store and process information in STM (Vernon, 1983); and apprehend and encode information (Nettelbeck, 1987; Nettelbeck & Lally, 1976). Results using measures of all of these different speed-of-processing variables have been fairly consistent: zero-order correlations with IQ scores are typically about -.30 but multiple correlations as high as .74 have been reported (Vernon, 1990). Thus, speed of information-processing typically accounts for about 10% but may account for as much as 50% of the variance in intelligence.

In a recent study, Vernon and Weese (1993) administered the MAB and four sets of speed of information-processing tasks to 152 University undergraduates. The sets of information-processing tasks were selected in an attempt to minimize intercorrelations between them and thereby to maximize their multiple correlation with MAB IQ scores. Factor analysis of the information-processing tests successfully yielded 4 orthogonal factors which in combination accounted for 40% of the variance in MAB full-scale IQs.

Vernon (1993) used one of Vernon and Weese's (1993) information-processing measures to examine in more detail its correlation with IQ, again measured by the MAB. In this study, 83 University undergraduates were administered the MAB and Der Zahlen-Verbindungs-Test (ZVT; Oswald & Roth, 1978): a trail-making test in which subjects draw lines to connect, in order, circled numbers from 1 to 90 which are positioned more or less randomly on pieces of paper. The original ZVT and 9 other versions of it (involving, for example, connecting alternating numbers and letters [1-A-2-B...] or upper and lower case letters [A-a-B-b...]) were administered in one of two ways: in one condition, subjects were allowed only 45 seconds to work on each ZVT task and were instructed to work as quickly as they could; in a second condition, subjects were again told to work quickly and the total time it took them to complete each ZVT was measured in seconds. Thus, subjects were assigned two scores: the average *n*umber of items they could complete in 45 seconds (ZVTN) and the average *t*ime it took them to complete all 90 ZVT items (ZVTT).

Both ZVTN and ZVTT proved to be quite highly correlated with full-scale MAB IQ scores: ZVTN/IQ correlations ranging from .45 to .71; ZVTT/IQ correlations ranging from -.44 to -.72. There was also some evidence that, after corrections for differences in their reliabilities, more difficult versions of the ZVT yielded higher correlations with IQs; a finding that has been reported in several other studies comparing the correlations with IQs of RT tasks varying in their relative complexity. Keeping in mind that the ZVT is a test that can be administered in 45 seconds, the fact that some versions of it account for over 50% of the variance in IQs is a quite remarkable finding; it supports previous studies which have identified speed of information-processing as an important component of general intelligence.

Miller and Vernon (1992) employed the MAB to test Spearman's notion of the generality of *g*: that essentially the same (or highly correlated) *g* factors could be extracted from any diverse collection of mental ability tests, no matter how different they might appear on the surface. Miller and Vernon administered a battery of 12 STM tests, a battery of 11 RT tests, and the MAB to 170 adult subjects. Tests within each battery, and the MAB subtests, were factor analyzed separately, yielding a general STM factor (STM*g*), a general RT factor (RT*g*), and a traditional general intelligence factor (IQ*g*), which accounted for 27%, 71%, and 37% of the variance in their respective batteries. Correlations between the three *g* factors were all significant: IQ*g*/STM*g* correlating .46, IQ*g*/RT*g* correlating -.26, and STM*g*/RT*g* correlating -.37 (all p < .001). Thus, some support was found for the generality of *g*.

Nettelbeck and Lally (1976) were the first researchers to use a measure termed *Inspection Time* (IT) as an information-processing correlate of general intelligence. IT is not a reaction time task *per se*: rather it measures the speed with which participants can apprehend and encode information into STM - typically by presenting visual information for very short durations by means of a tachistoscope.

Since Nettelbeck and Lally (1976), IT has been used in numerous studies investigating cognitive components of intelligence; Nettelbeck (1986) and Kranzler and Jensen (1989) have provided comprehensive reviews of the literature. More recently, Bates and Eysenck (1993a) studied relationships between IT, choice RT, and intelligence using the MAB. In this study, conducted with 88 adults, a very substantial -.62 correlation was reported between MAB Full-Scale IQs and IT, while IQ and RTs correlated -.36. The IT and RT measures were themselves correlated at .36. Employing a similar measure of IT, and also using the MAB as their measure of intelligence, Barrett, Petrides, and Eysenck (1998) reported an IQ/IT correlation of -.34.

In the final study to be mentioned in this section, Kranzler and Jensen (1991a) used the MAB in a study which was designed to assess whether Spearman's g factor of intelligence is in fact a unitary factor or whether it comprises a number of independent elemental processes. To decide this issue, Kranzler and Jensen (1991a) administered the MAB and the Raven Advanced Progressed Matrices (as their measures of g) as well as a large battery of elementary cognitive tasks (ECTs) to 101 University students. Principal components analysis of the ECTs yielded 10 orthogonal components which were then entered into a multiple regression analysis as predictors of g. This latter analysis showed that four of the orthogonal ECT components contributed significantly to the prediction of g (with an overall shrunken multiple R of .514), suggesting that g is not unitary; if it were, none of the other ECT components should have contributed significantly to its prediction over and above the first component. Note that this finding was replicated by the previously cited Vernon and Weese (1993), but see also Carroll (1991a,b) and Kranzler and Jensen (1991b) for additional comment.

BEHAVIOR GENETIC STUDIES OF COGNITIVE ABILITIES

Given that intelligence is quite highly related to measures of speed of information-processing, and given that the speed with which different cognitive processes can be executed must itself be dependent upon some property or properties of the brain and the neural system, one question which may be posed is: what underlying mechanisms regulate or are responsible for individual differences in speed-of-processing? That is, might it be possible to identify one or more biological or physiological variables to which individual differences in speed of information-processing, and hence perhaps in intelligence, can be attributed? As a first step towards addressing this question, behavior genetic studies will be described which have provided information about the heritability of different measures of speed-of-processing and which have estimated the genetic correlation between information-processing speed and intelligence.

In the first behavior genetic study of ECTs, McGue, Bouchard, Lykken, and Feuer (1984) reported that a general or overall speed of response factor had a heritability of .46. Similar results implicating the role of genetic factors in individual differences in speed-of-processing were found by Ho, Baker, and Decker (1988) and Vernon (1989), who reported heritabilities between .24 and .90 for different RT measures.

Closer examination of the heritabilities of the different speed-of-processing measures or parameters reported by McGue et al. (1984) and by Vernon (1989) reveals a sizeable variability in their magnitudes: ranging from .116 to .604 across nine parameters derived in McGue et al. (1984) and, as mentioned, between .24 to .90 across 11 RT measures in Vernon (1989). In both studies, there are also differences in the degree to which these different RT measures correlate with IQ, and of particular note is a positive relationship between the RT tests' heritabilities and their correlations with IQ: $r = .48$ in McGue et al. (1984) and $r = .61$ in Vernon (1989), in which the IQ measure was the MAB. Thus, the more heritable a RT measure, the stronger its correlation with IQ; alternatively, the more g-loaded a test - even if it is a relatively simple ECT or RT test - the more highly heritable it is.

Behavior genetics methodology allows one not only to compute heritabilities of variables but also to estimate the extent to which phenotypic correlations between two or more variables represent correlated genetic factors and/or correlated environmental factors (Neale & Cardon, 1992). That is, is it the case that IQ scores and RTs are correlated because both are dependent on the same genes – do the same biological or physiological factors operate on both intelligence and on speed of information-processing - and/or are there certain environmental factors that influence both an individual's IQ and the speed with which (s)he can process different kinds of information? Multivariate analyses of twin or other genetically-informative data allow these questions to be answered.

In Ho et al. (1988), phenotypic correlations between Full-Scale IQ scores and each of two speed-of-processing measures that they employed were approximately .40. For one of the speed measures – a rapid automatic naming task – multivariate biometrical analyses revealed that 70% of this phenotypic correlation with IQ could be explained by correlated genetic effects and the remaining 30% by correlated specific environmental effects. The phenotypic correlation between a second speed measure – the Colorado perceptual speed task – and IQ was entirely attributable to correlated genetic effects. Similarly, in a re-analysis of Vernon's (1989) twin data, Baker, Vernon, and Ho (1991) reported phenotypic and genetic correlations between Verbal and Performance MAB IQ scores and general speed-of-processing factor scores derived from 8 RT measures. In this study, phenotypic speed-VIQ and speed-PIQ correlations were both approximately .60 and a very sizeable proportion of these correlations was found to be attributable to correlated genetic factors: genetic correlations between Verbal IQ and RTs being 1.00 and between Performance IQs and RTs being .92.

These results indicate that genetic variations which lead to faster information-processing are highly associated with genetic variations important to high IQ scores. They further suggest that mental speed and IQ may share common biological mechanisms. Research that has sought to identify biological factors that correlate with either intelligence or with speed of information-processing or with both is discussed in the next section.

BIOLOGICAL CORRELATES OF INTELLIGENCE

Over the course of this century, various researchers have attempted to identify the biological basis of human intelligence. Some of these attempts have seemed fruitful at first but have either failed to replicate or have not been followed up for one reason or another, others have yielded a more consistent pattern of results. In this section, investigations of biological correlates of intelligence which have employed the MAB are described briefly; a fuller account of this field of research is given in Vernon (1993).

In the 1960's, a number of investigators looked at relationships between intelligence and *spontaneous* EEGs (e.g., Ellingson, 1966; Giannitrapani, 1969, Vogel & Broverman, 1964, 1966). The results of these studies were somewhat inconclusive (Gale & Edwards, 1983; but see also Anokhin & Vogel, 1996), prompting other researchers such as Ertl and his coworkers to study various parameters of *evoked* potentials (e.g., Chalke & Ertl, 1965; Ertl & Schafer, 1969).

As their name implies, evoked potentials refer to the electrical activity of the brain that is evoked by some external stimulus (e.g., a light flash or an auditory stimulus such as a beep or a click). Any individual potential may show considerable random fluctuations but over a large number of trials these fluctuations can be smoothed out, yielding an averaged evoked potential (AEP). Two parameters of AEPs have been studied extensively: their latencies – measuring the speed with which the brain responds to the stimulus – and their amplitude – measuring the amount of electrocortical activity that the stimulus evokes. A comprehensive review of recent studies of these parameters as correlates of intelligence is given in Vernon, Wickett, Bazana, & Stelmack (in press).

A number of recent studies have focused on what has become known as the "string measure" (A.E. Hendrickson, 1982; D.E. Hendrickson, 1982; Hendrickson & Hendrickson, 1980). This measure – essentially, the length of the contour perimeter of the AEP waveform – has yielded variable results: some studies reporting substantial correlations between it and intelligence (e.g., Blinkhorn & Hendrickson, 1982; Caryl & Fraser, 1985; Eysenck & Barrett, 1984; Haier,

Robinson, Braden, & Williams, 1983; D.E. Hendrickson, 1982; Stough, Nettelbeck, & Cooper, 1990), others reporting nonsignificant correlations or even correlations in the opposite direction to prediction (e.g., Barrett & Eysenck, 1992; Bates & Eysenck, 1993b; Shagrass, Roemer, Straunanis, & Josiassen, 1981). A recent study by Bates and Eysenck (1993), employing the MAB as its measure of intelligence, provides some resolution to the inconsistency of the results and argues that positive and negative correlations between intelligence and string length measures derived from different tasks can both be expected, depending upon the attentional demands of the task (see also Bates, Stough, Mangan, & Pellett, 1995).

Nerve conduction velocity (NCV) refers to the speed with which electrical impulses are transmitted along nerve fibers and across synapses. Reed (1984) proposed that individual differences in NCV might be attributable to genetic differences in the structure and amount of transmission proteins which, in turn, set limits on information-processing rates. Thus, faster NCV would be expected to correlate with faster RTs and higher intelligence.

Since Reed's 1984 paper, a number of researchers have investigated relationships between NCV, RTs, and IQ. Unfortunately, there has been no agreement in the results. Vernon and Mori (1992), for example, reported significant correlations between MAB IQs, RTs, and peripheral NCVs (measured in the median nerve of the arm) in two samples of University students. NCV-IQ correlations were .42 and .48; NCV-RT correlations were -.28 and -.18. Thus, as expected, faster NCVs were associated with higher IQs and faster speed of information-processing. Wickett and Vernon (1994), however, failed to replicate these results, despite using the same procedure to measure NCV and also using the MAB. In this study, two measures of NCVs correlated -.12 and .02 with IQs and .02 and .01 with RTs. Other investigators have also failed to find any correlation between IQs and NCV (e.g., Reed & Jensen, 1991; Barrett, Daum, & Eysenck, 1990; Rijsdijk, Boomsma, & Vernon, 1995), although two studies which measured brain NCV (rather than peripheral NCV) have reported positive correlations with IQ: Reed and Jensen (1992; $r = .26$) and Andres-Pueyo and Bonastre (1999; $r = .40$) A summary of the results of all NCV/IQ studies conducted to date is given in Vernon et al. (in press).

Interest in the possible relation between the size of the brain and intelligence dates back at least to the time of Paul Broca (1861) and was brought into the realm of psychology with the work of Galton (1888). Since then, numerous studies have reported correlations between intelligence, head size, and various *in vivo* estimates of brain size; the findings of all such studies to-date (49 studies, comprising 70 independent samples and over 57,000 subjects) are summarized in Vernon et al. (in press). The key finding in these studies is the absence of a single negative correlation between head size or *in vivo* brain-size and intelligence: head size/ability correlations range from .02 to .54 with an n-weighted mean of .19;

brain volume-IQ correlations range from .07 to .69 with an n-weighted mean of .35.

Two brain-volume/IQ studies have employed the MAB as their measure of intelligence. First, Wickett, Vernon, and Lee (1994) reported a correlation of .39 (p < .05) between MAB Full-Scale IQ scores and MRI estimates of brain volume among 40 adult females. Second, in Wickett, Vernon, and Lee (submitted), 34 pairs of adult male siblings (68 subjects) were administered an extensive battery of 22 paper-and-pencil or computerized intelligence, ability, and cognitive tests, including the MAB, in addition to undergoing MRI scans to assess right and left hemisphere and overall brain volume. Brain-volume and Full-Scale IQ correlated .35 in this study; this correlation rises to .51 after correction for restriction of range in IQ. Verbal and Performance IQs were equally highly correlated with left and right hemisphere volume; that is, no differential pattern of correlation emerged favoring PIQ and right hemisphere size or VIQ and left hemisphere size. Brain volume was also significantly correlated with digit span memory tests ($r = .41$ [forward span] and .27 [backward span]), a test of verbal closure (in which participants are required to complete words by filling in missing letters, $r = .27$), the ZVT ($r = .32$), and RT measures of speed of information-processing in short-term ($r = -.35$) and in long-term memory ($r = -.42$), but correlated non-significantly with tests of visualization, spatial rotation, perceptual speed, and flexibility of closure.

Scores on factors extracted from the 22 cognitive tests revealed a very interesting pattern of results: there was a high positive correlation ($r = .59$) between the g-loadings of the tests and the degree to which the tests correlated with brain volume, replicating Jensen, 1994, who found a .64 correlation. The same was true for the tests' loadings on a fluid ability factor ($r = .49$) and on a memory factor ($r = .45$). The tests' loadings on a spatial ability factor, however, were strongly *negatively* correlated with their correlations with brain volume ($r = -.84$). Thus, the more g-loaded, fluid ability-loaded, or memory-loaded a test, the higher its correlation with brain volume, but the more spatially-loaded a test, the lower its correlation with brain volume. If this finding replicates in future studies, it would be of considerable interest from both a psychological and an evolutionary perspective: suggesting as it does that the size of the brain has developed differentially with respect to the characteristics or demands of different tasks.

INTELLIGENCE AND PERSONALITY

Almost from as early as there were tests to measure intelligence and personality, psychologists have been interested in seeing whether relationships exist between these two broad dimensions of individual differences. Allport (1961), for example, suggested that intelligence and personality are interrelated and Cattell (1965) has long-argued that complete models of personality need to recognize the role of intelligence.

Studies have shown that certain dimensions of personality and intelligence are indeed correlated. Gormly and Gormly (1986), for example, reported a positive correlation between introversion and spatial abilities; other studies have shown positive correlations between introversion and verbal ability (Robinson, 1982, 1985; Saklofske & Kostura, 1990) and negative correlations between psychoticism and intelligence (Eysenck, 1993; Lynn, Hampson, & Agahi, 1989). Numerous other investigations have also examined intelligence-personality relationships (e.g., Ackerman & Heggestad, 1997; Allik & Realo, 1997; Austin, Deary, & Gibson, 1997; Baron, 1984; Bolton, 1980; Brand, 1994; Brebner & Stough, 1995; Chiu, Hong, & Dweck, 1994; Donahue & Sattler, 1971; Egan, 1989; Goff & Ackerman, 1992; Hakstian & Cattell, 1978; Holland, Dollinger, Holland, & MacDonald, 1995; Johnson, Nagoshi, Ahern, & Wilson, 1983; Ley, Spelman, Davies, & Riley, 1966; Mayer, Caruso, Zigler, & Dreyden, 1989; Sen & Hagtvet, 1993; Turner, Willerman, & Horn, 1976), typically finding low but significant correlations between the two.

As described above, there is a strong neurospsychological tradition in research on human intelligence. Similarly, several researchers have proposed that individual differences in personality traits may be traced back to underlying neuropsychological mechanisms. Zuckerman (1991), for example, attributes individual differences in introversion-extraversion to the ascending reticulocortical-activating system and its control of the level of stimulation of the central nervous system. Other influential theorists who have focused on the neuropsychological bases of individual differences in personality include Gray (1991), Strelau (1985), Robinson (1982), and Cloninger (1986). Excellent summaries of these and other neuropsychological approaches to personality may be found in Gonzalez, Hynd, and Martin (1994) and Matthews and Gilliland (1999).

A recent study by Harris, Vernon, and Jang (1998) employed the MAB and Jackson's Personality Research Form (PRF; Jackson, 1986) to provide a unique perspective on the neuropsychological basis of relationships between intelligence and personality. The PRF is a true-false personality inventory that measures 20 traits (e.g., aggression, dominance, endurance, impulsivity, succorance) and which has well-established, excellent psychometric properties (see Chapter 11 [this volume] for further description of the merits of the PRF). In Harris et al (1998), samples of adult monozygotic (MZ) and dizygotic (DZ) twins completed the MAB and the PRF; the twin data thus allowing both phenotypic and genetic correlations between intelligence and personality to be computed.

At the univariate level, both the MAB and the PRF scales showed fairly typical heritabilities (h^2s = .49, .28, and .77 for MAB Full-Scale, Verbal, and Performance IQs, respectively; h^2s ranging from 0 to .65, with a median of .45, for the 20 PRF traits). Small but significant phenotypic correlations were found between Full-Scale MAB IQs and the PRF scales Achievement ($r = .21$), Autonomy ($r = .15$), Dominance ($r = .25$), Endurance ($r = .14$), Harmavoidance ($r = -.25$), Order ($r = -.14$), Sentience ($r = .12$), Succorance ($r = -.14$), and Understanding ($r = .36$). Multivariate genetic analyses revealed genetic correlations similar to or greater in magnitude than the phenotypic correlations between these same variables (r_gs ranging from .10 to .43), while environmental correlations between them were much smaller (ranging from .05 to .26). Thus, for the majority of those personality traits that showed a phenotypic correlation with intelligence, these correlations appear to be largely attributable to common genetic factors. This in turn suggests that, from an evolutionary perspective, intelligence and certain personality traits may have been jointly selected for, and indeed high intelligence and such traits as autonomy, achievement, dominance, endurance, and harmavoidance would seem to be desirable characteristics that in combination would contribute strongly to survival.

Environmental Predictors of Personality Development

Behavior genetic studies of personality have consistently shown that *nonshared* environmental factors - those life experiences or circumstances not shared by twins or siblings from the same family - account for about as much, if not more, of the variance as do genetic factors. In contrast, *shared* environmental influences - those experiences and circumstances that twins and siblings have in common - typically account for none or only a negligible proportion of the variance in most traits (Plomin, DeFries, & McClearn, 1990)

Despite the importance of nonshared environmental factors, researchers have had limited success identifying them. Some early studies (e.g., Baker & Daniels, 1990; Daniels, 1986; Plomin & Daniels, 1987) employed the Sibling Inventory of Differential Experience (SIDE; Daniels & Plomin, 1985) as a measure of twins' perceptions of different experiences that they may have had. Correlations between SIDE scales and differences in personality were typically quite small: nonshared environmental factors accounting for no more than about 30% of the variance in personality.

A recent study by Vernon, Jang, Harris, and McCarthy (1997) administered the SIDE and three other environmental measures (the Environmental Response Inventory [ERI; McKechnie, 1974], the Family Environment Scale [FES; Moos & Moos, 1986], and the Classroom Environment Scale [CES; Trickett & Moos, 1974]) to samples of adult MZ and DZ twins and nontwin siblings (NT sibs). These subjects also completed Jackson's PRF (Jackson, 1986), which was factor analyzed to yield five factors: Extraversion, Conscientiousness, Autonomy, Neuroticism, and Openness. To examine the effects of nonshared environmental factors on differential personality development, differences between MZ and DZ twins and the nontwin siblings on the five PRF factors were correlated with their differences on factors derived from the several environmental measures.

Of the five PRF factors, Autonomy was found to be the least heritable and the most consistently predictable by nonshared environmental factors. Among MZs, DZs, and NT sibs, differences in Autonomy correlated significantly with differences on the ERI and the SIDE, showing that factors such as differential parental treatment and classroom experiences make some contribution to the differential development of Autonomy. With the exception of Extraversion, which proved to be one of the more highly heritable of the PRF factors, differences on each of the other personality factors extracted from the PRF were also found to be predictable by differences on one or more of the environmental measures. Among NT sibs, for example, differences in Neuroticism correlated positively with differences in an Acceptance-Rejection factor derived from the FES, and differences in Conscientiousness correlated positively with differences in parental affection and control.

Overall, by utilizing a wider range of measures of the nonshared environment than any previous studies, Vernon et al. (1997) were successful in demonstrating that differences between twins and siblings in several broad dimensions of personality can be accounted for to some extent (as much as 51% among NT sibs) by differences in the environments that they were exposed to while growing up. We are currently pursuing this line of enquiry among 3- to 6-year-old twins and sibs to see whether salient nonshared environmental effects can be identified in these earlier years when personalities are still very much in development.

CONCLUSION

In closing, it has been the intent of this chapter both to illustrate a number of directions that recent research in the area of human intelligence has taken - including investigations of its cognitive and biological correlates, behavioral genetic studies, and studies of relationships between intelligence and personality and of personality development - and, at the same time, to draw attention to the quite considerable body of work in these areas which has employed Jackson's MAB and/or his PRF. There is no question but that the MAB is becoming an increasingly popular tool among researchers interested in the study of human intelligence; its ease of administration to large samples of subjects and the fact that it provides a reliable and valid measure of *g* and other mental abilities contribute to its well-deserved acceptance by the research community. With the MAB, as with many of the other tests that he has developed, Jackson has made a valuable contribution to the scientific study of individual differences.

It should also be noted that the research described in this chapter is by no means an exhaustive account of all recent studies that have employed the MAB (and certainly not the PRF). Other MAB-based studies have focused on such topics as relationships between intelligence and problem-solving (Vernon & Strudensky, 1988), dynamic spatial skills (Jackson, Vernon, & Jackson, 1993), and statistical reasoning ability (Royalty, 1995); the use of intelligence tests in the selection and screening of air force officers and astronauts (Bishop, Faulk, & Santy, 1996; Carretta, Retzlaff, Callister, & King, 1998; King & Flynn, 1995; Retzlaff & Gibertini, 1987); comparisons of paper-and-pencil versus computerized administrations of the MAB (Harrell, Honaker, Hetu, & Oberwager, 1988; MacLennan, Jackson, & Bellantino, 1988); and studies of the intellectual characteristics of prison inmates and their likelihood of dropping out of school (Ahrens, Evans, & Barnett, 1990; Jones, Barnett, & McCormack, 1988; Tammany, Evans, & Barnett, 1990). Taken together with the work described in more detail above, these latter studies provide an additional indication of the theoretical and applied uses to which the MAB has been put, thereby illustrating its and its author's contribution to many areas of individual differences research.

REFERENCES

Ackerman, P. L., & Heggestad, E. D. (1997). Intelligence, personality, and interests: Evidence for overlapping traits. *Psychological Bulletin*, 121, 219-245.

Ahrens, J. A., Evans, R. G., & Barnett, R. W. (1990). Factors related to dropping out of school in an incarcerated population. *Educational and Psychological Measurement*, 50, 611-617.

Allik, J., & Realo, A. (1997). Intelligence, academic abilities, and personality. *Personality and Individual Differences*, 23, 809-814.

Allport, G. W. (1961). *Pattern and growth in personality*. New York: Holt, Rinehart, & Winston.

Andres-Pueyo, A., & Bonastre, R. M. (1999). *Nerve conduction velocity, MRI and intelligence: Preliminary data*. Paper presented at the 9th biennial meeting of the International Society for the Study of Individual Differences, Vancouver, Canada, July.

Anokhin, A., & Vogel, F. (1996). EEG alpha rhythm frequency and intelligence in normal adults. *Intelligence*, 23, 1-14.

Austin, E. J., Deary, I. J., & Gibson, G.J. (1997). Relationships between ability and personality: Three hypotheses tested. *Intelligence*, 25, 49-70.

Baker, L. A., & Daniels, D. (1990). Nonshared environmental influences and personality differences in adult twins. *Journal of Personality and Social Psychology*, 58, 103-110.

Baron, J. (1984). Personality and intelligence. In R.J. Sternberg (Ed.), *Handbook of human intelligence*. New York: Cambridge University Press.

Barrett, P. T., Daum, I., & Eysenck, H. J. (1990). Sensory nerve conduction and intelligence: A methodological study. *Journal of Psychophysiology*, 4, 1-13.

Barrett, P., & Eysenck, H J. (1992). Brain evoked potentials and intelligence: The Hendrickson paradigm. *Intelligence*, 16, 361-382.

Barrett, P. T., Petrides, K. V., & Eysenck, H. J. (1998). Estimating inspection time: Response probabilities, the BRAT IT algorithm, and IQ correlations. *Personality and Individual Differences*, 24, 405-419.

Bates, T. V., & Eysenck, H. J. (1993a). Intelligence, inspection time, and decision time. *Intelligence*, 17, 523-531.

Bates, T., & Eysenck, H. J. (1993b). String length, attention & intelligence: Focussed attention reverses the string length-IQ relationship. *Personality and Individual Differences*, 15, 363-371.

Bates, T., Stough, C., Mangan, G., & Pellett, O. (1995). Intelligence and complexity of the averaged evoked potential: An attentional theory. *Intelligence*, 20, 27-39.

Bishop, S. L., Faulk, D., & Santy, P. A. (1996). The use of IQ assessment in astronaut screening and evaluation. *Aviation, Space, and Environmental Medicine*, 67, 1130-1137.

Blinkhorn, S. F., & Hendrickson, D. E. (1982). Averaged evoked responses and psychometric intelligence. *Nature*, 295, 596-597.

Bolton, B. (1980). Personality (16PF) correlates of WAIS scales: A replication. *Applied Psychological Measurement*, **4**, 399-401.

Brand, C .R. (1979). The quick and the educable. *Bulletin of the British Psychological Society*, **32**, 386-389.

Brand, C. (1994). Open to experience - closed to intelligence: Why the 'big five' are really the 'comprehensive six'. *European Journal of Personality*, **8**, 299-310.

Brebner, J., & Stough, C. (1995). Theoretical and empirical relationships between personality and intelligence. In D.H. Saklofske & M. Zeidner (Eds.), *International handbook of personality and intelligence*. New York: Plenum.

Broca, P. (1861). Sur le volume et al forme du cerveau suivant les individus et suivant les races. *Bulletins et mémoires de la Société d'Anthropologie de Paris*, **2**, 139-207, 301-321, 441-446.

Carretta, T. R., Retzlaff, P. D., Callister, J. D., & King, R. E. (1998). A comparison of two U.S. air force pilot aptitude tests. *Aviation, Space, and Environmental Medicine*, **69**, 931-935.

Carroll, J. B. (1991a). No demonstration the g is not unitary, but there's more to the story: Comment on Kranzler and Jensen. *Intelligence*, **15**, 423-436.

Carroll, J. B. (1991b). Still no demonstration that g is not unitary: Further comment on Kranzler and Jensen. *Intelligence*, **15**, 449-453.

Caryl, P. G., & Fraser, I .C. (1985, September). *The Hendrickson string length and intelligence – a replication*. Paper presented at the Psychophysiology Society Scottish Conference, Edinburgh.

Cattell, R. B. (1965). *The scientific analysis of personality*. New York: Penguin.

Chalke, F., & Ertl, J. (1965). Evoked potentials and intelligence. *Life Science*, **4**, 1319-1322.

Chiu, C., Hong, Y., & Dweck, C. S. (1994). Toward an integrative model of personality and intelligence: A general framework and some preliminary steps. In R.J. Sternberg and P. Ruzgis (Eds.), *Personality and intelligence*. New York: Cambridge University Press.

Cloninger, C. R. (1986). A unified biosocial theory of personality and its role in the development of anxiety states. *Psychiatric Developments*, **3**, 167-226.

Daniels, D. (1986). Differential experiences of siblings in the same family as predictors of adolescent sibling personality differences. *Journal of Personality and Social Psychology*, **51**, 339-346.

Daniels, D., & Plomin, R. (1985). Differential experience of siblings in the same family. *Developmental Psychology*, **21**, 747-760.

Donahue, D., & Sattler, J. M. (1971). Personality variables affecting WAIS scores. *Journal of Consulting and Clinical Psychology*, **36**, 441.

Dugas, J. L., & Kellas, G. (1974). Encoding and retrieval processes in normal children and retarded adolescents. *Journal of Experimental Child Psychology*, **17**, 177-185.

Egan, V. (1989). Links between personality, ability and attitudes in a low-IQ sample. *Personality and Individual Differences*, **10**, 997-1001.

Ellingson, R. J. (1966). Relationship between EEG and test intelligence: A commentary. *Psychological Bulletin*, **65**, 91-98.

Ertl, J. P., & Schafer, E. W. P. (1969). Brain response correlates of psychometric intelligence. *Nature*, **223**, 421-422.

Eysenck, H. J. (1993). The relationship between IQ and personality. In G.L. Van Heck, P. Bonaiuto, I.J. Deary, & W. Nowack (Eds.), *Personality Psychology in Europe: Vol. 4* (pp. 159-181). Tilburg, The Netherlands: Tilburg University Press.

Eysenck, H. J., & Barrett, P. (1984). Psychophysiology and the measurement of intelligence. In C.R. Reynolds & V. Willson (Eds.), *Methodological and statistical advances in the study of individual differences*. New York: Plenum Press.

Gale, A., & Edwards, J. A. (1983). Cortical correlates of intelligence. In A. Gale & J.A. Edwards (Eds.), *Physiological correlates of human behaviour. Vol. 3: Individual differences and psychopathology*. London: Academic Press.

Galton, F. (1888). Head growth in students at the University of Cambridge. *Nature*, **38**, 14-15.

Giannitrapani, D. (1966). EEG average frequency and intelligence. *Electroencephalography and Clinical Neurophysiology*, **27**, 480-486.

Goff, M., & Ackerman, P. L. (1992). Personality-intelligence relations: Assessment of typical intellectual engagement. *Journal of Educational Psychology*, **84**, 537-552.

Goldberg, R. A., Schwartz, S., & Stewart, M. (1977). Individual differences in cognitive processes. *Journal of Educational Psychology*, **69**, 9-14.

Gonzalez, J. J., Hynd, G. W., & Martin, R. P. (1994). Neuropsychology of temperament. In P.A. Vernon (Ed.), *The neuropsychology of individual differences* San Diego, CA: Academic Press.

Gormly, J., & Gormly, A. (1986). Social introversion and spatial abilities. *Bulletin of the Psychonomic Society*, **24**, 273-274.

Gray, J.A. (1991). The neuropsychology of temperament. In J. Strelau and A. Angleitner (Eds.), *Explorations in temperament: International perspective on theory and measurement*. New York: Plenum.

Haier, R. J., Robinson, D. L., Braden, W., & Williams, D. (1983). Electrical potentials of the cerebral cortex and psychometric intelligence. *Personality and Individual Differences*, **4**, 591-599.

Hakstian, A. R., & Cattell, R. B. (1978). An examination of inter-domain relationships among some ability and personality traits. *Educational and Psychological Measurement*, **38**, 275-290.

Harrell, T. H., Honaker, L. M., Hetu, M., & Oberwager, J. (1988). Computerized versus traditional administration of the Multidimensional Aptitude Battery-Verbal scale: An examination of reliability and validity. *Computers in Human Behavior*, **3**, 129-137.

Harris, J. A., Vernon, P. A., & Jang, K. L. (1998). A multivariate genetic analysis of correlations between intelligence and personality. *Developmental Neuropsychology*, **14**, 127-142.

Hendrickson, A. E. (1982). The biological basis of intelligence. Part I: Theory. In H.J. Eysenck (Ed.), *A model for intelligence*. Berlin: Springer-Verlag.

Hendrickson, D. E. (1982). The biological basis of intelligence. Part II: Measurement. In H.J. Eysenck (Ed.), *A model for intelligence*. Berlin: Springer-Verlag.

Hendrickson, D. E., & Hendrickson A. E. (1980). The biological basis of individual differences in intelligence. *Personality and Individual Differences*, **1**, 3-33.

Ho, H. Z., Baker, L., & Decker, S. N. (1988). Covariation between intelligence and speed-of-processing: genetic and environmental influences. *Behavior Genetics*, **18**, 247-261.

Holland, D. C., Dollinger, S. J., Holland, C. J., & MacDonald, D. A. (1995). The relationship between psychometric intelligence and the five-factor model of personality in a rehabilitation sample. *Journal of Clinical Psychology*, **51**, 79-88.

Hunt, E. (1976). Varieties of cognitive power. In L.B. Resnick (Ed.), *The nature of intelligence*. Hillsdale, NJ: Erlbaum.

Jackson, D. N. (1984). *Multidimensional Aptitude Battery Manual*. Port Huron, MI: Research Psychologists Press.

Jackson, D. N. (1986). *Personality Research Form manual*. Port Huron, MI: Sigma Assessment Systems.

Jackson D. N. III, Vernon, P. A., & Jackson, D. N. (1993). Dynamic spatial performance and general intelligence. *Intelligence*, **17**, 451-460.

Jensen, A. R. (1979). g: Outmoded theory or unconquered frontier? *Creative Science & Technology*, **2**, 16-29.

Jensen, A. R. (1987). Individual differences in the Hick paradigm. In P.A. Vernon (Ed.), *Speed of information-processing and intelligence*. Norwood, NJ: Ablex.

Jensen, A. R. (1994). Psychometric g related to differences in head size. *Personality and Individual Differences*, **17**, 597-606.

Jensen, A. R. & Munro, E. (1979). Reaction time, movement time, and intelligence. *Intelligence*, **3**, 121-126.

Johnson, R. C., Nagoshi, C. T., Ahern, F. M., & Wilson, J. R. (1983). Correlations of measures of personality and intelligence within and across generations. *Personality and Individual Differences*, **4**, 331-338.

Jones, J. M., Barnett, R. W., & McCormack, J. K. (1988). Verbal/Performance splits in inmates assessed with the Multidimensional Aptitude Battery. *Journal of Clinical Psychology*, **44**, 995-1000.

Keating, D. P., & Bobbitt, B. (1978). Individual and developmental differences in cognitive processing components of mental ability. *Child Development*, **49**, 155-169.

King, R. E., & Flynn, C. F. (1995). Defining and measuring the "right stuff": neuropsychiatrically enhanced flight screening (N-EFS). *Aviation, Space, and Environmental Medicine*, **66**, 951-956.

Kranzler, J. H. (1991). The construct validity of the Multidimensional Aptitude Battery: A word of caution. *Journal of Clinical Psychology*, **47**, 691-697.

Kranzler, J. H., & Jensen, A. R. (1989). Inspection time and intelligence: A meta-analysis. *Intelligence*, **13**, 329-347.

Kranzler, J. H., & Jensen, A. R. (1991a). The nature of psychometric g: Unitary process or a number of independent processes? *Intelligence*, **15**, 397-422.

Kranzler, J.H., & Jensen, A.R. (1991b). Unitary g: Unquestioned postulate or empirical fact? *Intelligence*, **15**, 437-448.

Lally, M., & Nettelbeck, T. (1977). Intelligence, reaction time, and inspection time. *American Journal of Mental Deficiency*, **82**, 273-281.

Lee, M. S., & Wallbrown, F. H. (1990). Note on the construct validity of the Multidimensional Aptitude Battery. *Psychological Reports*, **67**, 1219-1222.

Ley, P., Spelman, M. S., Davies, A. D. M., & Riley, S. (1966). The relationships between intelligence, anxiety, neuroticism and extraversion. *British Journal of Educational Psychology*, **36**, 185-191.

Lynn, R., Hampson, S., & Agahi, E. (1989). Genetic and environmental mechanisms determining intelligence, neuroticism, extraversion and psychoticism: An analysis of Irish siblings. *British Journal of Psychology*, **80**, 499-507.

MacLennan, R. N., Jackson, D. N., & Bellantino, N. (1989). Response latencies and the computerized assessment of intelligence. *Personality and Individual Differences*, **9**, 811-816.

Matthews, G., & Gilliland, K. (1999). The personality theories of H.J. Eysenck and J.A. Gray A comparative review. *Personality and Individual Differences*, **26**, 583-626.

Mayer, J. D., Caruso, D .R., Zigler, E., & Dreyden, J. I. (1989). Intelligence and intelligence-related personality traits. *Intelligence*, **13**, 119-133.

McKechnie, G. E. (1974). *Environmental Response Inventory*. Palo Alto, CA: Consulting Psychologists Press.

McGue, M., Bouchard, T. J., Lykken, D. T., & Feuer, D. (1984). Information processing abilities in twins reared apart. *Intelligence*, **8**, 239-258.

Miller, L. T., & Vernon, P. A. (1992). The general factor in short-term memory, intelligence, and reaction time. *Intelligence*, **16**, 5-29.

Moos, R. H., & Moos, B. S. (1986). *Manual: Family Environment Scale*. Palo Alto, CA: Consulting Psychologists Press.

Neale, M. C., & Cardon, L. R. (1992). *Methodology for genetic studies of twins and families*. Dordrecht: Kluwer Academic Publishers.

Nettelbeck, T. (1987). Inspection time and intelligence. In P.A. Vernon (Ed.), *Speed of information-processing and intelligence*. Norwood, NJ: Ablex.

Nettelbeck, T., & Lally, M. (1976). Inspection time and measured intelligence. *British Journal of Psychology*, **67**, 17-22.

Oswald, W. D., & Roth, E. (1978). *Der Zahlen-Verbindungs-Test (ZVT)*. Gottingen, Germany: Hogrefe.

Plomin, R., & Daniels, D. (1987). Why are children in the same family so different from one another? *Behavioral and Brain Sciences*, **10**, 1-60.

Plomin, R., DeFries, J. C., & McClearn, G. E. (1990). *Behavioral genetics: A primer* (2nd ed.). New York: Freeman.

Reed, T. E. (1984). Mechanism for heritability of intelligence. *Nature*, **311**, 417.

Reed, T. E., & Jensen, A. R. (1991). Arm nerve conduction velocity (NCV), brain NCV, reaction time, and intelligence. *Intelligence*, **15**, 33-47.

Reed, T. E., & Jensen, A. R. (1992). Conduction velocity in a brain nerve pathway of normal adults correlates with intelligence level. *Intelligence*, **16**, 259-272.

Retzlaff, P. D., & Gibertini, M. (1988). Objective psychological testing of U.S. air force officers in pilot training. *Aviation, Space, and Environmental Medicine*, **59**, 661-663.

Rijsdijk, F. V., Boomsma, D. I., & Vernon, P. A. (1995). Genetic analysis of peripheral nerve conduction velocity in twins. *Behavior Genetics*, **25**, 341-348.

Robinson, D. L. (1982). Properties of the diffuse thalamocortical system and human personality: A direct test of Pavlovian/Eysenckian theory. *Personality and Individual Differences*, **3**, 1-16.

Robinson, D. L. (1985). How personality relates to intelligence test performance: Implications for a theory of intelligence, ageing research and personality assessment. *Personality and Individual Differences*, **6**, 203-216.

Royalty, J. (1995). Evaluating knowledge-based statistical reasoning. *Psychological Reports*, **77**, 1323-1327.

Saklofske, D. H., & Kostura, D. D. (1990). Extraversion-introversion and intelligence. *Personality and Individual Differences*, **11**, 547-551.

Sen, A. K., & Hagtvet, K. A. (1993). Correlations among creativity, intelligence, personality, and academic achievement. *Perceptual and Motor Skills*, **77**, 497-498.

Shagrass, C., Roemer, R. A., Straumanis, J. J., & Josiassen, R. C. (1981). Intelligence as a factor in evoked potential studies of psychopathology - 1. Comparison of low and high IQ subjects. *Biological Psychiatry*, **16**, 1007-1030.

Spearman, C. (1904). "General intelligence": Objectively determined and measured. *American Journal of Psychology*, **15**, 201-292.

Spearman, C. (1927). *The abilities of man*. New York: Macmillan.

Stough, C. K. K., Nettelbeck, T., & Cooper, C. J. (1990). Evoked brain potentials, string length and intelligence. *Personality and Individual Differences*, **11**, 401-406.

Strelau, J. (1985). Temperament and personality: Pavlov and beyond. In J. Strelau, F.H. Farley, and A. Gale (Eds.), *The biological bases of personality and behavior: Theories, measurement techniques, and development: Vol. 1*. Washington, DC: Hemisphere.

Tammany, J. M., Evans, R. G., & Barnett, R. W. (1990). Personality and intellectual characteristics of adult male felons as a function of offense characteristics. *Journal of Clinical Psychology*, **46**, 906-911.

Trickett, E. J., & Moos, R. H. (1974). *Classroom Environment Scale manual*. Palo Alto, CA: Consulting Psychologists Press.

Turner, R. G., Willerman, L., & Horn, J. M. (1976). Personality correlates of WAIS performance. *Journal of Clinical Psychology*, **32**, 349-354.

Vernon, P. A. (1983). Speed of information processing and general intelligence. *Intelligence*, 7, 53-70.

Vernon, P. A. (1989). The heritability of measures of speed of information-processing. *Personality and Individual Differences*, **10**, 573-576.

Vernon, P. A. (1990). An overview of chronometric measures of intelligence. *School Psychology Review*, **19**, 399-410.

Vernon, P. A. (Ed.) (1993). *Biological approaches to the study of human intelligence*. Norwood, New Jersey: Ablex.

Vernon, P. A., Jang, K. L., Harris, J. A., & McCarthy, J. M. (1997). Environmental predictors of personality differences: A twin and sibling study. *Journal of Personality and Social Psychology*, **72**, 177-183.

Vernon, P. A., & Mori, M. (1992). Intelligence, reaction times, and peripheral nerve conduction velocity. *Intelligence*, **16**, 273-288.

Vernon, P. A., & Strudensky, S. (1988). Relationships between problem-solving and intelligence. *Intelligence*, **12**, 435-453.

Vernon, P. A., Wickett, J. C., Bazana, P. G., & Stelmack, R. M. (in press). The neuropsychology and psychophysiology of human intelligence. In R. J. Sternberg (Ed.), *Handbook of intelligence*. Cambridge: Cambridge University Press.

Vogel, W., & Broverman, D. M. (1964). Relationship between EEG and test intelligence: A critical review. *Psychological Bulletin*, **62**, 132-144.

Vogel, W., & Broverman, D. M. (1966). A reply to "Relationship between EEG and test intelligence: A commentary. *Psychological Bulletin*, **65**, 99-109.

Wallbrown, F. H., Carmin, C. N., & Barnett, R. W. (1988). Investigating the construct validity of the Multidimensional Aptitude Battery. *Psychological Reports*, **62**, 871-878.

Wallbrown, F. H., Carmin, C. N., & Barnett, R. W. (1989). A further note on the construct validity of the Multidimensional Aptitude Battery. *Journal of Clinical Psychology*, **45**, 429-433.

Wechsler, D. (1981). *Manual for the Wechsler Adult Intelligence Scale-Revised*. Cleveland, OH: The Psychological Corporation.

Wickett, J. C., & Vernon, P. A. (1994). Peripheral nerve conduction velocity, reaction time, and intelligence: An attempt to replicate Vernon and Mori (1992). *Intelligence*, **18**, 127-131.

Wickett, J. C., Vernon, P. A., & Lee, D. H. (1994). *In Vivo* brain size, head perimeter, and intelligence in a sample of healthy adult females. *Personality and Individual Differences*, **16**, 831-838.

Wickett, J. C., Vernon, P. A., & Lee, D. H. (submitted). The relationships between the factors of intelligence and brain volume. *Personality and Individual Differences*.

Zuckerman, M. (1991). *Psychobiology of personality*. Cambridge, England: Cambridge University Press.

SECTION III: CONSTRUCT-ORIENTED ASSESSMENT OF INDIVIDUAL DIFFERENCES IN INDUSTRIAL/ORGANIZATIONAL PSYCHOLOGY

Since the inception of industrial/organizational (I/O) psychology, the assessment of individual differences has played an integral role. The decisions that are made as a result of assessing individual differences in I/O settings often have weighty consequences, meaning that tests applied in this area must be able to withstand a heavy burden of accountability. This section explores implications of the construct-oriented approach to assessment, as championed by Douglas Jackson and others, with respect to the measurement of personality, integrity/honesty, organizational commitment, and goal commitment within I/O settings.

Chapter 10 traces a program of research which has as it's goal the appropriate assessment of personality constructs within I/O settings. This odyssey began with Jackson and his colleagues in the 1970s, and continues to the present. Among other contributions, this chapter has much to say about personality traits and the employment interview; appropriate meta-analytic practices for the cumulation of criterion-related evidence of the validity of personality constructs; the problem of faking in personnel selection; and the advisability of using broad (i.e., "Big Five") versus narrow traits in the prediction of criteria.

Chapter 11 poses a heretofore untested question of clear relevance to modern I/O research involving personality assessment: Is the criterion-related validity of a given trait more or less invariant across different personality tests? New empirical evidence, collected using Jackson's (1984) *Personality Research Form* and the fourth edition of the *Sixteen Personality Factors test* (Cattell, Eber, & Tatsuoka, 1970), is presented to address this question. The implications of these findings for primary research and for meta-analytic investigations of the validity of personality assessment in the prediction of job performance are discussed.

In Chapter 12, Murphy explains that although the assessment of honesty or integrity has much to offer, there has been a general tendency in this area to overlook the basic conceptual and definitional issues that should ordinarily precede the operationalization of a construct. Consequently, much confusion exists as to what is being measured and how the research evidence involving these tests should be interpreted. In addition to providing a wealth of basic information relevant to both practitioners and researchers in this area, Murphy's chapter represents a systematic effort to review existing conceptual frameworks for honesty/integrity tests and chart out a path for the future.

Few work attitudes have generated as much interest as organizational commitment. The linkage of organizational commitment to turnover has particular relevance to many of today's organizations. In Chapter 13, Allen and Meyer chronicle the explication of this attitude as a three-dimensional construct, it's operation-alization, it's antcedents and consequences, cross-cultural issues, and the questions that remain to be explored. In so doing, these authors provide a practical model for the application of the construct approach within organizational behavior research.

Over the past three decades, organizational behavior researchers and practitioners have witnessed an explosion of evidence that goal setting has great efficacy as a motivational tool. Studies documenting the beneficial and often remarkable improvements in job performance that result from goal setting number in the hundreds (e.g., see Locke & Latham , 1990). In Chapter 14, Seijts and Latham highlight the key role that goal commmitment plays in goal setting. Current operationalizations of goal commitment are then critically evaluated. Consistent with Jackson's (1971, 1979, 1984) construct based approach to scale development, recommendations are provided for the further development of goal commitment measures.

REFERENCES

Cattell, R.B., Eber, H.W., & Tatsuoka, M.M, (1970). *Handbook for Sixteen Personality Factor Questionnaire (16PF)*. Champaign, IL: Institute for Personality and Ability Testing.
Jackson, D.N. (1971). The dynamics of structured personality tests: 1971. *Psychological Review*, 78, 229-248.
Jackson, D.N. (1979). Construct validity and personality assessment.   In: *Construct validity in psychological measurement. Proceedings of a colloquium on theory and application in education and employment*. Princeton, NJ: U.S. Office of Personnel Management.
Jackson, D.N. (1984). *Personality Research Form Manual*. (Third Edition). Port Huron, MI: Research Psychologists Press.
Locke, E.A., & Latham, G.P. (1990). *A theory of goal setting and task performance*. Englewood Cliffs, NJ: Prentice Hall.

10 THE ASSESSMENT OF PERSONALITY CONSTRUCTS IN INDUSTRIAL-ORGANIZATIONAL PSYCHOLOGY

Mitchell G. Rothstein
Richard D. Goffin

INTRODUCTION

In this chapter we will review the impact of the construct-oriented approach to the assessment of personality on several areas of research and practice in the field of industrial-organizational psychology. We provide an analysis of how the use of a deductive, construct-driven strategy in the assessment of personality has influenced a number of theoretical and methodological advances in this field. In particular, discussion will focus on the assessment of applicant personality traits in the employment interview, the use of personality measures in employee selection, the suppression of nuisance variance due to faking when using personality measures for selection purposes, and innovations in the use of meta-analysis to determine the validity of personality measures in employee selection. Although the focus of this chapter is on personality assessment in industrial-organizational psychology, much of this discussion draws on general principles of personality measurement that are relevant to many areas of psychology

Our general thesis is that the construct approach to test and scale construction and the measurement of individual differences, particularly as it applies to personality assessment, contributes a valuable perspective to measurement-related issues in industrial-organizational psychology. Just as construct-oriented test construction strategies have increased the reliability and validity of psychological measurement generally (Anastasi, 1988; Cronbach & Meehl, 1955; Wiggins, 1973), a construct-oriented approach to the assessment of personality in employee selection has contributed to demonstrating that personality constructs may be assessed for this purpose with high degrees of reliability and validity. In addition, the construct approach provides value to both researchers and practitioners in industrial-organizational psychology.   For researchers, such an approach contributes to the development of sound theories and enables greater linkages with other and/or more general theories of behavior in psychology. Practitioners benefit from the increased interpretability and understanding of personality constructs, as well as the greater ability to link these constructs to job requirements and make better predictions on the impact on job performance.

What is it about the construct approach to personality assessment that contributes to research and practice in industrial-organizational psychology? A detailed summary of the construct approach to psychological assessment is beyond the scope of this paper. In addition, critical features of this approach are well articulated in other chapters in the current volume (e.g., see Allen & Meyer, 1999;Goffin, Rothstein, & Johnston, 1999; Holden, 1999; Morey, 1999). However, several of these features should be highlighted as they are key to understanding the benefits provided to the area of industrial-organizational psychology of primary interest here, the assessment of personality in employee selection. These features are drawn from Jackson's (1971) theoretical rationale for the construct approach to personality assessment. First, the importance of using psychological theory to derive personality constructs is viewed as essential to ultimately determining the construct validity of measures of these constructs. Second, personality constructs must be clearly defined and consistent with the theoretical formulation of the construct. Third, the personality measure must demonstrate adequate levels of convergent and discriminant validity, thereby ensuring that the construct is theoretically and empirically distinct and not confounded with other measures or formulations of personality.   Finally, the personality measure must not be confounded with stylistic or method variance such as social desirability. In brief, clear, distinct, theoretically derived definitions of personality constructs enable researchers to develop theoretically sound hypotheses that are empirically verifiable. Practitioners also benefit from such clear construct definitions because they are more easily interpreted and understood in the context of predicting job performance.   Also, personality measures that demonstrate convergent and discriminant validity and are not confounded with stylistic or method variance enable both researchers and practitioners to have confidence in their research results and validation projects.   These benefits of a construct approach to personality assessment will be identified as a consistent theme as they apply to the discussion of each topic in industrial-organizational psychology in which they have had significant impact.

ASSESSING APPLICANT PERSONALITY TRAITS IN THE EMPLOYMENT INTERVIEW

In the early to mid 1980's Jackson and his colleagues (Jackson, Paunonen, & Rothstein, 1987; Jackson, Peacock, & Holden, 1982; Jackson, Peacock, & Smith, 1980; Rothstein & Jackson, 1980) undertook a series of experiments and field studies to investigate the assessment of applicant personality traits in the employment interview. That program of research was an integration of Jackson's inferential accuracy model of personality trait covariation and impression formation (Jackson, 1972; Jackson, Chan, & Stricker, 1979; Lay & Jackson, 1969; Lay, Burron, & Jackson, 1973; Reed & Jackson, 1975) and a body of research that may be characterized as psychological studies of the employment interview. It is of some historical interest that that program of research was quite controversial at the time.

There were two reasons for this. First, although the inferential accuracy of personality trait covariation was well known and accepted, the rationale for applying this model to the assessment of employability was vigorously challenged because personality traits were generally regarded as irrelevant to job performance (e.g., Guion & Gottier, 1965). Second, the employment interview was generally regarded by most industrial-organizational psychologists at the time as lacking acceptable levels of reliability and validity for personnel selection (e.g., Schmitt, 1976). Currently, relations between personality and job performance are well accepted (e.g., Barrick & Mount, 1991; Tett, Jackson, & Rothstein, 1991), as is the validity of the employment interview (Dipboye & Gaugler, 1993). However, it is worth reviewing the rationale for the research conducted by Jackson and his colleagues on assessing applicant personality traits in the employment interview because it illustrates to a considerable degree the impact of a deductive construct-driven research strategy on the development of an innovative research program.

Criticism of the employment interview prior to the 1980's followed a consistent theme (Rothstein & Jackson, 1984). Interviewer characteristics, interviewee characteristics, and/or contextual factors were experimentally manipulated or occasionally evaluated in a field study and invariably found to negatively affect the reliability and validity of the interview decision. This research had been reviewed qualitatively on numerous occasions and conclusions repeatedly focused on the number of variables that rendered selection decisions less reliable and valid (e.g., Schmitt, 1976). In contrast to identifying sources of error and bias in judgments of applicant suitability, Jackson and his colleagues sought to identify sources of accuracy in interview decisions. In this, they were guided by a considerable practitioner literature that specified applicant personality characteristics as critical job-related information that could be assessed most effectively in the employment interview (Black, 1970; Fear, 1978; Lopez, 1975; Peskin, 1971). This practitioner literature emphasized the importance of avoiding global socially desirable characteristics (e.g., Lopez, 1975) and evaluating specific traits for specific job requirements (e.g., Peskin, 1971).   Furthermore, interview practitioners demonstrated an awareness of the concept of trait covariation, specifically regarding the need to infer a number of job related traits from limited information based on statements made during the interview (Fear, 1978).   In addition, Jackson and his colleagues were guided by considerable theory and research in the area of person perception and trait inferential networks in developing hypotheses regarding potential sources of accuracy in interview judgments.   Thus, the rationale for Jackson's program of research investigating the assessment of applicant personality traits in the employment interview was very much linked to several of the principal features of the construct-driven approach to research: the use of psychological theory to derive hypotheses, an appreciation of the notion of convergent and discriminant validity with respect to linking specific traits to specific job requirements, and an understanding of the confounding effects of social desirability.

Although the role of personality in predicting job performance is much better understood today than it was in the 1980's (Tett et al., 1991), Jackson's interview research had to provide a rationale for assessing personality traits for job performance in the absence of meta-analytic evidence.   The prevailing wisdom at the time among the majority of industrial-organizational psychologists was that personality was not related to job performance (Campbell, Dunnette, Lawler, Weick, 1970; Gough, 1976; Guion, 1976; Korman, 1977; Landy & Trumbo, 1980), and the primary evidence cited for this conclusion was Guion and Gottier's (1965) influential review.   However, examination of Guion and Gottier's paper revealed that their conclusions were not cited accurately (Rothstein & Jackson, 1980).   In fact, the main conclusion from this review was that personality measures at that time had not demonstrated their general usefulness for personnel selection. Jackson and his colleagues interpreted this conclusion as entirely reasonable because, from a construct-oriented perspective, there were numerous problems with the research on personality-job performance relations reviewed by Guion and Gottier (1965).   In particular, over half (56%) of the studies reviewed involved measures that could not be considered as personality (e.g., biodata, vocational interest, psychopathology) or had no theoretical rationale for predicting job-related criteria (e.g., the Rorschach).   Of the remaining studies, most involved the use of personality measures that had well documented problems with (a) the inability to demonstrate convergent and discriminant validity, (b) measures confounded with social desirability and other stylistic or method variance, and/or (c) the absence of linkages to psychological theory.   Thus, from a construct-oriented perspective on personality assessment, it was not surprising that the studies reviewed by Guion and Gottier (1965) did not demonstrate the usefulness of personality measures for personnel selection.   Conversely, there was a strong rationale for investigating personality-job performance relations when personality measures were developed on the basis of psychological theory, the measures demonstrated adequate levels of convergent and discriminant validity, and the measures were not confounded with variance due to response styles. Furthermore, the rationale for investigating personality-job performance relations in the employment interview was based on strong support from the practitioner literature that personality can and should be assessed in the interview, as well as support from the person perception literature demonstrating that personality traits may be accurately inferred from observations of behavior (e.g., see Paunonen, 1989).

In a study conducted with professional employment interviewers, Jackson et al. (1982) investigated the degree that personality traits were perceived as differentially relevant for different occupations. A sample of 132 recruiting professionals was asked to imagine a typical person employed in each of 15 occupations and to judge how characteristic a series of personality traits would be of that person. Each occupation was defined by a one-paragraph job description and personality information was presented by a list of 20 traits and definitions taken from Jackson's (1974) Personality Research Form (PRF). Consistent with elements of the construct approach to measurement, clear definitions of personality traits developed to maximize convergent and discriminant validity and minimize confounding variance with social desirability were used to ensure that participants would be able to use reliable and valid personality information in their judgments. These definitions were based on the trait-based personality theory developed by Murray (1938).

Results from this study clearly indicated that these professional employment interviewers had highly differentiated and reliable implicit notions of the personality traits suitable for a number of different occupations. Using multidimensional scaling techniques, the personality traits were reduced to a more parsimonious set of eight bipolar dimensions on to which each occupation was projected reflecting the degree that each occupation was judged by interviewers to be identified with certain personality traits. For example, on the first dimension advertising executives were seen as thrill-seeking, impulsive, changeable, attention-seeking, and fun-loving, whereas on the opposite pole of this dimension accountants were seen as meek, seeking definiteness, and orderly. It has been suggested that these implicit theories of trait covariation are merely stereotypes. But Jackson et al. point out that stereotypes are generally regarded as oversimplified and inaccurate. In this study, the number of dimensions obtained by interviewers' judgments demonstrated a good deal of differentiation rather than simplification. In addition, the dimensional structure of interviewer judgments was highly consistent with the structure obtained from a multi-method factor analysis of self-report measures of personality and vocational interest (Siess & Jackson, 1970). Also, the purpose of the Jackson et al. (1982) study was not to demonstrate that these traits were valid predictors of job performance for this set of occupations, but rather to determine how differentiated and reliable were interviewers' judgments of which traits are suitable for different jobs. This was indeed verified with the help of a construct approach to the assessment of personality.

A number of additional studies were conducted by Jackson and his colleagues to determine how interviewers judge personality traits in a selection interview and to evaluate the extent to which these judgments could be used as a basis for suitability and selection decisions. In the first of these studies, Rothstein and Jackson (1980) used Jackson's (1972) inferential accuracy model of social perception in a simulated employment interview to determine how interviewers perceive and use personality information about job applicants to judge their suitability for two specific jobs. The model postulates that two distinct processes underlie inferential accuracy of trait covariation and that individuals vary with respect to these processes. The first process, sensitivity, refers to individual differences in awareness of the shared implicit network of trait covariation. The second process, threshold, refers to individual differences in readiness to attribute trait-related behaviors to others based on the implicit relations among behaviors.

For purposes of this discussion, we will limit our description of this experiment to the aspects most relevant to illustrating the influence of a construct orientation on the research strategy: measuring the trait inferential networks and selection decisions based on personality trait information in an employment interview. Subjects were asked to role play an employment interviewer seeking to hire either an engineer or an accountant. Subjects were given a description of the type of person well suited for the job. The descriptions were created from personality trait definitions for traits identified with these occupations by Siess and Jackson (1970). Subjects listened to excerpts from a simulated employment interview in which applicants made a number of self-referent statements based on trait adjectives taken from the PRF manual for the same traits used to create the job descriptions. Subjects then judged the suitability of the applicant for the job under consideration, and estimated the likelihood that the applicant would respond true to personality items from the PRF. The latter judgments were used to calculate sensitivity and threshold levels for each subject and to determine the reliability and accuracy of the subjects' perceptions of applicant personality.

Results from this study supported the use of the employment interview for obtaining reliable and accurate assessments of applicant personality characteristics. The inter-rater reliability of subjects' judgments of applicant personality traits was extremely high (0.99 for both applicant targets). Moreover, these reliabilities were not based on a global desirability impression: each judged applicant profile had negligible correlations with social desirability and was substantively unique. Analysis of sensitivity scores revealed that a substantial majority of subjects were aware of the shared implicit network of trait covariation in the target applicants. Threshold analysis revealed that subjects personality judgments were highly accurate: subjects attributed significantly different traits to the appropriate target and the pattern of these attributions accurately reflected the information given in the audiotape of the simulated interview. Finally, subjects rated the target whose personality characteristics were congruent with the occupation as more suitable, more likely to be satisfied with the work, and more likely to get hired than the target whose personality characteristics were incongruent with this occupation. Although there was no attempt in this study to argue for the criterion validity of these judgments of applicant personality, once again the judged applicant personality profiles were highly consistent with self-report measures obtained by Siess and Jackson (1970), as was found in the study by Jackson et al. (1982) discussed previously. Furthermore, there is some evidence to suggest that the mean personality profile of an actual occupational group is consistent with the implicit network of trait covariation obtained from judgments of personality (Jackson et al., 1982; Jackson et al., 1987). Although more research is necessary to support the validity of trait inferential networks, Rothstein and Jackson (1980) concluded that their results supported the use of the employment interview for assessing applicant personality traits with reliability and accuracy, as interview practitioners had long stated.

Several other experiments investigating the assessment of applicant personality traits in the employment interview were conducted by Jackson and his colleagues. These studies extended the findings reported by Rothstein and Jackson (1980) substantially and further illustrate the impact of a construct-orientation to research involving the measurement of personality. In particular, Jackson et al. (1980) reported the results from three studies in this area. In the first study, several different occupations were used, applicant information was presented to subjects as interview transcripts rather than an audiotape of the interview, and the statements reflecting personality characteristics made by the job applicants in the interview transcripts were actual PRF items rather than trait adjectives so that desirability of the applicants' statements could be controlled more rigorously. Although trait inferential judgments were not obtained in this study, results replicated Rothstein and Jackson's (1980) findings that applicant personality traits could be assessed in an interview context and used to make appropriate judgments of suitability for different occupations. In their second study, Jackson et al. used professional employment interviewers as subjects and varied the relevance of the personality trait information given about the applicants as well as the social desirability values of the self-referent statements made by the applicants. The most important findings were first, that when irrelevant personality information was presented to interviewers, their ratings of suitability for a job were higher than when the personality information was clearly inconsistent with the job, whereas the ratings based on inconsistent and irrelevant personality information were both lower than when the personality information was clearly consistent with the job. Secondly, although socially desirable statements made by applicants did generally increase their suitability ratings, interviewers looked for congruence first and were able to judge desirability as differentially relevant to different occupations. In their third study, Jackson et al. replicated the design of the first study, but manipulated applicant experience as well. The results of study one were replicated and there was no effect for applicant experience: subjects perceived congruence between applicant personality and the job as more critical in predicting suitability and expected job performance than actual past experience.

In summary, the program of research investigating the assessment of applicant personality traits in the employment interview conducted by Jackson and his colleagues in the 1980's contributed significantly to our understanding of how interviewers perceive and evaluate applicant personality characteristics. Interviewers were able to infer an implicit network of related traits from limited behavioral information with a high degree of reliability and accuracy. Judgments of job suitability were made that accurately reflected empirically derived personality profiles associated with occupational groups. These findings were replicated with different occupational groups and personality traits, and were found to be more important than applicant experience or general social desirability. This program of research also provides an excellent example of how a construct-oriented approach to personality assessment influences the design and conduct of the research, and ultimately the value of the research to theory development and practice. Jackson's interview research was grounded in psychological theory, first with regard to his use of implicit personality theory and impression formation theory, and secondly with regard to his use of theoretically derived constructs and measures of personality. The value of clearly defined personality constructs derived from sound psychological theory was apparent in the ability of subjects in these experiments to use the constructs to make appropriate decisions and identify broader inferential networks of related traits in an accurate manner. In addition, the use of personality constructs with demonstrated convergent and discriminant validity undoubtedly contributed to subjects' ability to understand the distinct meaning of each trait and make appropriate decisions as well. Finally, a concern for the potentially confounding effects of social desirability in personality measures provided the opportunity to demonstrate that this was not a problem when assessing construct valid traits in the employment interview.

More generally, research on the employment interview by Jackson and his colleagues has served to underline the viewpoint that, when used for personnel selection purposes, requisite personality traits can, and should, be closely linked to the requirements of the targeted job. As discussed in the following section, by incorporating this viewpoint into modern meta-analytic methods, the potential contribution of personality to the prediction of job performance has been greatly clarified.

THE INFLUENCE OF THE CONSTRUCT APPROACH ON META-ANALYTIC STUDIES OF PERSONALITY AND JOB PERFORMANCE

The advent of meta-analytic research methods in psychology has had a profound effect on a number of fields of research, not the least of which has been our understanding of relations between personality and job performance. Despite an early relatively unsophisticated (from a methodological viewpoint) quantitative review of personality-job performance relations undertaken by Ghiselli and Barthol (1953), in which an overall mean validity of .22 was reported, the prevailing "wisdom" of industrial-organizational psychologists until the mid-1980's was that the measurement of personality had no value for the prediction of job performance and therefore no usefulness for personnel selection. This view was reinforced by the influential qualitative review reported by Guion and Gottier (1965). In an early meta-analytic study of personality-job performance relations, Schmitt, Gooding, Noe, and Kirsch (1984) reported a sample-weighted mean correlation of .21, remarkably similar to results obtained by Ghiselli and Barthol (1953), although Schmitt et al. based their analysis on a limited sample of only 32 personality scale validities. However, a second more extensive meta-analytic study reported by Barrick and Mount (1991), in which personality scale validities were categorized in terms of the "Big Five" personality dimensions, obtained an overall corrected sample-weighted mean correlation of only .11, substantially lower than previous quantitative findings. On the basis of those inconsistent findings and a number of methodological problems with the earlier quantitative reviews, Tett, Jackson, and Rothstein (1991) undertook to conduct a new comprehensive meta-analysis of personality-job performance relations. Tett et al. obtained an overall sample-weighted mean correlation of .24 and substantially higher mean correlations when certain moderators were taken into account. Tett et al. concluded that, contrary to certain earlier reviews, there was grounds for optimism regarding the use of personality measures for predicting job performance in personnel selection.

The conceptual rationale for the Tett et al. (1991) study was fundamentally based on considerations of the principles associated with the construct-orientation to personality measurement. Although there were many objectives and features of the Tett et al. (1991) meta-analysis, they are too numerous to review here. Interested readers should consult the original sources for these details (Tett et al., 1991; Tett, Jackson, Rothstein, & Reddon, 1994; Tett, Jackson, Rothstein, & Reddon, 1999). For the purposes of this discussion, we will focus on three of their more critical objectives, which were initiated in response to the problems with previous meta-analyses, and which illustrate the value of applying principles of construct-oriented personality measurement to these problems; exploratory versus confirmatory research strategy as a moderator of validity; accommodating bidirectional relationships in meta-analysis; and, clarifying the relative importance of the Big Five personality variables in the prediction of job performance. We will first present the rationale for these three objectives, and then discuss the results obtained.

Exploratory versus Confirmatory Research Strategy as a Moderator of Validity Findings

Tett et al. (1991) distinguished between correlations derived from exploratory versus confirmatory research strategies and used this distinction as a moderator variable in their meta-analysis. One major problem Tett et al. identified with previous meta-analyses of personality-job performance relations was related to one of the earliest criticisms of personality-job performance research: the absence of a theoretical foundation for so much of the research in this area (Guion & Gottier, 1965). The primary research strategy was based solely on empirical considerations: typically, a personality inventory of convenience was administered to a group of job incumbents to determine if any scales correlated with measures of job performance. Using a theoretical or clear conceptual rationale for hypothesizing links between personality predictors and performance criteria directs researchers to think more clearly about the nature of the constructs under study and why they should be related, and therefore increases the likelihood of obtaining meaningful results. Conversely, studies of personality and job performance that lack any theoretical or conceptual rationale would be expected to underestimate the potential value of using personality measures in employee selection. Thus, meta-analyses of personality-job performance relations that ignore the distinction between exploratory and confirmatory research strategies can be expected to underestimate these relations. Tett et al. predicted that correlations based on a confirmatory strategy would yield a higher average validity than those based on an exploratory strategy and would provide a more meaningful estimate of the potential of personality measures for use in personnel selection.

Accommodating Bidirectional Relationships in Meta-analysis

The Tett et al. (1991) study broke new ground in addressing the problem of negative validities that they identified as being inherent to meta-analyses involving personality measures. Meta-analysis had previously been applied to psychological research examining relations between cognitive ability and job performance. Cognitive ability is unipolar in nature, and, in this realm, the adage "more is better" holds true. Consequently, correlations between cognitive ability and various work-related criteria are almost always positive. Accordingly, it was reasonable to assume that any negative correlations between cognitive ability and job performance criteria were attibutable to sampling fluctuations and should simply be averaged in "as is" with the positive values when computing the meta-analytic results. Personality traits, to the contrary, are almost always bipolar in nature, and, depending on the job in question, and the trait being studied, meaningful correlations may be either positive or negative. For example, affiliation has been shown to correlate positively with sales effectiveness but negatively with with creativity (Hough, 1992). Previous meta-analyses of personality-job performance ignored the issue of bidirectionality and averaged all negative and positive correlations, which as Tett et al. pointed out, would underestimate relations between these variables to an unknown degree.

In deriving a meta-analytic methodology to deal with the problem of bidirectional relationships, Tett et al. found that published source studies did not provide enough information regarding the nature of the job and/or the trait(s) being assessed to confidently decide whether a negative validity coefficient was conceptually meaningful and therefore veridical, or, obtained due to sampling error. It is well known that even when the population value of a correlation is positive, a certain proportion of negative values would be expected to occur due to sampling error. Thus, one could not simply assume that all observed negative validities were veridical and average their absolute values in with the obtained positive validities as this would upwardly bias the resulting estimates. Tett et al. therefore devised an innovation in the meta-analysis calculations whereby absolute values of correlations are averaged together, but a correction for upward bias is applied. This procedure is described in detail in Tett et al. (1991) with revisions reported in Tett, Jackson, Rothstein, and Reddon (1994, 1999). Tett et al. argued that without using absolute values and correcting for an upward bias when conducting meta-analyses with personality data, the results would fail to incorporate the inherent birectionality of personality-job performance relationships and would therefore be uninterpretable.

Clarifying the Relative Importance of the Big Five personality Variables

A third objective of the Tett et al. study was to clarify the relative importance of the Big Five personality content dimensions in predicting job performance. Barrick and Mount (1991) had previously sought to investigate the extent to which each of the Big Five personality traits (extroversion, emotional stability, agreeableness, conscientiousness, and openness to experience) were related to performance criteria. However, these authors failed to distinguish between exploratory and confirmatory research strategies, a factor that undoubtedly contributed to the relatively low overall mean validity (.11) they obtained. Tett et al. (1991) hypothesized that the average validity obtained from confirmatory studies only would exceed the validities reported by Barrick and Mount (1991) for the Big Five dimensions

What Does a Construct Approach Add to Meta-analysis of Personality-Job Performance Relations

All three of Tett et al.'s (1991) major objectives were conceptually based on principles associated with the construct approach to personality measurement. The emphasis on the value of confirmatory validation strategies is clearly related to the importance of psychological theory in personality measurement. Just as personality constructs should be derived from theory in order to enhance their meaningfulness and communicability (Burisch, 1984), theorizing about the relations between personality constructs and job performance is critical to further theory development and effective utilization of personality measures in personnel selection. Exploratory validation studies add little to our understanding of psychological theory, increase the likelihood of obtaining chance findings, are difficult to interpret and therefore use in personnel selection, and contribute to the underestimation of personality-job performance relations found in certain meta-analytic studies. Similarly, attempts to categorize personality constructs according to content dimensions such as the Big Five without considering the distinction between exploratory and confirmatory studies will also be of little value. Further problems inherent with the Big Five preoccupation that is evident in current personality research are discussed under "Broad versus Narrow Predictors of Job Performance." The second objective of the Tett et al. study, the accommodation of bidirectional relationships, may also be traced to a construct orientation. An appreciation of the meaning of negative validities with personality measures and their role in meta-analytic studies begins once again with understanding the theory underlying the measure as well as the research used in its development (e.g., demonstrations of its convergent and discriminant validity), which would illustrate meaningful negative relations with validation criteria. Thus, Tett et al.'s meta-analysis was fundamentally influenced by principles associated with the construct-orientation to personality measurement.

Results obtained by Tett et al. supported their main hypotheses and demonstrated the value of treating negative validities as meaningful data rather than random error in meta-analyses of personality-job performance relations. An overall sample-weighted corrected mean correlation of .24 was obtained, but mean validities derived from confirmatory studies were significantly greater (.29) than those derived from exploratory studies (.12). These results underscore the importance of a construct orientation to personality measurement generally and confirmatory validation strategies in particular. Exploratory validation strategies rely on chance findings, are less interpretable, and do not contribute to our understanding of the role of personality in predicting job performance. Clearly, including exploratory studies in meta-analyses of personality-job performance relations underestimates the value of personality measures for personnel selection. In addition, when confirmatory validation studies were classified according to the Big Five taxonomy, Tett et al. obtained overall stronger results than those reported by Barrick and Mount (1991). The overall mean validity obtained by Tett et al. for all Big Five dimensions was .24 compared to .11 reported by Barrick and Mount. Tett et al. concluded that the discrepancy between their results and those of Barrick and Mount must be attributable to combining exploratory and confirmatory studies and averaging positive and negative correlations in the Barrick and Mount meta-analysis. Tett et al. concluded further that studies of personality-job performance relations should be undertaken with careful consideration of potential trait-performance linkages using available psychological theory and trait-oriented job analysis. Only under these circumstances will the full potential of personality measures in personnel selection be realized.

Subsequent to the publication of Tett et al.'s meta-analysis, their findings were challenged by Ones, Mount, Barrick, and Hunter (1994) on both procedural and methodological grounds. Tett, Jackson, Rothstein, and Reddon (1994) replied to these criticisms and reanalyzed their data taking into consideration the methodological changes suggested by Ones et al. Although this resulted in a slightly lower overall mean validity (.24 in the reanalysis versus .29 in the original), Tett et al.'s (1991) main conclusions remained unchanged. The methodological issue involved revising the meta-analytic procedure to more accurately correct for the upward bias resulting from the use of absolute value correlations.

The most interesting part of the debate between Ones et al. and Tett et al. however, from the standpoint of discussing the impact of the construct-oriented approach to personality measurement, concerns the different perspectives taken on this issue in the debate. For example, Ones et al. argued that it was unnecessary to distinguish between exploratory and confirmatory research strategies. They believed that this distinction undermined the primary purpose of meta-anaysis, to test a hypothesis with adequate statistical power. Furthermore, they stated that the use of absolute value correlations and the statistical correction for upward bias were unnecessary. Ones et al. believed that negative values were statistically rare and should just be considered as normal sampling fluctuations. Tett et al. (1994) replied from the construct-oriented perspective. They argued that exploratory and confirmatory studies should not be combined solely to increase power and regardless of what such a procedure does to the interpretation of the results. Combining results from the two research strategies mixes spurious and potentially meaningless correlations with predicted, theoretically based findings, with the inevitable result of failing to test the hypothesis adequately that personality was related to job performance. Indeed, when such studies are combined, the result is a substantial underestimate of personality-job performance relations as demonstrated by Tett et al.'s (1991; 1994) results. In addition, Tett et al. (1994) argued both conceptually and empirically that negative validity coefficients could not all be considered due to sampling fluctuations. Tett et al. presented several concrete examples of meaningful negative correlations between personality and job performance measures effectively illustrating the need to understand the theoretical bipolarity of personality constructs. Empirically, Tett et al. demonstrated that in their meta-analysis, the number of observed negative validities exceeded the number expected by chance by a ratio of 2.5 to one. The corresponding ratio for significant negative correlations was 28.1 to one. Thus, Tett et al.'s meta-analysis demonstrated that the distinction between exploratory and confirmatory validation strategies, and an appreciation of the meaning of negative validity coefficients, were critical to determining accurately the nature and extent of personality-job performance relations. In doing so, Tett et al. also demonstrated the value of the construct orientation on the design and methodology of this research.

Tett, Jackson, Rothstein, and Reddon (1999a; 1999b) recently extended their meta-analytic investigations of personality and job performance by developing a modification of the standard meta-analysis procedure to account more accurately for bidirectional relationships. The procedure involved successive iterations of an initial estimate of the absolute correlation, accounting for sample sizes and the sampling distribution of the correlation, and resulted in a mean corrected validity coefficient of .30 for confirmatory studies, an increase over their previous estimate of .24 (Tett et al., 1994) but very close to their original estimate of .29 (Tett et al., 1991). Tett et al.'s modification of the meta-analysis procedure provides a more accurate estimate of personality-job performance relations and, has set the stage for a new generation of meta-analysis that accommodates the true bipolar nature of personality. Key principles underlying the construct orientation to personality assessment were critical contributions to the outcomes of this research.

Bidirectional Relationships as a Form of Trait-by-Situation Interaction

Tett et al. (1999b) point out that the existence of situational demands that moderate the direction of specific personality-job performance relations supports an interactionist framework for understanding how traits and situations combine to affect job behavior. An interactionist perspective could be used to predict when a particular personality trait would relate positively or negatively to different job performance criteria according to the work demands of the situation. Three levels of trait-relevant situational factors could determine work demands: task demands, work group demands, and organizational demands. Thus, a given personality trait may be relevant to either/or task, work group, or organizational demands. It is also possible that a trait that is relevant to one type of demand may also be a negative influence on a different type of work demand. This would complicate the validation process considerably and would require making a tradeoff in the selection decision.

Implications of Curvilinear Personality-Job Performance Relations

An additional potential complication with research in personality-job performance relations is that such relations may in some cases be curvilinear (Tett et al., 1999b). For example, if dominance is a trait relevant to managerial performance (e.g., Hogan, 1991), managers who are too low or too high in this trait may not achieve optimal levels of performance. The existence of potential situational demands and curvilinear relations, in addition to bidirectionality and type of research strategy, all contribute to the difficulty of interpreting meta-analyses of personality-job performance relations. These issues provide many challenges for future research in this area, but the construct orientation to personality measurement promises to continue to contribute conceptual insights and methodological rigor to this field.

An additional issue germane to the accurate meta-analytic estimation of the potential validity of personality variables in the prediction of job performance is the relative validity of different personality tests. This issue is discussed in detail, and an empirical demonstration is provided, in another chapter of this volume (Goffin et al., 1999).

We turn now to a discussion of issues of particular relevance to the conduct of primary research involving personality in personnel selection.

USING PERSONALITY MEASURES IN PERSONNEL SELECTION

Despite the considerable accumulated evidence for the validity of using personality measures for personnel selection, the practice of determining which measures to use and evaluating their validity for selection purposes has still attracted criticism from some researchers. In addition, even among those who accept that personality may be an important predictor of job performance, there has been a good deal of controversy regarding the most appropriate personality measures for use in personnel selection. In this section, we review some of the typical criticisms of personality testing for personnel selection and discuss a major controversy regarding the appropriateness of using broad versus narrow predictors of job performance. In doing so, we highlight once again the important role of the construct approach to personality measurement in answering these criticisms and providing a theoretically and empirically sound argument in support of using narrow rather than broad personality predictors of job performance.

Common Criticisms of Personality Testing

Criticisms of the use of personality measures for personnel selection often focus on one or more of the following concerns (e.g., Blinkhorn & Johnson, 1990;

Christiansen, Goffin, Rothstein, & Johnston, 1994): (1) certain personality measures or inventories are identified as psychometrically inadequate and therefore are incapable of predicting job performance criteria with any acceptable degree of reliability or validity; (2) validity coefficients for personality measures are too low to contribute in any meaningful way to the prediction of job performance; (3) validation research involving personality measures produces spurious validity coefficients due to capitalizing on chance factors including small sample sizes, the use of correlated predictors, and inappropriate statistical analyses; and (4) personality tests are susceptible to applicant faking, alternatively referred to dissimulation or motivated distortion, and this renders personality tests invalid. As discussed below, Jackson and Rothstein (1993) succinctly provided a response to the first three of these criticisms from the construct-oriented perspective, whereas the fourth criticism constitutes an ongoing area of research activity and will be addressed in a separate section.

First, Jackson and Rothstein (1993) pointed out that the identification of psychometric inadequacies in one, or a small number of personality measures, is insufficient evidence for drawing conclusions regarding the field as a whole. Certainly, personality measures must demonstrate independent evidence for acceptable levels of reliability and validity, and where such evidence is lacking, these personality measures would be inappropriate for use in personnel selection. In the Jacksonian tradition (Jackson, 1970, 1971), we believe that conclusions about personality-job performance relations must be based on personality measures that have first shown evidence for construct validity, including substantive links between items and the underlying theoretical construct, and evidence of convergent and discriminant validity (i.e., key principles of the construct orientation to personality assessment). Chapter 11 of this volume (Goffin et al., 1999) corroborates this viewpoint by providing empirical evidence that a personality test developed following Jacksonian principles may have superior levels of criterion-related validity.

The appropriate interpretation of a validity coefficient, in particular its magnitude, is critical to understanding the fallacy of the second criticism of personality measures used in personnel selection (Jackson and Rothstein, 1993). First, as Tett et al. (1991; 1994; 1999) have demonstrated, a number of meta-analyses of personality-job performance relations have substantially underestimated the magnitude of these relations due to averaging positive and negative correlations and failing to distinguish between exploratory and confirmatory validation strategies. Second, validity coefficients are attenuated by numerous artifacts (e.g., predictor and criterion unreliability, restriction of range) that realistically limit the ability of a validity study to obtain correlations of substantial magnitude. Third, the most meaningful evaluation of any selection system is based not solely on the validity of individual predictors, but rather on the combined incremental validity of the entire selection system and the utility of this system as measured in financial benefit (see Cascio, 1982) to an organization. In this regard it is relevant that validity coefficents of the magnitude found by Tett et al. (1991, 1994, 1999) can translate into substantial economic gains. Moreover, personality traits have been shown to provide significant incremental predictive variance when employed in combination with other commonly-used selection methods such as cognitive ability testing and the assessment center (see Goffin, Rothstein, & Johnston, 1996, for a review). Thus, low validity coefficients do not necessarily mean that personality assessment has no value in personnel selection. In fact, these correlations must be interpreted in the context of the above factors, the first of which could be largely remedied through greater consideration of the construct approach to personality assessment.

Notwithstanding the previous discussion, the possibility of spurious validity coefficients must be acknowledged. However, as Jackson and Rothstein (1993) have noted, this problem is simply not relevant to the research question of whether or not personality measures predict job performance. Evaluating the validity of personality measures for selection purposes requires appropriate statistical procedures.   There are well known statistical methods of correcting for capitalization on chance factors and the problem of multiple correlated predictors. In addition, the use of distinct personality constructs (demonstrated by evidence for convergent and discriminant validity) and a confirmatory validation strategy, again, key features of the construct orientation, will decrease the probability of obtaining spurious validity coefficients.

Faking and Personality Assessment in Personnel Selection

The possibility of applicants faking their responses to personality tests being used in personnel selection has been a major concern for quite some time (Christiansen et al., 1994; Hough, Eaton, Dunnette, Kamp, & McCloy, 1990). Supporting this sentiment, a survey of experienced I/O professionals revealled that 75% of the respondents would prefer to use personality scores that have been subjected to a correction for faking (Goffin, Christiansen, Johnston & Rothstein, 1994). To some extent, it is axiomatic that faking of personality test responses occurs in personnel selection. Given that (a) applicants are competing intensely for highly desired outcomes (e.g., employment); (b) many personality inventories are sufficiently transparent that the most beneficial responses to many items seem obvious to many applicants; and (c) there is typically no apparent means through which the honesty of applicants' personality item responses can be verified; faking might be construed as rational, although not commendable, goal-directed behavior. Although surprisingly little published field research has actually addressed the question of whether faking of personality tests does, indeed, occur in personnel selection, the research which does exist provides support for researchers' and practitioners' suspicions as to the severity of this problem (e.g., Rosse, Stecher, Levin and Miller, 1998).

Concerns about faking have motivated a wide-range of measurement innovations, which can be broadly categorized as descriptive, corrective or preventive.

Addressing the Problem of Faking: Descriptive Approaches

Descriptive approaches to addressing the faking problem involve trying to measure the degree to which faking has occurred. A variety of scales have been developed over the years in an effort to achieve this, or the related goal, of measuring the extent to which responses have been affected by socially desirable responding. Seminal work by Jackson and Messick (1958, 1961, 1962) was instrumental in providing a unifying framework for discussing the measurement of response styles such as socially desirable responding (see Chapter 2 in this volume for a detailed discussion of the social desirability issue). Work by Paulhus (1991), culminating in the development of the Balananced Inventory of Desirable Responding (BIDR), has done much to clarify the possible bidimensional nature of social desirability. Specificially, Paulhus has supported the contention that one facet of socially desirable responding can be termed self-deception (i.e., a *subconscious* tendency to describe oneself in favorable terms), whereas the second facet, referred to as impression management, refers to a tendency by test-takers to *deliberately* distort their responses in a manner that will enhance others' impressions of them. It is the latter facet that is presumed to underlie faking, whereas the former may be a personality trait in itself. Paulhus (1991) and Helmes (1999, chapter 2 of this volume) provide excellent summaries of this work so we will not replicate their efforts here. Interestingly, Holden and colleagues (1995; Holden & Kroner, 1992) have suggested a means of detecting faking that is based on test-takers' item response latencies. With few exceptions (e.g., Holden, 1995), personnel selection researchers appear to have largely overlooked the use of this approach. Presumably, if sufficiently valid measures of faking could be derived, personnel selection practitioners could at least be aware of who is, or is not, responding honestly and consider certain actions in the case of the latter group (e.g., not using their personality scores; or, informing them that they are suspected of faking their responses and asking them to retake the test). Nonetheless, even if scales that accurately measure the degree to which faking has occurred can be derived, this does not, in itself, completely solve the problem of faking. Consequently, interest has been focused on corrective and preventive measures that purport to attenuate the effects of faking.

Addressing the Problem of Faking: Corrective Approaches

Corrective measures consist of first trying to assess the extent to which faking has occurred using the descriptive approach. Next, trait scores are "corrected." Common "correction" formulas (e.g, Cattell, Eber, & Tatsuoka, 1970) are based on the premise that any variance trait scales share with scales purporting to measure faking should be partialled out in order to purify the respective scores. Unfortunately, existing empirical evidence suggests that the use of corrective faking measures in personnel selection fails to improve the validity of the personality scores (e.g., Christiansen et al., 1994; Ellingson, Sackett, & Hough, 1999). The failure of such measures is likely due to one or more of the following two factors. First, scales that are currently interpreted as measures of faking may not be valid. Arguably, it is only impression management that should be corrected for, whereas, many of the faking scales upon which corrections are based consist of a mixture of impression management and self-deception. As far as we are aware, no published work in the area of personnel selection has yet assessed the effect of basing a faking correction on the Paulhus (1991) impression management scale; thus, there is an important gap to be filled by future research. However, it is conceivable that even relatively pure impression management scales may not validly reflect the true degree of faking that has occurred due to a variety of reasons. For example, faking may be a complex behavior that is manifested in noticeably different patterns of responding depending upon individual differences among the applicants. Also, the nature of the job that applicants are applying for may affect the specific form that faking takes (e.g., Norman, 1967). Consequently, it is possible that the goal of a "universal" faking scale (e.g., impression management) that is suitable for use in any selection situation may be unattainable. Clearly, additional work studying and explicating the construct of faking as it relates to personality testing in personnel selection is necessary at this time.

A second possible reason for the failure of corrective faking measures to improve the validity of personality measures may be that common faking corrections (e.g., Cattell et al., 1970) treat faking much like a suppressor variable; however, statistically, it has been shown that the gain in predictive validity that can possibly be realized by taking suppressors into account is miniscule in the case of validity coefficients of the size that are typically seen in personnel selection, even if the suppressor correlates reasonably well with the predictor (Conger & Jackson, 1972). Supporting Conger and Jackson's (1972) conclusions, Christiansen et al. (1994) found that the faking correction used in the 16PF had essentially no effect on predictive validity. Interestingly, even though faking corrections appear to have a trivial effect on predictive validity, they can have consequential effects in determining who gets hired and who does not. (see Christiansen et al., 1994). A procedure that affects hiring decisions while not having sound empirical evidence to support its use could prove difficult to defend in today's litigious workplace.

Addressing the Problem of Faking: Preventive Approaches

Preventive approaches to dealing with faking seek to lower or eliminate respondents' tendency to dissimulate their item responses from the start rather than applying corrections.   We are aware of three primary preventive approaches, faking warnings, forced-choice items, and items with neutral levels of desirability.

The first approach to prevent faking within the context of personnel selection, the use of a faking warning, typically consists of informing test-takers that faking can be detected through sophisticated (but undisclosed) means.   Test-takers may also be warned that if evidence of faking is found in their responses, it could have a counterproductive effect with respect to their likelihood of being hired (Goffin & Woods, 1995).   Braun and Constantini's (1970) results suggested that a faking warning may aid in controlling the faking of personality test respones within a basic research context.   Schrader and Osburn's (1977) and Doll's (1971) conclusions were similar to Braun and Constantini's but pertained to biodata instruments rather than personality tests.   Jackson (1984) reported that no significant differences existed in PRF scores of groups that were instructed to fake good, respond honestly, and fake good with a faking warning, however, small sample sizes hinders a clear interpretation of his results.   To our knowledge only one published empirical work has assessed the efficacy of faking warnings in the control of faking on personality tests in a typical personnel selection scenario (Goffin & Woods, 1995).   Goffin and Woods found that a faking warning reduced but did not eliminate faking and suggested that much additional research is called for in order to explore different versions of the faking warning, and different target jobs, and to allow the generalization of their results to a variety of target jobs and respondent groups.   The paucity of published research on faking warnings is puzzling given its apparent success and the relative ease with which it can be applied.   One possible concern with the faking warning is the potential for deception.   It could be a violation of professional ethics to suggest to job applicants that faking can be detected, if, in fact, such a feat is impossible.   Thus, ethical application of the faking warning may ultimately be dependent upon the further development of the descriptive approach for addressing faking (described earlier).

The second approach taken to prevent faking, the use of forced-choice items, involves changing the usual format by which applicants respond to test items. Typically personality tests require test-takers to respond in terms of whether or not, or, to what extent, a single statement or adjective is descriptive of them.   By contrast, typical forced-choice items involve presenting statements in pairs, triplets, or quartets that have been matched in terms of desirability, but differ in terms of the traits that they are indicative of.   The respondent's task is then to indicate which statement is the most self-descriptive, and in the case of item quartets, the respondent is also asked to choose the least self-descriptive statement. Presumably, because the items have been matched in terms of desirability level, test-takers will see no advantage in faking their responses and will therefore respond honestly. Two well-known examples of the forced choice technique are the Edwards Personal Preference Schedule (1959) and the Gordon Personal Inventory (1956).

Unfortunately, thus far, forced-choice formats have failed to live up to their promise of eliminating faking (Anastasi, 1982). When instructed to do so, relatively naive participants are able to change their scores in desired directions on forced-choice inventories (Borislow, 1958; Dicken, 1959). The Achilles' heel of this approach appears to stem from the manner in which the desirability ratings, by which items are matched, are arrived at. Ordinarily, these ratings are obtained simply by asking a group of individuals to consider each statement, one at a time (i.e., each single statement or adjective used in the pairs or quartets of forced-choice items), in terms of how desirable (or undesirable) it is. Unfortunately, to say that two statements are matched in terms of general desirability level is not equivalent to saying that they are matched in terms of desirability with respect to a particular job. What is perceived to be a desirable for an engineer may not be so perceived with respect to a salesperson, and both may differ from what is perceived to be generally desirable in the population at large, which provides the benchmark for matching the statements. Any perceived lack of equivalence, by job applicants, in the desirability levels of the paired statements with respect to the particular job they are applying for, is likely to engender response distortion. Such distortion might be minimized through a modification of the standard forced-choice approach. Specifically, one could tailor the desirability matching of the statements to the specific job or occupation that the scale would eventually be used to make selection decisions for. To some extent, Jackson, Wroblewski, and Ashton (1999) incorporated this approach, and their results suggested that this method may serve to reduce faking and improve predictive validity beyond that which was achieved through using a non-forced-choice version of the same set of items. Carefully tailoring the desirability matching of forced-choice statements to a specific target job is worthy of further consideration by future researchers.

The fact that perceived desirability of statements can change as a function of the particular statements that they are paired with presents an additional challenge with respect to the accurate desirability matching of statements in forced-choice items (Anastasi, 1982). Perhaps more sophisticated desirability rating procedures that borrow from the tradition of multidimensional scaling could serve to ameliorate this problem.

The third approach taken to prevent faking involves the use of items with neutral levels of desirability. On the basis of several studies (e.g., Jackson, 1960; Jackson & Messick, 1961, 1962), Jackson and colleagues have been instrumental in demonstrating that one of the most predominant sources of variance in typical personality test scores is social desirability. Furthermore, although we do not believe that faking and socially desirable responding are one and the same, to the extent that personality test items elicit socially desirable responding, they are more likely to elicit faking (in addition to having lower construct validity). It follows that one way to attenuate motivated response distortion within personnel selection applications of personality testing would be to use personality test items that do not correlate highly, either positively or negatively, with measures of social desirability. Beginning with the PRF, Jackson (1970) devised an elaborate system of personality test construction that maximizes relevant trait saturation of personality test items while minimizing variance due to social desirability (see Chapter 2 of this volume for more details on this approach). We are aware of no published personnel selection studies that explicitly evaluate the use of items with neutral desirability levels in terms of the resistance to faking it gives rise to, however, the theoretical rationale supporting this approach should be sufficiently persuasive to motivate such work in earnest. An extension of this research could assess the possibility raised above that desirability ratings of items may, to some extent, be specific to the particular job that the applicants are being selected for.

In sum, as of yet, there is no single solution to the problem of faking in personnel selection applications of personality testing. Nonetheless, there is much to recommend both the descriptive and preventive approaches to addressing this problem. Ideally, preventive measures should be employed wherever possible, and their efficacy assessed using descriptive faking scales, provided that construct valid faking scales can be derived. With respect to preventive measures, the faking warning, presented in combination with forced-choice items or items of neutral desirability level would appear to be an effective strategy. Given that the development of effective forced-choice items can be an extremely laborious process, this approach might best be reserved for measuring traits that are inherently desirable, or undesirable, for which items of neutral desirability level are extremely challenging to derive (e.g., depression, anxiety, deviation, interpersonal problems, honesty). Based on existing research, (Christiansen et al., 1994; Ellingson et al., 1999) and relevant statistical considerations (Conger & Jackson, 1972) we are less sanguine as to the potential efficacy of using faking corrections.

It is important to point out at this juncture that the utility of personality testing for personnel selection applications would appear to be considerable *despite* the problem of faking. The meta-analyses discussed earlier (Barrick & Mount, 1991; Tett et al., 1991), which ultimately support the use of personality testing in personnel selection, included many predictive valildity studies in which the motivation to fake would clearly have been present. Sophisticated application of the faking countermeasures discussed above is likely to be rewarded by higher estimated validity coefficients in future meta-analyses. Additionally, as illustrated below, greater capitalization on the essential principles of the construct orientation to personality measurement could do much to enhance the utility of personality testing in personnel selection applications.

Recent I/O Studies Incorporating the Construct Orientation to Personality Assessment

Two recent studies illustrate how the essential principles derived from the construct orientation to personality measurement may be applied to studies of personality-job performance relations. In these two studies confirmatory strategies were used to guide the choice of personality measures such that the personality constructs and performance criteria could be explicitly linked in conceptual terms to maximize the probability of determining the validity of the personality measures. The formulation of conceptual links between predictors and criteria has been termed a "predictive hypothesis" by Guion (1991) who, in the context of arguing for the need to employ sound theoretical formulations to guide personnel selection research (see also Dunnette, 1982), particularly emphasized the importance of explicitly specifying the theoretical links between measures of personality constructs and job performance criteria in predictive research. The importance of using a predictive hypothesis in investigating personality-job performance relations is also a key component of the construct-oriented approach to personality scale development and validation, and has been empirically supported by Tett et al. (1991; 1994; 1999) who found substantially higher validities when confirmatory research strategies were used.

In both studies to be discussed, personality measures were used to predict behavior related to managerial performance criteria. A review of the research literature examining the contribution of personality traits to managerial job performance determined that there were theoretical and empirical grounds for hypothesizing that the personality traits of achievement, dominance, and extroversion would be related to general managerial performance (e.g., Brenner, 1982; Hanson & Harrell, 1985; Harrell, Harrell, McIntyre, & Weinberg, 1987; Hogan, 1991; Howard & Bray, 1988; Wertheim, Widom, & Wortzel, 1978). This constituted the predictive hypothesis in both research studies.

In the first study (Rothstein, Paunonen, Rush, & King, 1994), measures of cognitive ability and personality were obtained from 450 students enrolled in an MBA program. Students' GPA after the first year in the program was used as the performance criterion. Grade Point Average was determined by two distinct components. Evaluation of exams and written reports constituted one component of each course grade, and evaluation of students' contributions to class discussion constituted the other component of the grade. The written component of GPA was based on a demonstration of content knowledge and skill in analyzing business problems. It was hypothesized, therefore, that cognitive ability would be the best predictor of this component of GPA. Contributions to class discussion, rated independently by instructors in each course, was evaluated on the basis of students' ability to articulate their understanding of the business problem and to persuade others to accept their analysis and recommendations. This component of GPA was hypothesized to be related to the personality measures of achievement, dominance, and exhibition (a key facet of the broader trait of extroversion), which had been previously linked with managerial performance. The average interrater reliability of the classroom performance criterion was .88, indicating a high degree of agreement on how class contributions should be evaluated.

Results from this study supported the hypotheses. As predicted, cognitive ability was a better predictor of the written component of GPA, whereas the hypothesized personality traits were better predictors of classroom performance. A cross validation design was used to guard against interpreting spurious statistical effects. Specifically, although cognitive ability contributed to the prediction of classroom performance to some extent (.21), it was a better predictor of the written component of GPA (.37). Conversely, all three of the hypothesized personality variables were significantly related to classroom performance (achievement = .21; dominance = .23; exhibition = .33; all p < .001) whereas none of these personality traits were related to the written component of GPA.

In the second study illustrative of the construct orientation in research design (Goffin, Rothstein, & Johnston, 1996), assessment center (AC) evaluations, personality measures, and performance criteria were obtained from a sample of 68 first level supervisors in a large forestry products organization as part of a formal assessment program for these employees to determine their promotability. The AC consisted of five independent exercises and was designed and operated according to professional standards for assessment centers.   Candidates were evaluated against six AC dimensions: planning and organizing, coaching, results orientation, willingness to learn, team orientation, and communication skills. Participants had been selected into managerial positions from a larger group of 700 individuals assessed over a four year period.   Performance criteria consisted of supervisory ratings using Relative Percentile Method scales (Goffin, Gellatly, Paunonen, Jackson, & Meyer, 1996; Wagner & Goffin, 1997). An overall job performance score was obtained by summing ratings across all performance appraisal dimensions.   It was hypothesized that the stereotypical managerial personality traits of achievement, dominance, and exhibition would contribute significantly to the prediction of overall managerial performance, and that these personality measures would have incremental validity over that of the AC alone.

Results from this study indicated that the use of personality measures in predicting job performance resulted in significant incremental validity over that of the assessment centeralthough the converse was also true. In other words, Goffin et al. (1996) determined that personality and assessment center measures each predicted unique components of variance in the job performance ratings. Combining both sets of measures produced the best prediction of overall job performance (shrunken R^2 = .34).

Results from the two studies discussed illustrate the value of a construct orientation to personality assessment in a number of ways.   The personality measures used in both these studies were taken from Jackson's (1984) Personality Research Form (PRF), an inventory developed according to a construct-oriented strategy. PRF scales exhibit high levels of construct validity and allow a rigorous testing of hypotheses concerning personality-job performance relations.   As discussed previously, without the use of valid personality measures, attempts to predict job performance will inevitably underestimate the magnitude of the relations. In addition, these two studies demonstrate the importance of a predictive hypothesis and a confirmatory research strategy.   Rather than administer an inventory of many personality variables to "explore" relations with managerial job performance, previous theory and research was employed to hypothesize likely relations. This approach allowed the researchers to maximize the power of their statistical analyses and resulted in meaningful and interpretable findings that supported the theoretical formulations that were the basis of the original predictions. Finally, these results support the meta-analytic findings of Tett et al. (1991;   1994;   1999)   and   strongly   support   their   "construct-oriented" recommendations that a confirmatory research strategy (containing predictive hypotheses) is beneficial for examining personality-job performance relations in order to determine the full potential of personality traits for predicting job performance.

Having established that a confirmatory research strategy is beneficial, the next logical step is to derive a job analytic methodology by which the personality requirements of jobs can be determined. Although some traditional job analytic methods consider certain personality traits (e.g., Position Analysis Questionnaire; McCormick, Jeanneret, & Mecham, 1969; Threshold Traits Analysis; Lopez, Kesselman, & Lopez, 1981), such attempts have been limited in terms of their coverage of the domain of personality. Crediting Jackson for drawing attention to this issue, Raymark, Schmit, and Guion (1997) have undertaken an important first step in the development of a personality-oriented job analysis methodology. Much further development along these lines is required before the full potential of using personality testing in I/O psychology can be realized.

In addition to furthering the careful matching of personality traits to job requirements, as discussed in the following section, the construct-oriented viewpoint to personality assessment in I/O psychology also has much to say about the potential usefulness of broad versus narrow traits in the prediction of criteria.

Broad versus Narrow Personality Predictors

Most researchers and practitioners in industrial-organizational psychology now accept that personality can contribute to the prediction of relevant job performance criteria and therefore may be useful in personnel selection. No such consensus exists, however, on the type of personality traits that are most appropriate and useful for determining personality-job performance relations. In particular, a considerable debate has evolved concerning the relative merits of using broad versus narrow personality predictors of job performance. The construct-oriented perspective has been particularly relevant to this debate and has provided the framework for theoretical and empirically-based arguments in support of the position that narrow, specific personality traits are more appropriate for predicting job performance than broad, multidimensional personality factors. In this section, we review the key features of this debate and argue that principles underlying the construct orientation to personality measurement have had a significant impact on supporting the superiority of narrow, specific personality traits as predictors of job performance criteria.

Previously, we discussed the critical importance of using personality measures for predicting job performance only if these measures have demonstrated convincing evidence of construct validity. Where such evidence is lacking, these measures cannot be expected to correlate meaningfully with criterion measures of any kind. Personality measures found to be unreliable and/or confounded (theoretically or methodologically) with other variables will have limited value as predictors of job performance. Empirical validities obtained with such measures must also be unstable and/or uninterpretable. We contend that the Big Five personality dimensions, the most prevalent and widely cited taxonomy of broad personality constructs, has not demonstrated adequate independent evidence for construct validity. Therefore, empirical validities obtained with the Big Five cannot be interpreted as demonstrating meaningful relationships between personality and job performance.

Articulating the theoretical and methodological problems with the Big Five is critical to understanding why such broad personality constructs are inferior to specific traits as predictors of job performance. Block (1995) has provided a thorough review and critique of research underlying the Big Five and we summarize five critical problems from his analysis that pertain specifically to using the Big Five for personnel selection purposes:

> There has never been a theoretical basis for deriving the Big Five factors, or for interpreting them as the underlying structure of personality. No hypotheses guided the prediction of what factors would emerge, why these factors (as opposed to any other set), or why five (rather than any other number). Briggs (1989) concluded his

analysis of this issue by stating that "a coherent and falsifiable explanation for the five factors has yet to be put forward" (p. 249).

Justification for the Big Five taxonomy has relied on exploratory factor analytic studies. There has been no consistent basis for determining the number of factors to extract or the particular rotation method to apply. Researchers have employed different assumptions, preferences, and unstated decision rules to determine the factor structure of their data sets. Consequently, there has been wide disagreement on the number of factors underlying the structure of personality. Indeed, programmatic research, sometimes spanning decades, has been based on the "Big Two" (Wiggins, 1968), the "Big Three" (Eysenck, 1991), the "Big Six" (Hogan, 1986), the "Big Seven" (Jackson, 1984), and the "Big Nine" (Hough, 1992) – and this list is not exhaustive. There is no evidence to indicate that any of these taxonomies provide a better or worse theoretical explanation or empirical justification for an underlying structure of personality than the Big Five (Block, 1995).

An additional very serious problem with factor analytic studies used to identify the Big Five structure is the prior "prestructuring" of the variables used in the analyses. Block (1995) carefully reviewed all of the primary research studies purporting to identify the Big Five factors (Tupes & Christal, 1961; Norman, 1963; Goldberg, 1990; McCrae & Costa, 1985) and found that in all these studies certain personality variables were preselected for inclusion in the analyses and other variables were specifically excluded, or thrown out of the analyses if they could not be fit within the Five Factor structure, or simply ignored. Such systematic prestructuring has constructed or imposed a Five Factor solution on the data set. These methodological procedures cast serious doubt on the ability of the Big Five to represent the underlying structure of personality. For example, traits such as risk-taking, locus of control, and rugged individualism, all of which have demonstrated utility in predicting relevant criteria (Ashton 1998; Hough, 1992; Mikulay & Goffin, 1998) do not clearly map onto the Big Five.

Research underlying the development of the most widely cited Big Five inventory, the NEO-PI (Costa &McCrae, 1992), which was designed to measure the Big Five constructs directly rather than through factor analysis of specific traits, is also seriously flawed (Block, 1995). The scale construction strategy does not adequately assess or control for the potentially confounding effects of response biases such as social desirability, a problem that plagues a majority of personality measures (Hopkins, Stanley, & Hopkins, 1990).   In addition, the factor structure of the NEO-PI does not consistently fit the hypothesized dimensions, which are expected to be orthogonal. In fact, the NEO-PI factors are substantially intercorrelated (Costa & McCrae, 1992).   Thus, the research on the NEO-PI provides little evidence for the validity of the Big Five constructs.

To summarize, the Big Five personality taxonomy represents the most widely known and highly cited example of broad personality constructs. However, from the perspective of a construct-oriented critique, we contend that evidence for the existence of the Big Five is unreliable and confounded. There is no theoretical basis for postulating five particular factors underlying the structure of personality and there are many competing theories and equal empirical support for many other taxonomies. The empirically derived factor structure repeatedly fails to maintain its expected orthogonality or to replicate across subject samples. Identification of the Big Five factor structure has relied on repeated systematic prestructuring of the data set. If there is no theoretical basis for the Big Five, and evidence for this taxonomy is inadequate, clearly the use of Big Five constructs as predictors of job performance will have limited meaningfulness.

Previously, we argued that meta-analyses of personality-job performance relations that ignored bidirectionality and type of research strategy (i.e., confirmatory vs. exploratory) in the source studies (e.g., Barrick & Mount, 1991), produced results that were uninterpretable. Barrick and Mount (1991) employed the Big Five as an organizing framework for their meta-analysis in an attempt to draw conclusions as to which of the Big Five factors were better overall predictors of job performance. In light of the present discussion of the questionable value of the Big Five constructs as predictors of job performance, this is likely an additional reason for the substantially different results obtained from the meta-analyses performed by Barrick and Mount (1991) versus Tett et al. (1991; 1994; 1999). The explicit rationale underlying the Tett et al. meta-analyses, based fundamentally on principles associated with the construct approach to personality measurement, was that specific job requirements demand specific personality traits to maximize prediction, and that these specific relations, hypothesized in the context of a *confirmatory* research strategy, would be greater than relations with broad personality factors such as the Big Five, assuming the use of construct valid personality measures and reliable and differentiated performance criteria. Tett et al.'s meta-analytic results supported their contention that specific personality traits linked to specific performance criteria with a predictive hypothesis would be better predictors of job performance than would broad personality dimensions. Thus, although Tett et al. considered the Big Five in their research, this was done within the context of a demonstration that narrow traits were better predictors of job performance than broad measures such as the Big Five.

The rationale for Tett et al.'s approach to their meta-analysis of personality-job performance relations as well as their results concerning the superior predictability of specific versus broad personality measures, is further supported by measurement theory. Schonemann (1990) and Velicer and Jackson (1990) have demonstrated that it is theoretically possible for all of the predictive variance in a set of measures to be contained in the specificity and none in the common factor variance. These authors acknowledge that although this is an empirical question in each instance, the important point is that a single measure is not identical with a factor to which it might be related. When that variable is identified through conceptual analysis to be related to a criterion measure, there is good reason to evaluate its validity distinctly from the common factor. If it is assumed that the common factor variance is all that is important, valuable information regarding personality-job performance relations may be overlooked and/or the validity coefficient with a broad personality factor such as one of the Big Five dimensions will underestimate the role of personality. Similarly, meta-analyses using broad personality dimensions such as the Big Five taxonomy will aggregate validities from different traits because they load on a common factor, perhaps obscuring the unique or stronger variance that may be predicted from one of these traits. Whether or not individual personality traits may predict job performance better than the factor in which the trait is a part must be investigated further and empirically. In the study reviewed earlier regarding the prediction of performance in an MBA program, Rothstein et al. (1994) also compared the prediction of the classroom performance criterion with a single personality trait versus the Big Five factor in which the trait was related. For example, the trait of achievement correlated .21 (p < .001) with the criterion, whereas the factor of conscientiousness did not correlate significantly at all. Similarly, the trait of exhibition correlated .33 (p < .001) with classroom performance, and although the factor of extroversion also correlated .19 (p < .001) with the criterion, exhibition was significantly greater than extroversion in predictive ability. These results support the contention that narrow personality traits are superior to broad measures for personnel selection and the results are also consistent with the meta-analytic findings of Tett et al. Although clearly, considerably more research is needed in this area to determine the relative merits of broad versus narrow personality measures, some recently published studies have been highly supportive of the conclusion that narrow specific measures of personality are better predictors of job performance criteria than measures of broad multidimensional factors (Ashton, Jackson, Paunonen, Helmes, & Rothstein, 1995; Paunonen, 1998; Paunonen, Rothstein, & Jackson, 1999).

The debate on the relative merits of broad versus narrow personality predictors of job performance once again illustrates the value of the construct orientation to personality measurement. Research undertaken from the construct-oriented perspective is fundamentally driven by psychological theory. Personality measures used in construct-oriented research must be clearly defined and consistent with the theoretical formulation of the construct.   Such measures must demonstrate independent evidence of convergent and discriminant validity, and must not be confounded with stylistic or method variance.   Research undertaken with this perspective has contributed substantially to the evidence supporting the use of specific measures of personality rather than broad multidimensional measures to predict job performance. Broad measures of personality, in particular those based on the Big Five taxonomy, have been shown to have no compelling theoretical basis. Measures developed on the basis of broad constructs such as the Big Five have not been consistently defined, lack evidence for convergent and discriminant validity, and do not show adequate concern for the confounding effects of social desirability. Thus, construct-oriented research strongly supports the use of specific measures of personality for predicting job performance in personnel selection.

CONCLUSIONS

In this chapter we have reviewed the contributions of construct-oriented personality assessment to several areas of research and practice in industrial-organizational psychology. We have illustrated how construct-driven assessment strategies have: (1) increased our understanding of how employment interviewers perceive and evaluate applicant personality characteristics; (2) improved the accuracy of meta-analytic procedures for estimating the potential validity of personality-job performance relations; and (3) provided a more compelling theoretical rationale and rigorous methodological approach to determining the most appropriate personality measures and validation procedures for use in personnel selection. As research continues in these and other areas in industrial-organizational psychology, the construct approach promises to continue to contribute to theory development and more effective applications in this field.

REFERENCES

Allen, N. J., & Meyer, J. P. (1999). The construct approach in organizational behavior research: The case of organizational commitment. In R.D. Goffin and E. Helmes (Eds.) *Problems and Solutions in Human Assessment*. Norwell, MA: Kluwer Academic Press.

Anastasi, A. (1988). *Psychological Testing*. New York, NY: Macmillan.

Ashton, M.C. (1998). Personality and job performance: The importance of narrow traits. *Journal of Organizational Behavior, 19*, 289-303.

Ashton, M.C., Jackson, D.N., Paunonen, S.V., Helmes, E., & Rothstein, M.G. (1995). The criterion validity of broad factor scales versus specific facet scales. *Journal of Research in Personality, 29*, 432-442.

Barrick, M. R., & Mount, M. K. (1991). The big five personality dimensions and job performance: A meta-analysis. *Personnel Psychology, 44*, 1-25.

Black, J.M. (1970). *How to Get Results from Interviewing*. New York: McGraw-Hill.

Blinkhorn, S. & Johnson, C. (1990). The significance of personality testing. *Nature, 348*, 671-672.

Block, J. (1995). A contrarian view of the five-factor approach to personality description. *Psychological Bulletin, 117*, 187-215.

Braun, J. R., & Constantini, A. (1970). Faking and faking detection on the Personality Research Form, AA. *Journal of Clinical Psychology*, **26**, 516-518.

Brenner, D.C. (1982). Relationship of education to sex, managerial status, and the managerial stereotype. *Journal of Applied Psychology*, **67**, 380-383.

Briggs, S.R. (1989). The optimal level of measurement for personality constructs. In D.M. Buss & N. Cantor (Eds.), *Personality psychology: Recent trends and emerging directions* (pp.246-260). New York: Springer.

Campbell, J.P., Dunnette, M.D., Lawleer, E.E., & Weick, K.E. (1970). *Managerial Behavior, Performance, and Effectiveness*. New York: McGraw-Hill.

Cascio, W.F. (1982). *Costing human resources: The financial impact of behavior in organizations*. Boston: Kent.

Cattell, R.B., Eber, H.W., & Tatsuoka, M.M, (1970). *Handbook for Sixteen Personality Factor Questionnaire (16PF)*. Champaign, IL: Institute for Personality and Ability Testing.

Christiansen, N. D., Goffin, R.D., Johnston, N. G., & Rothstein, M. G. (1994). Correcting the 16PF for faking: Effects on criterion-related validity and individual hiring decisions. *Personnel Psychology*, **47**, 847-860.

Conger, A. J., & Jackson, D. N. (1972). Suppressor variables, prediction, and the interpretation of psychological relationships. *Educational and Psychological Measurement*, **32**, 579-599.

Costa, P.T. & McCrae, R.R. (1988). From catalog to classification: Murray's needs and the five-factor model. *Journal of Personality and Social Psychology*, **54**, 258-265.

Costa, P.T. & McCrae, R.R. (1992). *Revised NEO Personality Inventory (NEO-PI-R) and NEO Five-Factor Inventory (NEO-FFI) professional manual*. Odessa, FL: Psychological Assessment Resources.

Costa, P.T. & McCrae, R.R. (1993). Ego development and trait models of personality. *Psychological Inquiry*, **4**, 20-23.

Cronbach, L.J., & Meehl, P.E. (1955). Construct validity in psychological tests. *Psychological Bulletin*, **52**, 281-302.

Dipboye, R.L., & Gaugler, B.B. (1993). Cognitive and behavioral processes in the selection interview. In N. Schmitt & W.C. Borman (Eds.), *Personnel selection in organizations* (pp.135-170). San Francisco, CA: Jossey-Bass

Doll, R. E. (1971). Item susceptibility to attempted faking as related to item characteristics and adopted fake set. *Journal of Psychology*, **77**, 9-16.

Dunnette, M.D (1982). Critical concepts in the assessment of human capabilities. In M.D. Dunnette & E.A. Fleishman (Eds.), *Human performance and productivity: Vol. 1 Human capability assessment* (pp.1-11). Hilldale, NJ: Erlbaum.

Edwards, A. L. (1959). *Edwards Personal Preference Schedule manual*. New York: Psychological Corporation.

Ellingson, J.E., Sackett, P.R., & Hough, L.M. (1999). Social desirability corrections in personality measurement: Issues of applicant comparison and construct validity. *Journal of Applied Psychology*, **84**, 155-166.

Eysenck, H.J. (1991). Dimensions of personality: 16, 5, or 3? Criteria for a taxonomy paradigm. *Personality and Individual Differences*, **12**, 773-790.

Fear, R.A. (1978). *The Evaluation Interview*. New York: McGraw-Hill.

Ghiselli, E.E., & Barthol, R.P. (1953). The validity of personality inventories in the selection of employees. *Journal of Applied Psychology*, **37**, 18-20.

Goffin, R. D., Christiansen, N. D., Johnston, N. G., & Rothstein, M. R. (1994, April). *Correcting for faking: Effects on predictive validity of the 16PF*. Poster presented at the conference of the Society for Industrial and Organizational Psychology (Division 14 of APA), Nashville.

Goffin, R.D., Gellatly, I.R., Paunonen, S.V., Jackson, D.N., & Meyer, J.P. (1996). Criterion validation of two approaches to performance appraisal: The Behavioral Observation Scale and the Relative Percentile Method. *Journal of Business and Psychology*, **11**, 37-47.

Goffin, R. D., Rothstein, M. G., & Johnston, N.G. (1999). Personality and job performance: Are personality tests created equal? In R.D. Goffin and E. Helmes (Eds.) *Problems and Solutions in Human Assessment*. Norwell, MA: Kluwer Academic Publishers.

Goffin, R.D., Rothstein, M.G., & Johnston, N.G. (1996). Personality testing and the assessment center: Incremental validity for managerial selection. *Journal of Applied Psychology*, **81**, 746-756.

Goffin, R. D., & Woods, D. M. (1995). Using personality testing for personnel selection: Faking and test-taking inductions. *International Journal of Selection and Assessment*, **3**, 227-236.

Goldberg, L.R. (1990). An alternative "description of personality": The Big-Five factor structure. *Journal of Personality and Social Psychology*, **59**, 1216-1229.

Goldberg, L.R. (1992).   The development of marker variables for the Big-Five factor structure. *Psychological Assessment*, **4**, 26-42.

Goldberg, L.R. (1993). The structure of phenotypic personality traits. *American Psychologist*, **48**, 26-34.

Gordon, L.V. (1956). *Gordon Personal Inventory*. New York, NY: Harcourt, Brace & World.

Gough, H. (1976). Personality and personality assessment. In M.D. Dunnette (ed.) *Handbook of Industrial and Organizational Psychology*. Chicago: Rand McNally.

Guion, R.M. (1976).   Recruiting, selection, and job placement. In M. D. Dunnette (ed.) *Handbook of Industrial and Organizational Psychology*. Chicago: Rand McNally.

Guion, R.M. (1991).   Personnel assessment, selection, and placement. In M.D. Dunnette & C.M. Hough (Eds.), *Handbook of industrial and organizational psychology* (**Vol. 2**, pp.327-397).   Palo Alto, CA: Consulting Psychologists Press.

Guion, R.M., & Gottier, R.F. (1965). Validating of personality measures in personnel selection. *Personnel Psychology*, **18**, 135-64.

Hanson, B.A. & Harrell, T.W. (1985*).   Predictors of business success over two decades: an MBA longitudinal study* (Research paper No. 788).   Stanford, CA: Stanford University, Graduate School of Business.

Harrell, M.S., Harrell, T.W., McIntyre, S.H., & Weinberg, C.B. (1977).   Predicting compensation among MBA graduates five and ten years after graduation. *Journal of Applied Psychlogy*, **62**, 636-640.

Helmes, E. (1999). The construct of social desirability in personality test development. In R.D. Goffin and E. Helmes (Eds.) *Problems and Solutions in Human Assessment*. Norwell, MA: Kluwer Academic Publishers.

Hogan, R. (1986). *Hogan Personality Inventory manual*. Minneapolis, MN: National Computer Systems.

Hogan, R. (1991). Personality and personality measurement. In M.D. Dunnette & L.M. Hough (Eds.), *Handbook of industrial and organizational psychology* (**Vol. 2**, pp.873-919).   Palo alto, CA: Consulting Psychologists Press.

Holden, R. C. (1999). Application of the Construct Heuristic to the Screening of Psychopathology: The Holden Psychological Screening Inventory (HPSI). In R.D. Goffin and E. Helmes (Eds.) *Problems and Solutions in Human Assessment*. Norwell, MA: Kluwer Academic.

Holden, R.R. (1995). Response latency detection of fakers on personnel tests.*Canadian Journal of Behavioural Science, 27*, 343-355.

Holden, R.R., & Kroner, D.G. (1992). Relative efficacy of differential response latencies for detecting faking on a self-report measure of psychopathology. *Psychological Assessment: A Journal of Consulting and Clinical Psychology*, **4**, 170-173.

Hopkins, K.D., Stanley, J.C., & Hopkins, B.R (1990). *Educational and psychological measurement and evaluation*. Englewood Cliffs, NJ: Prentice Hall.

Hough, L.M. (1992). The 'Big Five' personality variables—construct confusion: Description versus prediction. *Human Performance*, **5**, 139-155.

Hough, L.M., Eaton, N.K., Dunnette, M.D., Kamp, J.D., & McCloy, R.A. (1990). Criterion-related validities of personality constructs and the effect of response distortion on those validities [Monograph]. *Journal of Applied Psychology*, **75**, 581-595.

Howard, A. & Bray, D.W. (1988). *Managerial lives in transition*. New York: Guildford Press.

Hunter, J.E., & Hunter, R.F. (1984). Validity and utility of alternative predictors of job performance. *Psychological Bulletin*, **96**, 72-98.

Jackson, D.N. (1960). Stylistic response determinants in the California Psychological Inventory. *Educational and Psychological Measurement*, **10**, 339-346.

Jackson, D.N. (1970). A sequential system for personality scale development. In C. D. Spielberger (Ed.), *Current topics in clinical and community psychology*, **Volume 2**. (pp. 61-96). New York: Academic Press.

Jackson, D.N. (1971). The dynamics of structured personality tests: 1971. *Psychological Review*, **78**, 229-248.

Jackson, D.N. (1972). A model for inferential accuracy. *Canadian Psychologist*, **13**, 185-95.

Jackson, D.N. (1974). *Personality Research Form Manual*. Port Huron, MI: Research Psycholgists Press.

Jackson, D.N. (1984). *Personality Research Form Manual.* (Third Edition). Port Huron, MI: Research Psychologists Press.

Jackson, D.N., Chan, D.W. & Stricker, L.J. (1979). Implicit personality theory: Is it illusory? *Journal of Personality*, **47**, 1-10.

Jackson, D.N., & Messick, S. (1958). Content and style in personality assessment. *Psychological Bulletin*, **55**, 243-252.

Jackson, D.N., & Messick, S. (1961). Acquiescence and desirability as response determinants on the MMPI. *Educational and Psychological Measurement*, **21**, 771-790.

Jackson, D.N., & Messick, S. (1962). Response styles on the MMPI: Comparison of clinical and normal samples. *Journal of Abnormal and Social Psychology*, **65**, 285-299.

Jackson, D.N., Paunonen, S.V., & Rothstein, M.G. (1987). Personnel executives: Personality, vocational interests, and job satisfaction. *Journal of Employment Counseling*, **24**, 82-86

Jackson, D.N., Peacock A.C. & Smith, J.P. (1980). Impressions of personality in the employment interview. *Journal of Personality and Social Psychology*, **39**, 294-307.

Jackson, D.N., Peacock A.C. & Holden, R.R. (1982). Professional interviewers' trait inferential structures for diverse occupational groups. *Organizational Behavior and Human Performance*, **29**, 1-20.

Jackson, D.N. & Rothstein, M.G. (1993). Evaluating personality testing in personnel selection. *The Psychologist*, **6**, 8-11.

Jackson, D.N., Wroblewski, V.R., & Ashton, M.C. (1999). *The impact of faking on employment test validity: Does forced-choice offer a solution?* Under review.

Korman, A.K. (1977). *Organizational Behavior.* Englewood Cliffs, N.J.: Prentice- Hall.

Landy, F.J. & Trumbo, D.A. (1980). *Psychology of Work Behavior.* Homewood, IL: Dorsey.

Lay, C.H. & Jackson, DN. (1969). Analysis of the generality of trait inferential relationships. *Journal of Personality and Social Psychology*, **12**, 12-21.

Lay, C.H., Burron, B.F., & Jackson, D.N. (1973). Base rates and information value in impression formation. *Journal of Personality and Social Psychology*, **28**, 390-395.

Lopez, F.M. (1975). *Personnel Interviewing.* New York: McGraw-Hill.

Lopez, F.M., Kesselman, G.A., & Lopez, F.E. (1981). An empirical test of a trait-oriented job analysis technique. *Personnel Psychology*, **34**, 479-502.

McCormick, E.J., Jeanneret, P.R., & Mecham, R. C. (1969). *Position Analysis Questionnaire.* West Lafayette, IN: Purdue Research Foundation.

McCrae, R.R., & Costa, P.T. (1985). Updating Norman's "adequate taxonomy": Intelligence and personality dimensions in natural language and in questionnaires. *Journal of Personality and Social Psychology*, **49**, 710-721.

Mikulay, S. M., & Goffin, R. D. (1998). Predicting counterproductivity in the laboratory using integrity and personality testing. *Educational and Psychological Measurement*, **58**, 768-790.

Morey, L. C. (1999). The challenge of construct validity in the assessment of psychopathology. In R.D. Goffin and E. Helmes (Eds.) *Problems and Solutions in Human Assessment.* Norwell, MA: Kluwer Academic.

Murray, H.A. (1938). *Explorations in Personality.* Cambridge: Harvard University Press.

Norman, W. T. (1963). Personality measurement, faking, and detection: An assesment method for use in personnel selection. *Journal of Applied Psychology*, **47**, 225-241.

Norman, W.T. (1963). Toward an adequate taxonomy of personality attributes: Replicated factor structure in peer nomination personality ratings. *Journal of Abnormal and Social Psychology*, **66**, 574-583.

Ones, D.S., Mount, M.K., Barrick, M.R., & Hunter, J.E. (1994). Personality and job performance: A critique of the Tett, Jackson and Rothstein (1991) meta-analysis. *Personnel Psychology*, **47**, 147-156.

Paulhus, D.L. (1991). Measurement and control of response bias. In J. P. Robinson, P. R. Shaver, & L. S. Wrightsman (Eds.), *Measures of personality and social psychological attitudes.* Vol.1. (pp. 17-59). San Diego: Academic Press.

Paunonen, S.V. (1989). Consensus in personality judgments: Moderating effects of target-rater acquaintanceship and behavior observability. *Journal of Personality and Social Psychology*, **56**, 823-833.

Paunonen, S.V. (1998). Hierarchical organization of personality and prediction of behavior. *Journal of Personality and Social Psychology*, **74**, 538-556.

Paunonen, S.V., Rothstein, M.G., & Jackson, D.N. (1999). Narrow reasoning about the use of broad personality measures for personnel selection. *Journal of Organizational Behavior*, **20**, 389-405.

Peabody, D., & Goldberg, L.R. (1989).   Some determinants of factor structure from personality-trait descriptors. *Journal of Personality and Social Psychology*, **57**, 552-567.

Peskin, D.B. (1971).   *Human Behavior and Employment Interviewing*, New York: American Management Association.

Raymark, P. H., Schmit, M. J., & Guion, R. M. (1997). Identifying potentially useful personality constructs for employee selection. *Personnel Psychology*, **50**, 723-736

Reed, P.C., & Jackson, D.N. (1975).   Clinical judgment of psychopathology: A model for inferential accuracy. *Journal of Abnormal Psychology*, **84**, 475-82.

Rosse, J. G., Stecher, M. D., Miller, J. L., & Levin, R. A. (1998). The impact of response distortion on preemployment personality testing and hiring decisions. *Journal of Applied Psychology*, **83**, 634-644.

Rothstein, M.G., & Jackson, D.N. (1980).   Decision-making in the employment interview: An experimental approach. *Journal of Applied Psychology*, **65**, 271-283.

Rothstein, M.G., & Jackson, D.N. (1984).   Implicit personality theory and the employment interview. In M. Cook (Ed.), *Issues in person perception* (pp.167-201). New York: Methuen.

Rothstein, M.G., Paunonen, S.V., Rush, J.C., & King, G.A. (1994).   Personality and cognitive ability predictors of performance in graduate business school. *Journal of Educational Psychology*, **86**, 516-530.

Schmit, M.J., & Ryan, A.M. (1993).   The Big-Five in personnel selection: Factor structure in applicant and non-applicant populations. *Journal of Applied Psychology*, **78**, 966-974.

Schmitt, N. (1976).   Social and situational determinants of interview decisions: Implications for the employment interview. *Personnel Psychology*, **29**, 79-101.

Schmitt, N., Gooding, R.Z., Noe, R.A., & Kirsch M. (1984).   Meta-analyses of validity studies published between 1964 and 1982 and the investigation of study characteristics. *Personnel Psychology*, **37**, 407-421.

Schönemann, P.H. (1990).   Facts, fictions, and common sense about factors and components. *Multivariate Behavioral Research*, **25**, 47-51.

Schrader, A. D., & Osburn, H. G. (1977).   Biodata: Effects of induced subtlety and position specificity. *Personnel Psychology*, **30**, 395-404.

Siess, T.F. & Jackson, D.N. (1970).   Vocational interests and personality: An empirical integration. *Journal of Counseling Psychology*, **17**, 27-35.

Tett, R.P., Jackson, D.N., & Rothstein, M.G. (1991).   Personality measures as predictors of job performance: A meta-analytic review. *Personnel Psychology*, **44**, 703-742.

Tett, R.P., Jackson, D.N., Rothstein, M.G., & Reddon, J.R. (1994).   Meta-analysis of personality-job-performance relations: A reply to Ones, Mount, Barrick, and Hunter (1994). *Personnel Psychology*, **47**, 157-172.

Tett, R.P., Jackson, D.N., Rothstein, M.G., & Reddon, J.R. (1999a).   Meta-analysis of bi-directional relations in personality-job-performance research. *Human Performance*, **12**, 1-29.

Tett, R.P., Jackson, D.N., Rothstein, M.G., & Reddon, J.R. (1999b).   Bi-directionality in personality-job-performance relations.   In S.L. McDaniel & K.R. Brinkmeyer (Co-chairs), Using personality for workplace applications: More is not always better.   Symposium conducted at the 14th Annual Conference of the Society for Industrial and Organizational Psychology, Atlanta, GA.

Tupes, E.C., & Christal, R.E. (1961).   Recurrent personality factors based on trait ratings, (USAF ASD Tech. Rep. No. 61-97).   Lackland Air Force Base, TX: U.S. Air Force; republished in *Journal of Personality*, **60**, 225-251.

Velicer, W.F., & Jackson, D.N. (1990).   Component analysis versus common factor analysis: Some further observations. *Multivariate Behavioral Research*, **25**, 97-114.

Wagner, S.H., & Goffin, R.D. (1997).   Differences in accuracy of absolute and comparative performance appraisal methods. *Organizational Behavior and Human Decision Processes*, **70**, 95-103.

Wertheim, E.G., Widom, C.S., & Wortzel, L.H. (1978).   Multivariate analysis of male and female professional career choice correlates. *Journal of Applied Psychology*, **63**, 234-242.

Wiggins, J.S. (1968).   Personality structure. *Annual Review of Psychology*, **19**, 293-350.

Wiggins, J.S. (1973).   *Personality and Prediction: Principles of Personality Assessment*.   Reading, MA: Addison-Wesley.

11 PREDICTING JOB PERFORMANCE USING PERSONALITY CONSTRUCTS: ARE PERSONALITY TESTS CREATED EQUAL?

Richard D. Goffin
Mitchell G. Rothstein
Norman G. Johnston

As a result of recent research (e.g., Barrick & Mount, 1991; Goffin, Rothstein, & Johnston, 1996; Hough, 1992; Hough, Eaton, Dunnette, Kamp, & McCloy, 1990; Robertson & Kinder, 1993; Tett, Jackson, & Rothstein, 1991), little doubt remains as to the potential usefulness of personality tests in predicting job performance. Recent meta-analyses (e.g., Barrick & Mount, 1991; Hough, 1992; Robertson & Kinder, 1993; Tett et al., 1991) have been particularly effective in reviving interest in the use of personality assessment for personnel selection.

However, one important question that has yet to be addressed is whether or not different personality tests may give rise to important differences in criterion-related validities. If substantial differences in validity are associated with the use of different personality measures, independently of differences due to variability in jobs, performance criteria, or sample, then the common meta-analytic practice of cumulating results across studies that used different personality tests (e.g., Barrick & Mount, 1991; Hough, 1992; Tett et al., 1991) may obscure important inter-test differences in validity. It follows that if a given personality test has demonstrably superior validity to that of other tests, then the average validity of personality tests, as determined in past meta-analytic work, provides an inaccurate picture of the *potential* validity achievable using optimal tests.

There is reason to believe that the particular test development strategy championed by Douglas Jackson (e.g., Jackson, 1970) in the development of the Personality Research Form (Jackson, 1984) and other tests (e.g., the Jackson

Personality Inventory, Jackson, 1994) may have important advantages in the assessment of personality. In particular, it has been shown that the test development strategy underlying the PRF may be advantageous to that of the California Psychological Inventory (CPI; Megargee, 1972) in terms of criterion-related validity (Ashton & Goldberg, 1973).

Burisch (1984) distinguished between three predominant categories of personality test development strategies, external, inductive, and deductive. External (also referred to as "empirical") strategies assume that tests should be composed of items that best discriminate between known criterion groups. Following an external strategy, if one wished to develop a scale measuring dominance, one would start with a large heterogeneous set of items and choose those items that best differentiate a group of dominant individuals from other groups. Inductive strategies begin with a large pool of items, then assemble items into scales on the basis of data analytic tools such as factor analysis. Finally, deductive strategies, which include the Jacksonian approach, call for the assembling of items according to a priori definitions of the respective traits. Ultimately, Burisch (1984, p. 214) concluded that "deductive scales normally communicate information more directly to an assessor, and they are definitely more economical to build and administer." Burisch (1984, p. 214) further states that "wherever there is a genuine choice, the simple deductive approach is recommended." Notwithstanding the above, deductive scales were not found to be advantageous with respect to what might be considered the "gold standard" with respect to personnel selection, that is, criterion-related validity (Burisch, 1984). However, a large majority of the research reviewed by Burisch in which the criterion-related validity associated with the three strategies was compared, involved the use of a restrictive form of the deductive approach whereby the item pool was fixed. Arguably, the use of a fixed item pool, in effect, "handcuffs" the deductive strategy. Whereas the external and inductive strategies are routinely limited to a fixed item pool, a key step in Jackson's (1970, 1984) particular operationalization of the deductive strategy (described in more detail below) involves the careful *generation* of pools of items that conform as precisely as possible to the definitions of the respective traits.

Importantly, to our knowledge, most published comparative evaluations of personality tests have compared criterion validities within the domain of basic personality research and none have dealt specifically with personnel selection applications. Furthermore, the above discussion highlights the fact that existing comparative evaluations of the three main personality test development strategies have often failed to adequately operationalize the deductive strategy as it is employed by Jackson. In fact, although it is possible to roughly divide existing developmental strategies into external, inductive and deductive, such broad categories do not adequately describe the wide diversity of personality tests that currently exist. For example, the category of deductively derived tests includes some tests comprised of forced-choice items (e.g., the Edwards Personnal Preference Schedule; EPPS; Edwards, 1959) and others comprised of true-false items (e.g., the PRF; Jackson, 1984). The unique nature of forced-choice items (see Anastasi, 1982 for a discussion) is likely to result in important differences in the performance of the EPPS and the PRF despite the fact that both tests share the same general developmental strategy. Additionally, although most personality tests can ultimately be pidgeonholed according to the predominant triarchy, many, such as the MMPI-2 (Butcher, 1990), the ABLE (Hough, 1993), the 16PF, and the PRF are, in reality, a product of more than one strategy. In sum, we suggest that attempts to make accurate inferences about criterion-related validities of personality tests on the basis of which of the three test development strategies they embody is unlikely to produce meaningful results.

Nonetheless, because each personality test potentially represents a unique combination of test development strategies, the specific personality test that is used in a given study may, indeed, be a moderator of validity that is worthy of consideration. In fact, Tett et al. (1991) and Barrick and Mount (1991) found that estimates of the percentage of variance in personality tests' validity coefficients that was collectively accounted for by sampling error, test unreliability, criterion unreliability, and range restriction, tended to fall well short of the 75% meta-analytic rule of thumb (Hunter & Schmidt, 1990) in many cases.

Interestingly, there may be an important limitation to the use of standard meta-analytic methodology in pursuing the use of different personality tests as a moderator of validity. James, Demaree, Mulaik, and Ladd (1992) and Russell and Gilliland (1995) have shown that when true moderators correlate with statistical artifacts, such as test reliability, that are routinely corrected for in meta-analysis, the effect of such moderators will tend to be spuriously attenuated. It is likely that different personality tests give rise to scores with differing levels of reliability. For example, scores from the Sixteen Personality Factors, fourth edition[1] (16PF, Cattell, Eber, & Tatsuoka, 1970) would appear to suffer from low reliability (Zuckerman, 1989), whereas scores from the Personality Research Form (PRF; Jackson, 1984), typically have high reliability (Kelley, 1972). Therefore, as a result of correcting for predictor unreliability, meta-analysis might underestimate the potential moderating influence attributable to the specific test. We suggest that this problem might be overcome by simply not correcting for predictor unreliability in meta-analyses of personality test validity. This approach would allow personality test to be more effectively examined as a potential moderator, and, although the resulting validity estimate would be a downwardly biased estimate of "true" validity, it would provide a plausible estimate of "operational" validity.

Unfortunately, the following concern is not amenable to simple statistical correction. It would appear that an insufficient number of validity studies exists to allow the meta-analytic pursuit of personality test as a moderator of validity. We reviewed the prevalence of specific personality tests as they appeared in the research summarized in the Tett et al. (1991) meta-analysis. We were quickly led to the conclusion that it was not meaningful to meta-analytically summarize validity results according to different personality tests because there were typically insufficient numbers of studies and insufficient total N's to allow meaningful cumulation of results obtained for many, if not most, specific tests. Consequently, at present, appropriate primary research would appear to be the only viable approach to investigating whether or not the specific personality test that is used can appreciably influence criterion-related validity. The current primary research is aimed at evaluating the relative predictive validity of the PRF (Jackson, 1984) and the 16PF (see Note 2).

The PRF and the 16PF may be expected to differ in criterion-related validity due to differences in their respective psychometric properties, but also, theoretically, due to differences in scale construction strategies. Both inductive and deductive personality test construction strategies, as used in the development of the 16PF and PRF respectively, have their proponents (e.g., see Kelly, 1972, and Schuerger, 1992). Moreover, both the PRF and the 16PF have been successfully related to job performance (e.g., Christiansen, Goffin, Johnston, & Rothstein, 1994; Day & Silverman, 1989; Furnham, 1991; Gellatly, Paunonen, Meyer, Jackson, & Goffin, 1991; Goffin, Rothstein et al., 1996; Lamont & Lundstrom, 1977). However, we believe that divergence in test construction strategies and the resulting psychometric properties of these two tests will result in important discrepancies in their applicability for personnel selection. For example, independent reviews of the PRF and 16PF have produced dramatically different profiles of the psychometric properties of the two instruments. The PRF has been evaluated as "...among the most methodologically sophisticated personality inventories presently available. Careful attention to issues of substantive, structural, and external validity during the scale construction phase has resulted in an inventory of commendable psychometric properties" (Wiggins, 1972, p. 301). Similarly, Anastasi (1972) has pointed out the careful control of response bias and evidence for both convergent and discriminant validity in the PRF, concluding that "technically, the PRF appears to be exemplary" (p. 298). Kelly (1972) has also reviewed the test construction strategy and psychometric qualities of the PRF and concluded that it is "an instrument which would make possible the measurement of personality traits with levels of precision and validity formerly associated only with intellectual abilities and scholastic achievement" (p.298). In contrast to these evaluations of the PRF, Zuckerman's (1989) review of the 16PF points out that its level of internal consistency reliability and criterion validity are unacceptable, and that even these low criterion validities, as well as the factor structure of the test, do not replicate across samples. Butcher (1989) similarly raises questions concerning the lack of demonstrated validity for 16PF profile interpretations. Despite these negative reviews, Ryan and Sackett (1987) found the 16PF to be one of the most commonly-used personality tests for individual assessment.

This discrepancy in the psychometric properties of the PRF and 16PF suggests a high likelihood that differences in criterion validity between the two tests would emerge. An opportunity to compare these two specific tests in terms of their ability to predict the same job performance criterion would add to our understanding of differences in personality-job performance validities and the potential impact on meta-analytic studies and selection practices. In the following sections we outline key differences between the test construction strategies of the PRF and 16PF, which may underlie differences in personality-job performance validities. Next, the degree to which the two tests may uniquely predict important aspects of job performance is investigated using a sample of managerial candidates.

The 16PF's Developmental Strategy

As outlined by Cattell et al. (1970), and Cattell (1989), the starting point for development of the 16PF was a comprehensive list of approximately 4,000 descriptors of human behavior compiled from dictionaries by Allport and Odbert (1936). Observers were asked to rate subjects on these adjectives, and a series of factor analyses was carried out on the ratings. Twelve factors were developed through these initial analyses, that is, those factors which the 16PF fourth edition labels A, B, C, E, F, G, H, I, L, M, N, O. Items utilizing a self-report format were then written to represent these factors, and additional data were collected and factor analyzed. On the basis of the latter analyses, four more factors were added (Q1 through Q4). Finally, two validity scales were later derived from the existing items.

A key tenet of the inductive strategy employed in the 16PF was that important personality traits could best be identified on the basis of factor analysis. Thus, rather than starting with a priori ideas concerning personality traits, Cattell and colleagues used factor analysis to uncover groupings of apparently homogeneous items, and inferred the existence of sixteen specific personality traits corresponding to these groupings. Nonetheless, the item-writing which occurred after the identification of the original 12 factors appears to have been deductively driven.

The PRF's Developmental Strategy

The deductive, construct-driven strategy adopted in the development of the PRF contrasts sharply with the above approach. On the basis of a theoretical framework for personality developed by Murray (1938), Jackson (1984) began with explicit definitions of a comprehensive set of presumed personality traits. Thus, the dimensions of personality were mapped out *a priori* on the basis of substantive considerations. Jackson then proceeded to carefully generate large pools of items corresponding to each of these traits. Going beyond the basic requirements of the deductive strategy, an exhaustive series of analyses was then carried out in order to select the most promising items, refine the psychometric characteristics of the trait scales, and maximize trait saturation while minimizing variance due to response styles. The final version of the PRF consists of 20 trait scales and two validity scales.

Research Issues

Given that both the 16PF and PRF have empirical support for the measurement of personality, it is not surprising that both have been successfully applied in the prediction of job performance (e.g., Christiansen et al., 1994; Day & Silverman, 1989; Furnham, 1991; Gellatly et al., 1991; Goffin, Rothstein, et al., 1996; Lamont & Lundstrom, 1977). However, as discussed above, to the best of our knowledge, there are no published studies that specifically compare any personality tests in terms of their validity in predicting job performance. We believe there is a substantive rationale for hypothesizing that higher levels of predictive validity may be obtained from the PRF versus the 16PF in personnel selection. The rationale is based on the fundamental differences between the particular deductive, construct-oriented strategy to personality scale development employed in the PRF, and the inductive, factor-analytic strategy employed in the 16PF. These differences in scale development strategies seem to have had a significant impact on the psychometric properties of the two tests (e.g., see Anastasi, 1972; Butcher, 1989; Kelly, 1972; Wiggins, 1972; Zuckerman, 1989), which also should contribute to a difference in predictive validity.

In the current study we evaluated the PRF and the 16PF in terms of their intercorrelations and their ability to predict job performance and promotability in a sample of candidates for managerial positions. The three main issues under investigation in this research were: (1) the extent to which job-relevant personality traits measured by the PRF and 16PF converge; (2) the comparability of the two tests in terms of their ability to predict job performance; (3) the extent to which the variance that is predicted by the PRF may be incremental to that of the 16PF, and vice versa.

METHOD

Participants and Procedure

Participants in this study were 487 (267 males, 23 females, 197 undeclared) managerial assessment center (AC) candidates in a large forestry products organization who completed the 16PF Form A (Cattell et al., 1970) and the PRF Form E (Jackson, 1984) as part of an assessment of their managerial potential. Their mean age was 38 ($sd = 7.4$) with a range of 25 to 59 years. Eighty-three of the participants (76 males, 7 females) were selected for promotion on the basis of the AC evaluation. In addition to 16PF and PRF scores, performance ratings collected after one year on the job were available for this subsample of 83 participants.

Personality Measures

Personality Research Form

As described earlier, the Personality Research Form-E (Jackson, 1984) was used. The PRF is a self-report personality test consisting of 22 16-item scales (20 primary trait scales plus two validity scales; see Jackson, 1984, for descriptions). Following, Jackson's (1984) instructions, raw scores on PRF primary traits were converted to T-scores (M=50, SD=10 in the population). Additionally, six second-order factors can be derived from the PRF by summing the appropriate triads of primary trait scores (see Jackson, Paunonen, Fraboni, & Goffin, 1996).

Sixteen Personality Factors Test

The 16PF, fourth edition (Cattell et al., 1970; see Note 2), as discussed earlier, was also employed in this research. The 16PF is a self-report personality test providing 16 primary trait scales and two validity scales (see Cattell et al., 1970, for descriptions). Following Cattell et al.'s instructions, 16PF raw scores were converted to sten scores (M=5, SD=2 in the population). Five replicatable second-order trait scales for the 16PF can be computed based on formulas derived from Krug and Johns (1986).

A Priori Selected Personality Traits

Twenty PRF primary trait scales and six PRF second-order trait scales were available for study. Similarly, 16 16PF primary trait scales and five second-order trait scales were available. With such an abundance of available scales we could have chosen personality traits purely on the basis of their observed empirical relations with performance. However, we believed it was important to select specific personality traits on the basis of *a priori* considerations because this research strategy is less likely to capitalize on chance and has been identified as optimal for determining valid relations between personality and job performance

(Tett et al., 1991; Tett, Jackson, Rothstein, & Reddon, 1994). Therefore, a subset of personality traits identified as being crucial to the performance of managers, namely, dominance and extraversion, were used as predictors in a series of validational analyses. These traits were chosen on the basis of considerable previous empirical support for their ability to predict meaningful aspects of managerial performance (e.g., Brenner, 1982; Hanson & Harrell, 1985; Harrell, Harrell, McIntyre, & Weinberg, 1977; Hogan, 1991; Howard & Bray, 1988; Wertheim, Widom, & Wortzel, 1978) and their availability in *both* the PRF and 16PF. Extraversion was measured as a second-order trait in the case of both tests whereas dominance, referred to as "Factor E" in the 16PF, was a first-order trait. Beyond extraversion and dominance, additional job-relevant personality traits (e.g., achievement) could have been used, but all such additional traits were available only through one or the other of the two tests and thus direct comparisons could not have been made when assessing the relative validities of the PRF and 16PF.

Performance Measures

Ten supervisory ratings, including eight different performance dimensions determined through job analysis, an overall performance rating, and a promotability rating, were used as criterion variables. The eight different performance dimensions were work practices and procedures, planning and problem solving, group cooperation and cross-functional management, promoting safety, communication, personnel development, customer and supplier relations, and personal work style. Raters were informed that these ratings were being done for research purposes only and that they would not influence the ratees' careers in any manner or be made available to anyone other than the researchers except in aggregated form. All ratings were made using the Relative Percentile Method (RPM, Goffin, Gellatly, Paunonen, Jackson, & Meyer, 1996). The RPM approach requires that ratings be made on 101-point scales, where a rating of 50 is considered average for workers in that job (Goffin, Gellatly, et al., 1996). For each dimension, all the ratees of a given supervisor are considered relative to one another and rated on a zero-to-100 scale. Wagner and Goffin's (1997) laboratory research found that the comparative rating format used in the RPM tends to result in higher levels of accuracy than does the more common "absolute" or "individual" rating format used in many performance ratings whereas Goffin, Gellatly et al.'s (1996) field study suggested that the RPM approach has relatively high criterion-related validity. Supervisors carried out the performance ratings one year after the ratees' were hired. At no time did the supervisors see the scores from the 16PF or PRF.

RESULTS

Preliminary Analyses

The eight performance dimensions and the overall performance rating were highly intercorrelated. Moreover, a principal components analysis revealed that only one eigenvalue exceeded unity and it explained 62% of the variance. Therefore, a total performance measure was formed on the basis of an equally-weighted composite of the eight performance dimensions and the rating of overall performance. The rating of promotability was kept separate because promotability and performance would appear to be differentially predictable (Turnage & Muchinsky, 1984). The maximum possible score was 900 on the total performance composite and 100 on the promotability scale.

Convergence of PRF and 16PF Scales

Based on the entire sample (N=487), correlations between extraversion and dominance, measured using the PRF and the 16PF, are displayed in Table 1. As shown in the table, the correlation of the 16PF second-order scale of extraversion with the corresponding second-order PRF scale was 0.73, indicating 53% shared variance between the two measures, and a relatively high degree of convergence. However, the correlation of the 16PF primary scale measuring dominance (Factor E) evidenced only a 0.25 correlation with the corresponding PRF scale, suggesting a low degree of convergence of the two scales and only 6% shared variance.

Correlations of PRF and 16PF Scales with Criteria

These results were based on the subsample of 83 managers for whom both personality and criterion data were available.[2] As shown in Table 1, all four criterion relationships involving the PRF were moderate in magnitude and significant. In the case of the 16PF, three of four criterion relations were significant and they ranged in magnitude from weak to moderate.

Incremental Validity Analyses

In phase one of these analyses, the 16PF scales of dominance and extraversion were entered as the first block of predictors in a multiple regression equation, and the incremental validity of the corresponding PRF traits was then assessed by entering them as the second block. However, assuming correlated predictors, it is well known that the order of entry of variables in a multiple regression analysis is crucial (Pedhazur,1982). Accordingly, groups of variables that are entered in a

Table 1. Convergence of PRF and 16PF Scales

	PRF		16PF		Criteria	
	Extraversion	Dominance	Extraversion	Dominance	Tot. Perform.	Promot.
PRF						
Extraversion	1.00					
Dominance	.61**	1.00				
16PF						
Extraversion	.73**	.36**	1.00			
Dominance	.25**	.25**	.19**	1.00		
Criteria						
Total performance	.39**	.41**	.32*	.25*	1.00	
Promotability	.32*	.30*	.16	.19*	.64**	1.00
M	161.98	56.00	6.24	6.35	591.08	62.46
SD	16.92	6.32	2.03	1.95	95.64	18.13

Note. For correlations between personality trait scales, $N=487$, for correlations involving criteria, $N=83$. PRF=Personality Research Form; 16PF=Sixteen Personality Factors; Tot. Perform.=the total performance score; Promot.=the promotability rating.
$*p < .05$ (one-tailed). $**p < .001$ (one-tailed).

later step are much less likely to contribute significant predictive variance. Therefore, in order to gain a fuller appreciation of the relative importance of PRF and 16PF scales in predicting performance and promotability, a second phase of the analysis was conducted in which the selected PRF scales were entered into the equation first, followed by the 16PF scales.

It should be noted that a "forced entry" approach was used in these analyses to insure that independent variables remained in the equation regardless of the significance level of their beta weights. Although it would be possible to use a stepwise strategy in order to select only those predictors that are statistically significant, this was not done for three main reasons. First, experts in multiple regression have cautioned that the significance tests of R^2 values from regression analyses in which the selection of predictors takes advantage of prior knowledge are likely to be biased in favor of giving significant results (Darlington, 1990; Pedhazur, 1982). Second, the emphasis in the present analyses was to assess how well personality traits that were chosen on the basis of *a priori* considerations regarding the target job would perform. Third, an additional problem with the use of strategies whereby only significant predictors remain in the equation is that when predictors are correlated, as is currently the case, the standard errors of the tests of significance of individual beta weights are increased. As a result of this increase in standard errors, the power of the significance tests of beta weights is reduced and there is an increased possibility that predictors which are important in the population may be overlooked.

As shown in Table 2, when the 16PF scales were entered first, total performance was significantly predicted and, based on the shrunken R^2, in the population at large an estimated 10% of the variance in this criterion was predicted. Promotability was not significantly predicted by the 16PF scales. Table 2 also shows that when the PRF scales were entered first into the equation, total performance and promotability were both significantly predicted. Moreover, in the population it is estimated that 17% and 9% of the variance in total performance and promotability, respectively, would be predicted by the PRF measures (see shrunken R^2s, presented in brackets in Table 2). Further, Table 2 shows that the combination of the PRF measures of dominance and extraversion evidenced significant incremental variance over corresponding 16PF scales in the case of both criterion measures, the average shrunken incremental variance equaling 5.5%. Conversely, the 16PF failed to contribute significant incremental variance in the case of both criteria. In fact, adding the 16PF scales to the equation in which the PRF scales had already been entered only served to reduce the shrunken R^2 values associated with both criterion measures.

Table 2. Hierarchical Regressions

I. 16PF scales entered first, PRF scales entered second

	Squared Multiple Correlations		
Performance Criterion	16PF	16PF + PRF	ΔR^2_{PRF}
1. Total Performance	.12**(.10)	.19**(.15)	.07* (.05)
2. Promotability	.04 (.02)	.13* (.08)	.09* (.06)

II. PRF scales entered first, 16PF scales entered second

	Squared Multiple Correlations		
Performance Criterion	PRF	PRF + 16PF	ΔR^2_{16PF}
1. Total Performance	.19**(.17)	.19**(.15)	.01 (-.02)
2. Promotability	.11**(.09)	.13* (.08)	.02 (-.01)

Note. N=83. Values in brackets are shrunken R^2s (see Pedhazur, 1982, p. 148). 16PF= the 16PF (Cattell et al., 1970), traits of dominance and extraversion, each entered as a predictor. PRF=The PRF (Jackson, 1984) traits of dominance and extraversion, each entered as a predictor. ΔR^2_{PRF}=change in R^2 as a result of adding the PRF dominance and extraversion measures to the regression equation. ΔR^2_{16PF}=change in R^2 as a result of adding the 16PF dominance and extraversion scales to the regression equation. *$p<.05$. **$p<.01$

DISCUSSION

In sum, these results suggest that the PRF may have advantages over the 16PF (see Note 2) in predicting the performance of the managers in our sample. At the zero-order level, the PRF scales of extraversion and dominance evidenced somewhat stronger criterion relations than did the corresponding 16PF scales (Table 1). Where the trait of dominance is concerned, the PRF scale exhibited notably stronger criterion relations with both criteria than did the 16PF counterpart (Table 1). The low correlation between 16PF-Dominance and PRF-Dominance (Table 1) suggests that dominance, as it is embodied in these two tests, may entail quite different things. The results reviewed above suggest that the PRF's measurement of dominance is distinguished from that of the 16PF by its greater relevance to the domain of managerial performance. Substantively, there are many similarities in the descriptions of dominance which appear in the PRF (Jackson, 1984) and 16PF (Cattell et al., 1970) documentation. Quite reasonably, both the PRF and 16PF appear to operationalize dominance in terms of assertiveness and a domineering tendency. However, in addition to these core dominance elements, the 16PF's operationalization of dominance also includes aspects of autonomy, social recognition, and value orthodoxy (e.g., see Cattell et al., 1970, p. 86). It is conceivable that this blending of dominance with autonomy, social recognition, and value orthodoxy detracts from the 16PF's measurement of dominance and is partially to blame for the lower criterion relationships of this scale relative to the PRF dominance scale.

Hierarchical regression analyses further reinforced the view that the PRF may be advantageous. As shown in Table 2, the PRF traits, by themselves, predicted a larger percentage of performance and promotability variance than did the 16PF and exhibited more incremental variance than did the 16PF. In fact, the PRF was able to predict a significant proportion of variance over and above that predicted by the 16PF in the case of both criteria, whereas the 16PF consistently failed to predict significant variance beyond that predicted by the PRF.

Our comparison of the 16PF and PRF was based only on the traits of dominance and extraversion. One might argue that if we had based our comparison on some other choice of traits this might possibly have changed the results. However, dominance and extraversion were chosen based on relevant *a priori* considerations regarding their ability to predict managerial performance (e.g., Brenner, 1982; Hanson & Harrell, 1985; Harrell, Harrell, McIntyre, & Weinberg, 1977; Hogan, 1991; Howard & Bray, 1988; Wertheim, Widom, & Wortzel, 1978) and their availability in *both* the PRF and 16PF. Tett et al. (1991) have suggested that choosing personality traits on an a priori basis is preferable. Moreover, to afford a fair comparison of the relative predictive ability of the PRF and 16PF it was necessary that the same set of traits be used from both tests. Nonetheless, it is instructive to consider what might have happened if an empirically chosen set of traits had been used. To address this issue we conducted one series of step-wise regressions in which all traits from the PRF were made available as potential predictors and the final choice of traits was based solely on empirical concerns (i.e., the multiple regression computer program was set up to choose traits as predictors based solely on their contribution to the prediction of the criteria). A corresponding series of regressions was carried out using the 16PF. Throughout these analyses, the PRF retained its predictive edge over the 16PF. In fact, the proportions of variance predicted by the 16PF and PRF respectively did not differ meaningfully from the values reported in Table 2. Thus, it appears that even if sets of traits chosen purely on the basis of empirical priorities had been used as predictors, the PRF would still have been advantageous.

Although we are aware of no other studies which explicitly compared the criterion-related validity of different personality tests within the realm of personnel selection, previous basic research in personality has compared the PRF to the CPI. Specifically, Ashton and Goldberg (1973) found the PRF to be superior to the CPI in predicting peer rankings. Thus, although gathered in a different context, our results are consistent with Ashton and Goldberg's in supporting the effectiveness of the PRF over other personality scales. Similarly, Jackson (1975) found that his particular approach to the deductive, construct-oriented strategy to personality scale development, which underlies the PRF, is superior to that of external development strategies. Because Jackson's deductive, construct heuristic strategy begins with the precise definition of traits and the generation of large pools of items which are later subjected to intense scrutiny, it facilitates the development of highly homogeneous trait measures which are comparatively free of extraneous variance from response styles.

Our results, in concert with those of Ashton and Goldberg (1973), and Jackson (1975), suggest that there may be distinct predictive advantages associated with the PRF (Jackson, 1984). Unfortunately, only a relatively small percentage of the existing research on personality assessment in personnel selection has been carried out using this test (e.g., in Tett et al.'s, 1991, meta-analysis, only three of the 97 independent samples that were employed used the PRF). Thus, it is quite conceivable that existing meta-analyses may have underestimated the levels of validity that would be achievable using a test such as the PRF. Regrettably, as we discussed at length in the introduction of this article, it is unlikely that meta-analysis can overcome this problem by treating personality test as a moderator because of limitations in the existing base of primary research. Thus, more primary research evaluating the criterion-related validity of various personality tests is called for.

The present study dealt only with a managerial job and only two specific personality tests, thus, additional research is required for greater generalization. Eventually, through the gradual accumulation of relevant primary research, sufficient data will be available to allow the meta-analytic comparison of validities associated with different personality tests. As discussed earlier, in such meta-analyses it would be pertinent to address the possibility that the moderating effect of the specific personality test that is used on criterion validity may possibly be obfuscated to the extent that different tests give rise to systematic differences in a statistical "artifact" (i.e., predictor unreliability) that is routinely corrected for.

NOTES

[1]This research was supported by a grant from the Social Sciences and Humanities Research Council of Canada to Richard D. Goffin. A preliminary version of these results was presented at the Annual Meeting of the Society for Industrial and Organizational Psychology, Orlando, May, 1995. Requests for reprints should be sent to Richard D. Goffin, Department of Psychology, Social Science Centre, The University of Western Ontario, London, Ontario, Canada N6A 5C2.

[2]In meta-analyses of the validity of personality testing (e.g., Barrick & Mount, 1991; Tett et al., 1991) it is the *fourth* edition of the 16PF which has predominated, and it is in regards to the results of these meta-analyses that the current work is particularly relevant. Therefore, the results reported here, the reviews of the 16PF which we cite (e.g., Butcher, 1989; Zuckerman, 1989), and the statements which are made regarding the 16PF refer to the *fourth* edition of the 16PF. At the time this article was written, the fourth edition is still administered frequently and is still available for purchase, however, a substantially revised *fifth* edition of the 16PF (Conn & Rieke, 1994) has recently been made available.

[3]As in past research (e.g., Borman, 1982; Bray & Grant, 1966; Crawley, Pinder, & Herriot, 1990; Hinrichs, 1978; Tziner & Dolan, 1982) the personality predictors used in this work were largely orthogonal to the assessment center scores. Consequently, the personality scores of the subsample of 83 managers who were selected on the basis of their AC evaluation did not differ substantially from the scores of the 404 who were not selected.

REFERENCES

Allport, G. W., & Odbert, H. S. (1936). Trait names: A psycholexical study. *Psychological Monographs, 47*, (1, Whole No. 211).

Anastasi, A. (1972). Review of the Personality Research Form. In O.K. Buros (Ed.). *The Seventh Mental Measurements Yearbook* (pp. 297-298). Highland Park, NJ: The Gryphon Press.

Anastasi, A. (1982). *Psychological Testing*. New York, NY: MacMillan.

Ashton, S. G., & Goldberg, L. R. (1973). In response to Jackson's challenge: The comparative validity of personality scales constructed by the external (empirical) strategy and scales developed intuitively by experts, novices, and laymen. *Journal of Research in Personality, 7*, 1-20.

Barrick, M.R. & Mount, M.K. (1991). The big five personality dimensions and job performance: A meta-analysis. *Personnel Psychology, 44*, 1-26.

Borman, W. C. (1982). Validity of behavioral assessment for predicting military recruiter performance. *Journal of Applied Psychology, 67*, 3-9.

Bray, D. W., & Grant, D. L. (1966). The assessment center in the measurement of potential for business management. *Psychological Monographs, 80* (17, Whole No. 625).

Brenner, D.C. (1982). Relationship of education to sex, managerial status, and the managerial stereotype. *Journal of Applied Psychology, 67*, 380-383.

Burisch, M. (1984). Approaches to personality inventory construction. *American Psychologist, 39*, 214-227.

Butcher, J. N. (1989). Review of the Sixteen Personality Factor Questionnaire. In J. C. Conoley & J.J. Kramer (Eds.) *The Tenth Mental Measurements Yearbook* (pp. 1391-1392). Lincoln, NE: Buros Institute of Mental Measurements of the University of Nebraska.

Butcher, J.N. (1990). *MMPI-2 in psychological treatment*. New York, NY: Oxford University Press.

Cattell, H. B. (1989). *The 16PF: Personality in depth.* Champaign, IL: Institute for Personality and Ability Testing.

Cattell, R.B., Eber, H.W., & Tatsuoka, M.M, (1970). *Handbook for Sixteen Personality Factor Questionnaire (16PF).* Champaign, IL: Institute for Personality and Ability Testing.

Christiansen, N. D., Goffin, R. D., Johnston, N. G., & Rothstein, M. G. (1994). Correcting the Sixteen Personality Factors test for faking: Effects on criterion-related validity and individual hiring decisions. *Personnel Psychology, 47,* 847-860.

Conn, S. R., & Rieke, M. L. (1984). *16PF Fifth Edition: Technical manual.* Champaign, IL: Institute for Personality and Ability Testing.

Crawley, B., Pinder, R., & Herriot, P. (1990). Assessment centre dimensions, personality and aptitudes. *Journal of Occupational Psychology, 63,* 211-216.

Darlington, R. B. (1990). *Regression and linear models.* New York: McGraw-Hill.

Day, D.A. & Silverman, S.B. (1989). Personality and job performance: Evidence of incremental validity. *Personnel Psychology, 42,* 25-36.

Edwards, A.L. (1959). *Edwards Personal Preference Schedule.* New York, NY: The Psychological Corporation.

Furnham, A. (1991). Personality and occupational success: 16PF correlates of cabin crew performance. *Personality and Individual Differences, 12,* 87-90.

Gellatly, I. R., Paunonen, S. V., Meyer, J. P., Jackson, D. N., & Goffin, R. D. (1991). Personality, vocational interests, and cognitive predictors of managerial job performance and satisfaction. *Personality and Individual Differences, 12,* 221-231.

Goffin, R. D., Gellatly, I. R., Paunonen, S. V., Jackson, D. N., & Meyer, J. P. (1996). Criterion validation of two approaches to performance appraisal: The Behavioral Observation Scale and the Relative Percentile Method. *Journal of Business and Psychology, 11,* 37-47.

Goffin, R. D., Rothstein, M. G., & Johnston, N. G. (1996). Personality testing and the assessment center: Incremental validity for managerial selection. *Journal of Applied Psychology, 81,* 746-756.

Hanson, B.A. & Harrell, T.W. (1985). *Predictors of business success over two decades: An MBA longitudinal study* (Research paper No. 788). Stanford, CA: Stanford University, Graduate School of Business.

Harrell, M.S., Harrell, T.W., McIntyre, S.H., & Weinberg, C.B. (1977). Predicting compensation among MBA graduates five and ten years after graduation. *Journal of Applied Psychology, 62,* 636-640.

Hinrichs, J. R. (1978). An eight-year follow-up of a management assessment center. *Journal of Applied Psychology, 63,* 596-601.

Hogan, R.T. (1991). Personality and personality measurement. In M.D. Dunnette & L.M. Hough (Eds.), *Handbook of industrial and organizational psychology, 2,* pp. 873-919). Palo Alto, CA: Consulting Psychologists Press.

Hough, L.M. (1992). The "Big Five" personality variables - construct confusion: Description versus prediction. *Human Performance, 5,* 139-155.

Hough, L.M. (1993). Development of "Assessment of Background and Life Experiences (ABLE): A temperament inventory.Unpublished manuscript.

Hough, L.M., Eaton, N.K., Dunnette, M.D., Kamp, J.D., & McCloy, R.A. (1990). Criterion-related validities of personality constructs and the effect of response distortion on those validities [Monograph]. *Journal of Applied Psychology, 75,* 581-595.

Howard, A. & Bray, D.W. (1988). *Managerial lives in transition.* New York: Guilford Press.

Hunter, J. E., & Schmidt, F. L. (1990). *Methods of meta-analysis: Correcting error and bias in research findings.* Newbury Park, CA: Sage.

Jackson, D.N. (1970). A sequential system for personality scale development. In C. D. Spielberger (Ed.), *Current topics in clinical and community psychology, 2.* (pp. 61-96). New York: Academic Press.

Jackson, D. N. (1975). The relative validity of scales prepared by naive item writes and those based on empirical methods of personality scale construction. *Educational and Psychological Measurement, 35,* 361-370.

Jackson, D. N. (1984). *Personality Research Form manual.* Port Huron, MI: Research Psychologists Press.

Jackson, D.N. (1994). *Jackson Personality Inventory - Revised manual.* Port Huron, MI & London, Ontario: Sigma Assessment Systems.

Jackson, D. N., Paunonen, S. V., Fraboni, M., & Goffin, R. D. (1996). A five-factor versus six-factor model of personality structure. *Personality and Individual Differences, 20,* 33-45.

James, L. R., Demaree, R. G., Mulaik, S. A., & Ladd, R. T. (1992). Validity generalization in the context of situational models. *Journal of Applied Psychology*, **77**, 3-14.

Kelly, E.L. (1972). Review of the Personality Research Form. In O.K. Buros (Ed.), *The seventh mental measurements yearbook* (p. 298). Highland Park, NJ: Gryphon Press.

Krug, S. E., & Johns, E. F. (1986). A large-scale cross-validation of second-order personality structure as determined by the 16PF. *Psychological Reports*, **59**, 683-693.

Lamont, L. M., & Lundstrom, W. J. (1977). Identifying successful industrial salesmen by personality and personal characteristics. *Journal of Marketing Research*, **14**, 517-529.

Megargee, E. I. (1972). *The California Psychological Inventory handbook*. San Francisco: Jossey-Bass

Murray, H. A. (1938). *Explorations in personality*. Cambridge, MA: Harvard University Press.

Pedhazur, E. J. (1982). *Multiple regression in behavioral research*. New York: Holt, Rinehart and Winston.

Robertson, I. T., & Kinder, A. (1993). Personality and job competencies: The criterion-related validity of some personality variables. *Journal of Occupational and Organizational Psychology*, **66**, 225-244.

Russell, C. J., & Gilliland, S. W. (1995). Why meta-analysis doesn't tell us what the data really mean: Distinguishing between moderator effects and moderator processes. *Journal of Management*, **21**, 813-831.

Ryan, A.M., & Sackett, P.R. (1987). A survey of individual assessment practices by I/O psychologists. *Personnel Psychology*, **40**, 455-488.

Schuerger, J. M. (1992). The Sixteen Personality Factor Questionnaire and its junior versions. *Journal of Counseling and Development*, **71**, 231-244.

Tett, R. P., Jackson, D. N., & Rothstein, M., (1991). Personality measures as predictors of job performance: A meta-analytic review. *Personnel Psychology*, **44**, 703-742.

Tett, R.P., Jackson, D.N., Rothstein, M., & Reddon, J.R. (1994). Meta-analysis of personality-job performance relations: A reply to Ones, Mount, Barrick, and Hunter (1994). *Personnel Psychology*, **47**, 157-172.

Turnage, J. J., & Muchinsky, P. M. (1984). A comparison of the predictive validity of assessment center evaluations versus traditional measures in forecasting supervisory job performance: Interpretive implications of criterion distortion for the assessment paradigm. *Journal of Applied Psychology*, **69**, 595-602.

Tziner, A., & Dolan, S. (1982). Validity of an assessment center for identifying future female officers in the military. *Journal of Applied Psychology*, **67**, 728-736.

Wagner, S. H., & Goffin, R. D. (1997). Differences in accuracy of absolute and comparative performance appraisal methods. *Organizational Behavior and Human Decision Processes*, **70**, 95-103.

Wertheim, E. G., Widom, C.S., & Wortzel, L.H. (1978). Multivariate analysis of male and female professional career choice correlates. *Journal of Applied Psychology*, **63**, 234-242.

Wiggins, J. S. (1972). Review of the Personality Research Form. In O.K. Buros (Ed.). *The Seventh Mental Measurements Yearbook* (pp. 301-303). Highland Park, NJ: The Gryphon Press.

Zuckerman, M. (1989). Review of the Sixteen Personality Factor Questionnaire. In J. C. Conoley & J.J. Kramer (Eds.). *The Tenth Mental Measurements Yearbook* (pp. 1392-1394). Lincoln, NE: Buros Institute of Mental Measurements of the University of Nebraska.

12 WHAT CONSTRUCTS UNDERLIE MEASURES OF HONESTY OR INTEGRITY?

Kevin R. Murphy

The problem of assessing peoples' honesty or integrity, predicting their trustworthiness and dependability, detecting their efforts to deceive others, etc. has long been the focus of research, speculation, and debate (Ekman, 1975; Ekman & O'Sullivan, 1991; Kleinmuntz & Szucko, 1984; Lykken, 1981; Murphy, 1993). Methods of addressing this problem run the gamut from those used in criminal investigations (e.g., forensic science, interrogation methods) to those used by most of us in everyday life (e.g., using nonverbal behaviors as clues that a person might be insincere when giving a compliment). Assessments of honesty, integrity, and dependability are of particular interest to organizations, for a number of reasons. In particular, there is evidence that workplace dishonesty, including theft, fraud, embezzlement, etc. is both widespread and costly.

Murphy and Luther (1997) and Murphy (1993) discuss a number of methods used by organizations to measure honesty or integrity or to detect deception, including: (1) integrity tests, (2) interviews and other self-reports, and (3) graphological analyses, (4) polygraph analyses, (5) voice stress analyses, (6) drug and alcohol tests, and (7) assessments of behavioral cues to deception. The current chapter focuses on paper-and-pencil measures that purport to measure peoples' honesty, integrity, dependability, or reliability, that is, integrity tests. However, before discussing this class of tests in detail, it is useful to describe the relationships between the various measures used by organizations, as well as some of the constructs different classes of measures are designed to tap.

The tests and assessment techniques listed above are all designed to provide information about honesty, but they differ substantially in their focus. It is useful to distinguish first between deception and integrity or dependability. Measures of integrity or dependability are used to make inferences about an individual's past or future behavior. For example, integrity tests are typically used to forecast future workplace dishonesty (sometimes on the basis of admissions of previous misdeeds). Similarly, integrity interviews, application blanks, and a variety of self-report measures are used to make predictions about an individual's likely level of honesty and dependability. These inferences might be based on information about past behavior, or on measures of specific traits and attributes thought to be relevant to workplace honesty, but in all cases, the focus is on predicting future behavior rather than drawing inferences about the truthfulness of specific claims or statements.

Assessments of deception are designed to determine whether an individual is telling or withholding the truth in a particular context. For example, polygraph examinations are structured to support inferences about whether a subject's responses to a specific set of questions are truthful. Similarly, voice stress analyses are designed to determine whether answers to specific questions are truthful. Drug and alcohol tests are used to determine whether individuals are withholding information about their use of alcohol, drugs, or other substances of abuse. In all of these cases, these tests are used to draw inferences about the probability that individuals are attempting to deceive or withhold information from the examiner.

The distinction between tests of deception and predictions of future honesty is often blurred in practice. For example, it is common practice in many American firms to use drug or alcohol tests in pre-employment screening. These tests may do little more than indicate whether an individual has ingested alcohol or drugs within the last few hours to days, and might be more suited to detecting and deterring deception (e.g., in determining whether drugs or alcohol were involved in an accident) than to predicting whether a job applicant is likely to be a good prospect for employment (Murphy & Wright, 1996). In general, tests or assessment methods that provide valid information about deception in specific contexts might nevertheless prove useless in predicting future dishonesty (Ben-Shakhar & Furedy, 1990; U.S. Congressional Office of Technology Assessment [OTA], 1983). Similarly, measures of integrity or dependability may provide little information about the truthfulness of a specific statement or claim.

Although the terms honesty, integrity and dependability are often used interchangeably in this literature, a useful distinction should be drawn between them. Honesty refers to a particular respect for truthfulness, whereas integrity and dependability imply slightly broader conceptions, including a willingness to comply with rules, internalized values, norms and expectations. Tests that are used to infer future behavior in the workplace are likely to draw upon this broader conception rather than focusing narrowly on honesty per se. Integrity tests vary considerably in their content and focus, but for the most part, they have been developed with the goal of assessing this broad conception of "integrity" or with the goal of predicting behaviors related to this conception (e.g., theft, counterproductivity, abiding by rules and norms).

Jackson (1970, 1971) has been a strong proponent of construct-oriented methods of test development - i.e., methods that depend on a careful definition of the constructs to be measured and of the relationships between specific test items and those constructs. These methods have rarely been applied in the development of integrity tests (although the emphasis on defining key constructs has varied considerably across tests), and the result is considerable confusion about what these tests actually measure. For example, "integrity" is often a poorly defined or poorly understood construct (e.g., it is not clear whether "integrity" means the same thing as "dependability", even though these two terms are often used interchangeably), and claims that specific tests actually measure this construct must be examined with a critical eye. A theme to be developed in this chapter is that the failure to attend to the definition of key constructs and the relationships between those constructs and the various types of items that define integrity tests has hampered our ability to make sense of research evidence showing links between scores on these tests and organizationally-relevant criteria.

INTEGRITY TESTS

Until the late 1980's, polygraph examinations (often called "lie detector tests") were widely used in organizations as a means of dealing with workplace dishonesty, and were often an important consideration in decisions to hire or fire specific individuals. However, their examinations were highly controversial, both because of lingering doubts about their validity and because of concerns over invasions of the privacy and dignity of examinees (Murphy, 1993). The Employee Polygraph Protection Act of 1988 placed such severe restrictions on the use of the polygraph in the workplace that this method was abandoned by most employers. Employers who had relied on polygraph examinations and other potentially invasive methods sought alternatives for dealing with workplace dishonesty, and integrity tests have been embraced by many organizations either as a replacement for the polygraph or as a selection tool in its own right.

Paper-and pencil integrity tests have been in existence since at least the 1950's, and even prior to federal laws restricting the use of the polygraph in the workplace, they were used in a number of industries. O'Bannon, Goldinger and Appleby (1989) report that in the 1980's these tests were used by 10-15% of all U.S. employers, concentrated in the retail sales, banking, and food service industries, and that shortly after the passage of laws regulating the use of the polygraph, over 2.5 million tests were being given by over 5,000 employers each year. More recent estimates of integrity test use suggest that over 5 million tests are given per year (Ones and Viswesvaran,1998b). Many of these tests make only indirect references to theft, dishonesty, deviance, etc., and it is likely that many job applicants are unaware that decisions about them are based in part on tests that claim to measure honesty, integrity, or dependability.

Characteristics of integrity tests

There are over 40 published integrity tests, and at least 15-20 of these are in widespread use (O'Bannon et al., 1989; Ones & Viswesvaran, 1998b). Although the individual tests differ in a number of specifics, there are a number of features common to virtually all integrity tests. In particular, integrity tests usually include items that refer to one or more of the following areas: (a) direct admissions of illegal or questionable activities, (b) opinions regarding illegal or questionable behavior, (c) general personality traits and thought patterns thought to be related to dishonesty (e.g. the tendency to constantly think about illegal activities), and (d) reactions to hypothetical situations that may or may not feature dishonest behavior.

A distinction is usually drawn between tests that inquire directly about integrity, asking for admissions of past theft, or asking about the degree to which the examinee approves of dishonest behaviors, and tests that indirectly infer integrity on the basis of responses to questions that are not obviously integrity-related. Several authors (e.g. Sackett, Burris & Callahan, 1989) refer to the former as "overt" tests, and to the latter as "personality based" tests. The labels "clear-purpose" and "veiled-purpose" are also used (Murphy, 1993); these labels might be preferable because they highlight the fact that the purpose of testing is sometimes obvious and sometimes hidden from examinees.

Many integrity tests seem similar in terms of the dimensions or characteristics they purport to measure. Examples of the dimensions that appear to underlie the items included on many integrity tests are presented in Table 1 (for reviews, see Cunningham & Ash,1988; Harris & Sackett, 1987; O'Bannon et al., 1989). There are several themes common to these dimensions. First, individuals who receive low scores (i.e., scores indicating low levels of integrity) are likely to see dishonest behavior as relatively frequent and acceptable. Second, they tend to think about and rationalize these behaviors (e.g. they may claim that taking things from a large company is not "really" stealing, because the company will never miss the objects taken). Finally, they tend to act on impulse.

The characteristics summarized above may help explain why some people are willing to admit wrongdoing on overt integrity tests. Individuals who believe that wrongdoing is common, acceptable, and easily rationalized may see nothing wrong with admitting a little larceny. If you believe that everyone else steals $500 a year, admitting that you steal "only" $300 may make you appear relatively virtuous. I will return to this theme later in this chapter.

Examples of tests usually classified as either clear-purpose or veiled-purpose integrity tests, together with descriptions of dimensions measured by the tests (in some cases, these refer merely to the labels attached to scale scores reported) are presented in Table 2; O'Bannon et. al. (1989) present detailed descriptions of the dimensions measured by forty-three integrity tests. As this table suggests, the distinction between clear-purpose and veiled-purpose tests is not always a simple one (O'Bannon et al., 1989; OTA, 1990). Many clear-purpose tests include items, scales, etc. that are not obviously related to honesty, and many veiled purpose tests contain items that might alert the respondent to the true purpose of the test.

There is considerable debate over what, in fact, is measured by integrity tests (Ash, 1991; Murphy, 1993; O'Bannon et al., 1989). These tests are far from homogeneous, and it is possible that they measure several distinct constructs. While there is evidence that tests that infer dishonesty from responses to items similar to those on standard personality measures share common factors (Woolley & Hakstian, 1992), it is also clear that these personality-based tests do not measure precisely the same thing as is measured by tests that ask for direct admissions of wrongdoing (Sackett et al., 1989). Debates about what integrity tests measure are complicated further by the fact that these tests often produce a variety of scores, some of which might have only limited links with the concept "integrity".

Table 1. Dimensions Often Reported in Analyses of Integrity Tests

1. Perceived Incidence of Dishonesty - less honest individuals are likely to report a higher incidence of dishonest behavior

2. Leniency Toward Dishonest Behavior - less honest individuals are more likely to forgive or excuse dishonest behavior

3. Theft Rationalization - less honest individuals are likely to come up with more excuses or reasons for theft

4. Theft Temptation or Rumination - less honest individuals are likely to think about theft

5. Norms Regarding Dishonest Behavior - less honest individuals are likely to view dishonest behavior as acceptable

6. Impulse Control - less honest individuals are likely to act on their impulses

7. Punitiveness Toward Self or Others - less honest individuals are likely to have more punitive attitudes

Table 2. Examples of Integrity Tests

Test	Scores Reported	Remarks
Reid Report	Honesty Attitude, Social Behavior Substance Abuse, Personal Achievements, Service Orientation, Clerical/Math Skills	measures both attitudes and direct admissions
Stanton Survey	Honesty Attitude, Admissions of previous dishonesty	measures both attitudes and direct admissions
Hogan Reliability Index	Score from Hogan Personality Inventory (HPI)	HPI is general purpose personality inventory
PDI	Productive Behavior, Tenure Employment Inventory	measures attitudes, self-description

Scoring integrity tests

As you can see from Table 2, integrity tests sometimes yield a wide range of scores. For example, the PDI Employment Inventory yields scores designed to predict both productive vs. counterproductive behavior on the job and tenure or turnover. The Reid Report yields scores for Honesty Attitude and Substance, both of which are arguably relevant to integrity, but it also yields scores for Service Orientation and Clerical/Math skills. Evidence that the scores reported for these tests mean what they claim to mean (e.g., claims that scores on a scale such as "drug Abuse" really measure that dimension rather than a dimension of general deviance are hard to test, much less prove; See Normand, Lempert and O'Brien, 1994) varies widely across tests, and claims that different tests measure either comparable constructs (e.g., scales with similar names) or that they measure meaningfully different constructs (e.g., scales with substantially different names) cannot always be accepted at face value (Camara & Schneider, 1994).

Scoring schemes for integrity tests are often proprietary, making it difficult to independently judge the measurement properties of these tests. During the first few decades of integrity testing, independent researchers often had limited opportunities to gain access to data about these tests, which contributed to an air of skepticism, secrecy, and even paranoia about what these tests measured. In the last 10-15 years, reputable test publishers have cooperated extensively with the research community, and many of the old suspicions about the legitimacy of this type of testing are starting to fade (e.g., Murphy, 1993, described codes of conduct that have been adopted by many integrity test publishers). Nevertheless, the use of proprietary scoring schemes, together with a tendency to produce diverse labels for scores that are probably comparable across tests (e.g., what is labeled "Honesty" in one test might be labeled "Productivity" in another) does greatly complicate the interpretation of integrity tests and of reviews and general discussions of this class of tests. Integrity tests are sufficiently diverse that some of the general statements about this class of testing encountered in the literature sometimes fall apart on close analysis.

Reliability and criterion-related validity of integrity tests

Sackett and his colleagues have conducted several reviews of research on the reliability, validity, and usefulness of integrity tests (Sackett, 1985; Sackett, Burris & Callahan, 1989; Sackett & Decker, 1979; Sackett & Harris, 1984; Sackett & Wanek, 1996 ; See also Goldberg, Grenier, Guion, Sechrest & Wing, 1991; Jones & Terris, 1991; Murphy, 1993; OTA, 1990). Ones et al. (1993) conducted a large-scale meta-analysis that quantitatively summarized the outcomes of multiple validity studies (See also Ones & Viswesvaran, 1998b). These reviews usually focus on general honesty or integrity scores produced by these tests (to the extent these are available), although bottom-line recommendations that are provided along with test scores (e.g., hire vs. do not hire) are sometimes used as proxy measures of general integrity. Conclusions about the reliability and validity of integrity tests as a class do not necessarily extend to specific scale scores (e.g., "Drug Abuse") that are reported on many of these tests.

   Several of the older reviews of integrity tests lamented the shortcomings of research on these measures, but the general conclusion of the more recent reviews has been more positive. Goldberg et al. (1991) suggest that these tests should be judged by the same standards used to evaluate standard personality inventories, and by these standards, integrity tests more than hold their own. There is now a substantial body of evidence showing that: (1) scores on integrity tests are reliable and stable across time, (2) integrity tests show consistent evidence of validity for predicting a variety of criteria that are relevant to organizations, and (3) these correlations have been replicated across a wide range of settings (Ones et al., 1993). This research does not say that tests of this sort will eliminate theft or dishonesty at work, but it does suggest that individuals who receive poor scores on these tests tend to be less desirable and less productive employees.

In discussing validity evidence, it is important to identify the specific criteria used in different studies.   Some studies have validated integrity tests against measures of counterproductive behavior, sometimes correlating scores on integrity tests with direct admissions criteria (i.e., measures involving direct admissions of wrongdoing).   Many integrity tests include questions dealing with direct admissions of wrongdoing, so it should come as no surprise that tests of this sort show very high correlations with direct admissions criteria.   However, even studies involving broad behavioral criteria suggest that integrity tests are consistently correlated with a fairly wide range of important outcome variables.   For example, scores on integrity tests show average corrected correlations of .34 and .47 with measures of overall job performance and counterproductivity, respectively (Ones et al., 1993).   Validities vary somewhat as a function of factors such as the type of integrity test (i.e., clear-purpose vs. veiled-purpose tests), the criterion measure (e.g., job performance measured in terms of either supervisory ratings or production) and job complexity (validities for predicting performance in complex jobs are generally higher), etc., but for most types of tests, criterion measures, jobs, etc., scores on integrity tests predict performance and counterproductivity on the job.   It is also important to note that the quality and and the number of validity studies included in the meta-analyses referred to above varies tremendously across tests.   The bulk of the available evidence comes from studies of a few well-researched tests, and caution must be observed in generalizing validity to all integrity tests.

Job performance and counterproductivity are clearly not independent; employees who engage in a wide variety of counterproductive behavior are unlikely to be good performers.   As a result, it is not surprising that integrity tests predict both criteria.   Nevertheless, this pattern of findings has led to a broader appreciation of the potential usefulness of these tests.   It seems clear that integrity tests are not simply a tool for investigating theft, fraud, of other specific aspects of workplace crime, but rather are a potentially useful tool in identifying individuals who are likely to perform well in their jobs and who are relatively unlikely to engage in a fairly broad range of counterproductive behaviors.

The consistent success of integrity tests in predicting broad-based criteria begs the question of why these tests work.   That is, how can we explain the success of tests that seem narrow in their focus (e.g., overt integrity tests), that appear to vary widely in their characteristics (e.g., clear-purpose tests are very different in their design, content, and scoring than veiled-purpose tests), and that produce such a wide range of specific scores, in predicting broad-based criteria such as overall job performance?   Much of the recent research on integrity testing has focused on understanding what these tests measure and why they work.

INTEGRITY AND CONSCIENTIOUSNESS

Much of the initial speculation about what integrity tests measure and why they are useful in predicting criteria such as overall job performance centered on the construct "conscientiousness". Most veiled-purpose tests include items that directly measure conscientiousness, or some closely related personality construct (Sackett, et al., 1989). One widely-used test (e.g. the Employee Reliability Index) was designed explicitly to tap conscientiousness, along with several other theoretically relevant traits. Overt integrity tests are not necessarily designed to measure this personality characteristic, but even these tests are probably influenced by the respondent's level of conscientiousness. Highly conscientious individuals are probably less likely to commit illegal or questionable acts, which means that they simply have less to admit when responding to tests that call for admissions of past thefts, crimes, or other questionable behaviors.

Three reasons have been cited for believing that integrity tests measure conscientiousness. First, examinations of the items and subscales included in commercially-developed integrity tests show strong similarities to the items used in some measures of conscientiousness (Hogan & Hogan, 1989; Johnson, 1991; O'Bannon et al., 1989; Sackett et al., 1989). Hogan and Ones (1997) recently reviewed different theoretical perspectives on the conscientiousness construct and noted that several of these perspectives could be linked to the construct "integrity". Second, the descriptions of individuals who exhibit high levels of either integrity or conscientiousness (e.g. dependable, responsible, careful) show striking similarity. That is, peoples' behavior often leads to inferences about their integrity and their conscientiousness, and these inferences often closely parallel one another. Third, several studies have reported significant correlations between measures of integrity and conscientiousness (Collins & Schmidt, 1993; Hogan, 1986; Jones & Terris, 1983; Woolley & Hakstian, 1992). Murphy and Lee (1994a) showed that the average correlations between measures of conscientiousness and scores on two integrity tests were higher than correlations between integrity and most other personality dimensions.

While it is tempting to view integrity tests as surrogate measures of conscientiousness, there are a number of problems with this explanation for what these tests measure and why they work. First, conscientiousness is a complex construct. Costa and McCrae (1992) suggest six facets for conscientiousness (competence, order, dutifulness, achievement striving, self discipline, deliberation), whereas other authors (e.g., Hogan, 1991) suggest that only some of these are part of the conscientiousness construct. Given the continuing debate over exactly what constitutes conscientiousness, linking integrity to conscientiousness may not help all that much in understanding what integrity tests really measure. Second, most integrity tests are factorially complex (Murphy, 1993; Ones & Viswesvaran, 1998b), and generally reflect several factors that are not obviously linked to conscientiousness (e.g. punitiveness, thrill-seeking, intolerance for dishonesty; see also O'Bannon et al., 1989; Woolley & Hakstian, 1992). Although many integrity tests are partially based on conscientiousness measures, evidence from a variety of studies and methods does not support the hypothesis that they are surrogate measures of conscientiousness (Woolley & Hakstian, 1992, 1993). There is evidence that a general factor may pervade many of these tests (Harris & Sackett, 1987; Ones, Viswesvaran & Schmidt, 1993), but it is far from clear whether this general factor is conscientiousness.

Even if integrity tests measure factors other than conscientiousness, it is possible that the links between integrity tests and conscientiousness explain why integrity tests "work" as predictors of broad-based criteria such as overall job performance. Conscientiousness is consistently correlated with job performance and other broad criteria of this sort (Barrick & Mount, 1991), and it also correlated with scores on many integrity tests. The hypothesis that conscientiousness explains the relationship found between integrity test scores and measures of job performance can be tested by the simple expedient of partial correlation. If this hypothesis is true, statistically controlling for conscientiousness should substantially diminish the relationship between integrity and performance.

Conscientiousness as an explanation for why integrity tests "work"

Murphy and Lee (1994b) used the strategy outlined above - i.e., examining the semi-partial correlation between integrity and performance, controlling for the effect of conscientiousness on integrity. This study, which was based on a meta-analysis of selected published research on integrity tests, suggested that removing conscientiousness from integrity tests has little influence on the validity of these tests as predictors of job performance. The average zero-order correlation between integrity and performance is approximately .34; when conscientiousness is removed from integrity, this correlation changes only slightly (the semi-partial correlation is .27). Hogan and Ones (1997) report similar results from a more comprehensive meta-analysis of integrity tests.

An alternative method for examining the relative contribution of integrity and conscientiousness to the prediction of job performance is to examine their multiple correlation with performance. Murphy and Lee (1994b) reported that the multiple R for predicting performance on the basis of conscientiousness and integrity was .36, which is only slightly larger than the zero-order correlation between integrity and performance (i.e., r = .34). The results of this study and studies discussed above suggest that: (1) integrity test scores are consistently correlated with measures of overall job performance, (2) conscientiousness cannot explain the correlation between integrity and job performance, and (3) conscientiousness adds little, over and above integrity test scores, to the prediction of job performance.

Although conscientiousness is clearly an important component of integrity, it seems clear that conscientiousness is not the only factor, and perhaps not even an important factor in explaining why scores on tests that appear to be so narrow and specific in their focus (i.e., tests that focus on honesty, theft, deviant behavior) should consistently correlate with broad measures of performance on the job. Recent studies of the validity and meaning of integrity tests have attempted to explain their success by arguing that integrity is in fact a higher-order construct that subsumes many facets of personality.

Is Integrity a Higher-Order Construct ?

Analyses of integrity tests consistently show that these tests measure several aspects of personality and behavior (Cunningham & Ash, 1988; O'Bannon et al., 1989; Ones & Viswesvaran, 1998b). For example, Woolley and Hakstian (1992, 1993) discuss four factors common to many integrity tests: (1) conventional commitment, (2) intolerance for dishonesty, (3) socialized control, and (4) active conscientiousness.   Ones and her colleagues have suggested that scores on integrity tests are substantially related to measures of several of the "big five" personality factors (Digman, 1990; See Murphy and Lee, 1994a, for further discussions of correlations between integrity and big five measures). In general, this research suggests that scores on integrity tests are correlated with personality dimensions such as agreeableness and emotional stability, and these correlations are nearly as large as the correlation between integrity and conscientiousness (Ones and Viswesvaran, 1998). Scores on these tests are also correlated with measures of Extroversion, but these correlations are substantially smaller than for conscientiousness, agreeableness or emotional stability. In an attempt to account for this pattern of relationships, several authors have labeled integrity as a higher-order construct (Ones & Viswesvaran, 1998a, 1988b; Ones, Viswesvaran, & Schmidt, 1993; Sackett & Wanek, 1996).

There has been considerable speculation about what this higher-order construct might represent. Collins and Schmidt (1993) note that measures of Socialization and scores on integrity tests show similar correlations to measures of conscientiousness, agreeableness and emotional stability, suggesting that socialization may function as a higher-order trait that overlaps with integrity. Others have suggested that integrity might function as the "g" factor in personality (perhaps here "g" might stand for "good"). Hogan and Ones (1997) note that it is possible to draw inferences about what integrity tests measure (and therefore about the nature of this higher-order construct) on the basis of the known correlates of these tests. For example, individuals with low scores on the Hogan Reliability Scale are rated as tense, moody, worrying and self-pitying, and as hostile, insensitive and impulsive. Individuals with high scores on these scales are rated as mature, thoughtful, responsible, and inhibited. A theme running through this list of attributes is that people who receive high scores on integrity tests tend to have "good" characteristics, at least in the sense that these characteristics make it more likely that they will function smoothly in society.

The fact that integrity tests show substantial correlations with such a wide range of personality variables is both a blessing and a curse to researchers interested in determining what these tests measure. On the one hand, integrity tests seem to correlate with just about every major facet of personality other than Openness to Experience (scores on integrity tests are essentially uncorrelated with this personality dimension or with measures of general cognitive ability; Murphy, 1993). This supports the notion that integrity is indeed a higher-order factor, perhaps one that comprises a good deal of the domain of normal personality. On the other hand, there are good reasons to question the claim that integrity is a higher-order construct of this sort. If integrity is not a higher-order construct, this pattern of relatively large correlations between such a wide range of personality dimensions and integrity tests could present a significant problem for determining what "integrity" really means.

There are several reasons to doubt the claim that integrity is a higher-order construct, in any meaningful sense of the word. First, it is not clear whether there is any well-defined higher-order personality factor for these tests to measure. Higher-order constructs have been identified in analyses of several domains, most notably in analyses of performance on cognitive ability tests (Carroll, 1993; for opposing views, see Sternberg, 1977; Sternberg & Wagner, 1993). In the ability domain, a general factor appears to underlie performance on a wide range of cognitively demanding tasks, and factors can be defined at several levels of specificity (e.g., verbal vs. spatial groupings are often reported) to describe the structure of this domain. General factors of this sort have not typically been found in analyses of personality inventories (Murphy, 1996, contrasts analyses of cognitive and personality domains), and while the "big five" might be thought of as higher-order factors that each summarize specific facets of personality, there is no clear evidence that meaningful factors exist at any higher level of analysis. That is, there is no clear evidence that there is any meaningful "g" in the domain of personality.

Second, assuming that there is some meaningful higher-order personality factor, it seems unlikely that the developers of integrity tests happened upon a general factor that has evaded other personality researchers for decades. There is no evidence that integrity tests were developed with the goal of providing a summary measure of the "g" underlying personality (if such a thing exists), and it is hard to believe that this happened by accident. As I will note below, the approach typically used to develop integrity tests has focused more on predicting future behavior than on understanding the constructs measured by these tests, and it begs belief to argue that a group of tests developed in such a way stumbled on a fundamental aspect of the personality domain that has evaded virtually all other personality researchers.

The alternative to arguing that integrity is a higher-order construct that encapsulates much of the domain of normal personality is the argument that these tests don't measure any well-defined construct at all, but rather contain a hodgepodge of items that span large portions of the domain of personality. That is, it is possible that these tests might sample many aspects of personality and behavior that are generally desirable (or that are generally deviant), with relatively little regard for tying these themes together into a general but interpretable construct. This characterization is hardly fair to some tests (e.g., the PDI Employment Inventory and the Hogan Reliability Index are examples of tests that were developed based on a well-articulated theory or rationale), but it may be a reasonable summary of integrity tests as a class. As I will note below, the strategies used to develop these tests argue against developing a coherent definition of the construct "integrity".

CRITERION VS. CONSTRUCT-ORIENTED TEST DEVELOPMENT: IMPLICATIONS FOR UNDERSTANDING THE INTEGRITY CONSTRUCT

Literature describing the development of integrity tests is somewhat spotty, and it is often necessary to make guesses and inferences about the exact strategy for developing these tests. When you consider how and why these tests were developed, it is easy to see why there is less material describing the constructs, the research strategies, the ideas, etc. underlying these tests than there is for other personality inventories. Integrity tests were originally developed to address a practical need (reducing theft, deviance, counterproductive behavior, etc.), and they were typically developed for commercial purposes rather than for research purposes. As a result, there are aspects of the development of integrity tests that are still not well-documented, and the discussion below of test development strategies is necessarily somewhat speculative. Nevertheless, it is useful to consider how and why these tests were developed, and what this might mean for identifying the constructs measured by these tests.

On the whole (with exceptions noted above), the strategy involved in developing these tests has focused more strongly on the pragmatic uses of these tests than on the question of what these tests might measure. That is, more emphasis had been placed on developing tests that would predict counterproductivity than on developing tests that measure a well articulated construct (i.e., integrity). This emphasis makes sense for several reasons, most notably because there is still little agreement about what construct(s) integrity tests should measure (Camara & Schneider, 1994; Murphy, 1993). There has been a longstanding debate about the nature of the "honesty" construct (Burton, 1963; Hartshorne & May, 1928; Hollinger & Clark, 1982), and to this day it is not clear whether honesty, integrity, or dependability are characteristics of the individual, the situation, or some interaction between the two (Murphy, 1993). There is little argument with the fact that scores on integrity tests are useful predictors of counterproductive behavior, job performance, and other organizationally-relevant criteria, but there is still no clear consensus about what high or low scores on these tests really mean. To a large extent, the problem is probably a reflection of the way in which many of these tests were developed.

Approaches to developing integrity tests

There appear to be three distinct strategies that have been followed developing integrity tests, none of which involve a careful explication of the constructs these tests are thought to measure (again, some measures, including the Hogan Reliability Index and the PDI Employment index are exceptions.   First, many items, scales, and tests appear to be based on the well-known principle that past behavior predicts future behavior.   Thus, many clear-purpose tests have used admissions of past theft, counterproductivity, etc. to predict similar behavior in the future - with considerable success.   At first glance, this approach to test development seems almost too simplistic to be practical.   Indeed, some of the skepticism surrounding integrity tests (especially clear-purpose tests) revolves around the idea that people will not be so stupid as to admit past transgressions, especially when applying for a job.   However, the logic of clear-purpose tests is more subtle than it first appears, because many of these tests also draw on a second conceptual underpinning that both allows one to predict dishonesty, counterproductivity, etc. and explains why people might be willing to make admissions - i.e., the idea that dishonesty in the workplace is tied to a state of relative normlessness (Murphy, 1993).

It is possible that people differ substantially in their beliefs about what behaviors are or are not acceptable in particular contexts, and that it is the people who believe that dishonest behavior is normatively acceptable (in a particular setting or directed against a particular target) who engage in this behavior. Explanations of dishonest behavior that involve the concept of normlessness run something like this: (1) most people believe that they are honest, at least in the sense that they abide with current norms regarding respect for the truth, for others' property, etc., (2) people vary considerably in their beliefs about what these norms really call for, (3) some people believe that theft, dishonesty, etc. is in fact acceptable, because it is part of "how things really work" in a particular setting, whereas others believe that norms regarding honesty and dependability are much less flexible, (4) people who believe that their own dishonest behavior is in fact well within the norm will engage in dishonesty and will be less concerned about admitting dishonest behavior. Murphy (1993) argues that people are often willing to admit wrongdoing when responding to clear-purpose tests because they believe that their behavior is in fact quite acceptable (i.e., it conforms to workplace norms), and that they are at least as honest as most people in their same situation.

The idea that dishonesty springs from normlessness is not only a basis for tests involving direct admissions, it also serves as a conceptual basis for many of the items found on clear-purpose and even veiled-purpose tests. Many items ask about your beliefs, opinions, and attitudes toward dishonesty, and it is a reasonable bet that people who think that dishonest behavior is common, is not really sanctioned, is in keeping with the norm, etc. will be at risk for engaging in these same behaviors.

Tests based on the principle of behavioral consistency or on the concept of normlessness imply a partial definition of what integrity is, but these definitions are quite limited. For example, you might define integrity in terms of not engaging in dishonest behaviors (this is what the behavioral consistency concept suggests). This is true almost by definition, but it does not help us much in understanding what integrity is. Tests developed on the basis of the normlessness concept provide a somewhat clearer definition of integrity, but even here, there are difficulties. According to the normlessness explanation, people high on integrity accept a relatively narrow and restrictive set of norms, whereas those low on integrity abide by a much more flexible set of norms. This notion ties in nicely with the suggestion that integrity is strongly linked to the Socialization trait (Collins & Schmidt, 1993), but it still leaves the question of why some people believe that workplace norms are strict while others in the same setting believe that norms are more tolerant of dishonesty, counterproductivity, etc.. That is, arguing that people who are dishonest or undependable abide by a different set of norms than people who are scrupulously honest leads directly to the question of why they differ so much in their perceptions of what behaviors are or are not normative.

The development of veiled-purpose integrity tests sometimes starts with a hypothesis or theory about the personality characteristics that might be linked to honesty in the workplace; a number of veiled purpose integrity tests have been developed to measure these personality traits. Tests developed on the basis of some theory about the reasons for dishonest behavior in the workplace have the advantage of being tied into a network of other constructs, some of which (e.g., conscientiousness) are likely to be well-researched. However, these tests are not particularly strong examples of construct-oriented tests, for two reasons. First, these tests usually leave the construct of "general integrity","honesty", etc. undefined, or at best poorly defined. That is, many tests have been developed on the basis of hypotheses about why people engage in dishonest or deviant behavior, but few have been developed explicitly to measure a well-articulated concept of integrity. To complicate matters further, different tests that have been developed on the basis of some model or theory of honesty vs. dishonesty in the workplace are rarely based on theories that are identical or even similar in their nature. The theories or models that underlie many integrity tests tend to be ad hoc, untested networks of ideas that vary widely from author to author. There is not yet any single well-accepted theory of honesty in the workplace, and those tests that are based on some theory or model may not be any better than the underling theories. Because the theories underlying many tests are not tested or fully developed, it is often difficult to determine whether theory-based tests are in fact any more interpretable than tests designed simply to maximize predictive efficiency.

Some inferences about the constructs that underlie integrity tests

The focus on criterion-related rather than construct-oriented questions in developing integrity tests has left us with a difficult state of affairs. We know that these tests "work", but we still do not know why. In particular, there is still no clear, widely-accepted definition of the integrity construct, and still no good sense of what scores on these tests really tell you about a person. However, we can draw from the available research to make some inferences about what these tests are likely to measure, and possibly about ways that these tests could be improved.

First, it is reasonable to infer that these tests do not measure honesty. People who receive favorable scores on integrity tests may be less prone to engage in dishonest behavior, or may be willing to engage in this behavior in a more narrow range of situations than people with less favorable scores, but there is little to be gained by thinking of these as "honesty" tests. These tests cover a wider range of behaviors and attitudes that would be expected in a measure of honesty (which would logically focus on truthfulness, but not necessarily on impulsiveness, thrill-seeking, likelihood of goldbricking or some other form of counterproductive behavior, etc.)

Second, these tests clearly relate to concepts such as Socialization (Collins & Schmidt, 1993) and normlessness (Murphy, 1993). Interviews, self-reports, and other assessments of peoples' beliefs about their own behavior consistently indicate that people who engage in dishonest or counterproductive behavior often believe that they have done nothing wrong. There may be some self-delusion, face-saving, or defensiveness in these assessments, but peoples' willingness to make obviously damaging admissions in so many settings argues that many of the people who engage in workplace dishonesty honestly believe that what they have done is normal, common, and acceptable. The hypothesis that these tests relate to the ability to identify those behaviors that are socially desirable and the tendency to endorse those behaviors might also help to explain the pattern of correlations between measures of the "big 5" and integrity tests. Most of the "big 5" factors have a strong current of social desirability, in the sense that there is no doubt about which end of most dimensions is the "good" one (e.g., a person who is dependable, stable, and agreeable is almost always preferable to a person who is unreliable, neurotic and mean).

Third, the fact that conscientiousness cannot explain the validity of these tests as predictors of overall performance, counterproductivity, etc. should not cause us to lose sight of the unique status of conscientiousness for understanding these tests. Measures of this personality attribute are consistently among the strongest correlates of scores on integrity tests, and any adequate theory about what these tests measure must start with an explanation of the links between integrity tests and measures of conscientiousness.

Finally, statements about this class of tests (including many such statements made in this chapter) can be confusing because these tests are far from homogeneous. Scores on most integrity tests are likely to be correlated, but they are rarely substitutable. These tests differ in terms of the item types they include, in terms of their focus, and even in terms of the criteria they are designed to predict. There are some tests that were developed with considerable attention to construct explication, and others in which there is no serious attempt to determine what the scores really mean. Statements of any sort about integrity tests as a class are likely to require extensive footnotes (e.g., the statement that the underlying constructs are not at all defined applies to some tests but not to others). Much of what you read about integrity tests, starting with promotional material and going right through reviews published in leading journals needs to be examined with a critical eye.

Integrity tests occupy a niche that is both familiar and slightly depressing for applied psychologists - i.e., tests that seem to work well, without anyone knowing exactly why (measures based on biodata sometimes occupy this same niche). That is, these tests fill a real need, and they will continue to fill that need even if debates over precisely what they measure are never resolved. On the other hand, there is a powerful pragmatic argument for pursuing questions about the construct validity of these tests. It is a good bet that if we knew precisely what they measured and why they worked, we would be able to improve on existing measures (which work pretty well even now; see Jackson, 1970, 1971). Indeed, in the end, the strongest argument for pushing questions of construct validity to the forefront is likely to be the very practical argument that this is the likeliest road toward improving on the current generation of integrity tests. These tests are useful now, but with a clearer understanding of the dynamics of integrity testing, it might be possible to improve the tests and improve peoples' willingness to use these tests as aids in making decisions in organizations.

REFERENCES

Ash, P. (1991). *The construct of employee theft proneness.* Chicago: SRA/London House.

Barrick, M.R. & Mount, M.K. (1991). The big five personality dimensions and job performance: A meta analysis. *Personnel Psychology,* **44,** 1-26.

Ben-Shakhar, G. & Furedy, J.J. (1990). *Theories and applications in the detection of deception.* New York: Springer-Verlag.

Burton, R.V. (1963). Generality of honesty reconsidered. *Psychological Review,* **70,** 481-499.

Camara, W. J. & Schneider, D. L. (1994). Integrity tests: Facts and unresolved issues. *American Psychologist,* **49,** 112-119.

Carroll, J.B. (1993) *Human cognitive abilities: A survey of factor-analytic studies.* Cambridge, UK: Cambridge University Press.

Collins, J. & Schmidt, F. (1993). Personality, integrity, and white collar crime. *Personnel Psychology,* **46,** 295-311.

Costa, P.T. and McCrae, R.R. (1992). *Manual for the Revised NEO Personality Inventory* (NEO- PI-R). Odessa, Florida: Psychological Assessment Resources, Inc.

Cunningham, M.R. & Ash, P. (1988). The structure of honesty: Analysis of the Reid Report. *Journal of Business and Psychology,* **3,** 54-66.

Digman, J.M. (1990). Personality structure: Emergence of the five-factor model. *Annual Review of Psychology,* **41,** 417-440.

Ekman, P. (1975). *Telling lies: Clues to deceit in the marketplace, politics, and marriage.* New York: Norton.

Ekman, P. & O'Sullivan, M. (1991). Who can catch a lie? *American Psychologist,* **46,** 913-920.

Goldberg, L.R., Grenier, J.R., Guion, R.M., Sechrest, L.B. & Wing, H. (1991). *Questionnaires used in the prediction of trustworthiness in preemployment selection decisions.* Washington, DC: American Psychological Association.

Harris, M.M. & Sackett, P.R. (1987). A factor analysis and item response theory analysis of an employee honesty test. *Journal of Business and Psychology,* **2,** 122-135.

Hartshorne, H. & May, M.A. (1928). *Studies in deceit.* New York: MacMillan.

Hogan, R. (1986). *Manual for the Hogan Personality Inventory.* Minneapolis: National Computer Systems.

Hogan, J. & Hogan, R. (1989). How to measure employee reliability. *Journal of Applied Psychology,* **74,** 273-279.

Hogan, R. (1991). Personality and personality measurement. In M. D. Dunnette and L. M. Hough (Eds). *Handbook of Industrial and Organizational Psychology* (Vol. **2,** pp.327-398). Palo Alto, CA: Consulting Psychologists Press.

Hogan, J. & Ones, D. (1997) Conscientiousness and integrity at work. In R. Hogan and J. Johnson (Ed.s). *Handbook of personality psychology* (pp. 849-870). San Diego: Academic Press.

Hollinger, R.C. & Clark, J.P. (1983). *Theft by employees. Lexington,* MA: D.C. Heath.

Jackson, D.N. (1970). A sequential system for personality scale development. In. C.D. Spielberger (Ed.), *Current Topics in clinical and community psychology* (Vol. **2,** pp 61-96). New York: Academic Press.

Jackson, D.N. (1971). The dynamics of structured personality tests: 1971. *Psychological Review,* **78,** 29-248.

Johnson, J.A. (1991). PDI Employment Inventory. In D. Keyser and R. Sweetland (Eds.), *Test critiques* (vol. **8**). Kansas City: Test Corporation of America.

Jones, J.W. & Terris, W. (1991). Integrity testing for personnel selection: An overview. *Forensic Reports,* **4,** 117-140.

Kleinmuntz, B. & Szucko, J. (1984). Lie detection in ancient and modern times: A call for contemporary scientific study. *American Psychologist,* **39,** 766-776.

Lykken, D.T. (1981). *A tremor in the blood: Uses and abuses of the lie detector.* New York: McGraw-Hill.

McKee, T.E. & Bayes, P.E. (1987). Why audit background investigations . *Internal Auditor,* **44** (5), 53-56.

Murphy, K. (1993). *Honesty in the workplace.* Monterey, CA: Brooks/Cole.

Murphy, K. (1996). Individual differences and behavior in organizations: Much more than g. In Murphy, K. (Ed). *Individual differences and behavior in organizations.* (pp. 3-30). San Francisco: Jossey-Bass.

Murphy, K. & Lee, S. (1994a). Does conscientiousness explain the relationship between integrity and performance? *International Journal of Selection and Assessment*, **2**, 226-233.

Murphy, K. & Lee, S. (1994b). Personality variables related to integrity test scores: The role of conscientiousness. *Journal of Business and Psychology*, **8**, 413-424.

Murphy, K. & Luther, N. (1997). Assessing and inferring honesty, integrity and deception. In N. Anderson and P. Herriot (Eds.), *International handbook of selection and appraisal:Second Edition* (pp. 369-392). Chichester, UK: Wiley.

Murphy, K. & Wright, K. (1996). Accounting for the apparently limited validity of preemployment drug and alcohol tests: States versus traits as predictors of future performance and suitability. *Human Performance*, **9**, 331-347

Normand, J., Lempert, R. & O'Brien, C. (1994). *Under the influence ?: Drugs and the American workforce.* Washington, DC: National Academy Press.

O'Bannon, R.M., Goldinger, L.A. & Appleby, J.D. (1989). *Honesty and integrity testing: A practical guide.* Atlanta: Applied Information Resources.

Office of Technology Assessment (1990). *The use of integrity tests for pre-employment screening.* Washington, DC: U.S.Congress Office of Technology Assessment.

Ones, D. & Viswesvaran, C. (1998a). Gender, age and race differences on overt integrity tests: Results across four large-scale job applicant data sets. *Journal of Applied Psychology*, **83**, 35-42.

Ones, D. & Viswesvaran, C. (1998b). Integrity testing in organizations. In R. Griffen and A. O'Leary-Kelly (Eds.) *Dysfunctional behavior in organizations: Violent and deviant behavior.* Monographs in Organizational Behavior and Industrial Relations. Vol. **23**, parts A & B (pp. 243-276). Stamford, CT: JAI Press.

Ones, D.S., Viswesvaran, C. & Schmidt, F.L (1993). Comprehensive meta-analysis of integrity test validities. *Journal of Applied Psychology* (Monograph), **78**, 679-703.

Sackett, P.R. (1985). Honesty research and the person-situation debate. In W. Terris (Ed.), *Employee theft .* Chicago: London House Press.

Sackett, P.R., Burris, L.R. & Callahan. C. (1989). Integrity testing for personnel selection: An update. *Personnel Psychology*, **42**, 491-529.

Sackett, P.R. & Decker, P.J. (1979). Detection of deception in the employment context: A review and critique. *Personnel Psychology*, **32**, 487-506.

Sackett, P.R. & Harris, M.M (1984). Honesty testing for personnel selection: A review and critique. *Personnel Psychology*, **37**, 221-245.

Sackett, P. R., & Wanek, J. E. (1996). New developments in the use of measures of honesty, integrity, conscientiousness, dependability, trustworthiness, and reliability for personnel selection. *Personnel Psychology*, **49**, 787-829.

Sternberg, R.J. (1977). *Intelligence, information processing, and analogical reasoning: The componental analysis of human abilities.* Hillsdale, NJ: Erlbaum.

Sternberg, R.J. & Wagner, R.K. (1993). The g-ocentric view of intelligence and performance is wrong. *Current Directions in Psychological Science*, **2**, 1-5.

Woolley, R.M. & Hakstian, A.R. (1992). An examination of the construct validity of personality-based and overt measures of integrity. *Educational and Psychological Measurement*, **52**, 475-489.

Woolley, R.M. & Hakstian, A.R. (1993). A comparative study of integrity tests: The criterion- related validity of personality-based and overt measures of integrity. *International Journal   of Selection and Assessment*, **1**, 27-40.

13 CONSTRUCT VALIDATION IN ORGANIZATIONAL BEHAVIOR RESEARCH: THE CASE OF ORGANIZATIONAL COMMITMENT

Natalie J. Allen
John P. Meyer

Several years ago, in a paper entitled "Construct validity and personality assessment" Jackson (1979) argued that the greatest impact of the construct approach to psychological measurement had been felt in the area of personality. In describing his own work, and that of others, he demonstrated the value of this approach for understanding personality and for personality scale construction. As in personality assessment work, much of the research conducted by organizational psychologists relies on questionnaire measures developed to assess complex constructs. It is interesting to note that, around the same time as Jackson's comments, Schwab (1980, p.34) lamented that "organizational behavior has suffered" from a lack of attention to construct validation. In the intervening 20 years, attention to the construct and its measurement has increased in organizational research. Nonetheless, one could not argue that the construct approach has gained center stage in this area or that concerns about conceptual and measurement adequacy in organizational research have been ameliorated dramatically. Indeed, in recent discussions of questionnaire measures developed for use in organizations, Hinkin (1995, 1998) suggested that concerns about adequate construct measurement represented "perhaps the greatest difficulty in conducting survey research" (Hinkin, 1995, p. 967).

In this chapter, our overall objective is to illustrate the use, and demonstrate the value, of the construct approach within organizational psychology. To do so, we focus particular attention on the conceptualization and measurement of organizational commitment. We begin with a short history of research on organizational commitment. This is followed by an overview of our program of organizational commitment research and a discussion of construct issues that remain to be explored more fully.

ORGANIZATIONAL COMMITMENT: A SHORT RESEARCH HISTORY

Very generally speaking, organizational commitment refers to a psychological state that characterizes an employee's relationship with the organization for which s/he works and which has implications for the employee's intention to remain with the organization. Of the several "work attitude" variables studied by organizational psychologists, only job satisfaction has received more research attention than organizational commitment. Much of this interest was prompted by (a) an interest in better understanding, and an ability to predict, employee turnover and (b) the belief that strongly committed employees would outperform those with weak commitment.

"Early" Organizational Commitment Research

Organizational psychologists have been interested for some time in understanding how and why people become psychologically attached to various aspects of the work they do and the various contexts in which they do this work. By the mid-1980s, a great deal of research had been conducted on "commitment" to several work-related foci including unions, occupations, one's career, the job itself, and the organization. In her 1983 review of the existing work commitment literature, Morrow identified 30 forms of work commitment and called for a moratorium on new commitment constructs until these various concepts, and their associated measures, could be evaluated systematically. Reflecting on the state of the research that existed at the time of their 1986 review, Griffin and Bateman wrote that "depending on one's point of view, the study of work commitment may be characterized by either (a) healthy eclecticism, or (b) schizophrenic fragmentation" (p.165).

Although this "early research" focussed on psychological attachment to various work domains, commitment to the organization was most extensively studied. This body of research, which spanned the 60s, 70s, and early 80s, is characterized by three important features that, arguably, have served to shape subsequent thinking about the organizational commitment construct and its measurement.

Perhaps the most striking characteristic of the early research on organizational commitment is the wide variety of definitions that researchers gave to the term "commitment." Although there is consensus that commitment serves to reduce the likelihood that the employee will choose to leave the organization, researchers described the psychological nature of commitment quite differently. The various definitions correspond, some more closely than others, to three general themes. For several researchers, commitment represents a positive emotional response to the organization, its goals, and values. For example, Buchanan (1974) described commitment as a "partisan, affective attachment to the goals and values, to one's role in relation to goals and values, and to the organization for its own sake, apart from its purely instrumental worth" (p. 533). Kanter (1968) referred to the "attachment of an individual's fund of affectivity and emotion toward the group" (p. 507). Other researchers focussed on the difficulties – or costs – associated with leaving the organization. Most influential among these was Becker (1960) who described commitment as "consistent lines of activity" (p. 33) that come about when individuals make, and accumulate, side bets that would be lost if the activity were discontinued. In a similar vein, Kanter (1968) used the term "calculative commitment" to refer to "profits associated with continued participation and a "cost" associated with leaving" (p. 504). Finally, still other researchers described commitment as a feeling of obligation to remain with the organization. Marsh and Mannari (1977) argued, for example, that "the committed employee considers it morally right to stay in the company" (p. 59). Similarly, Wiener and Vardi (1980) suggested that commitment to an organization stems from "values of loyalty and duty toward the organization" and that an employee continues to contribute to an organization "because he believes he "should" behave this way, since this is the "right" and expected behavior" (p. 84).

Until the early 1980s, these various definitions were used somewhat interchangeably in the research literature. Needless to say, this created considerable conceptual and interpretive confusion within the study of organizational commitment.

A second feature of this research is that very little attention was given by researchers to explicating the commitment construct (as they saw it) and to developing and validating measures of commitment within a systematic program of research. An important exception to this is the work done by Mowday and his colleagues (for a summary see Mowday, Porter, & Steers, 1982). Consistent with the first theme described above, they conceptualized organizational commitment in terms of the employee's identification with, involvement in, and desire to stay with the organization. On the basis of this definition, they developed the Organizational Commitment Questionnaire (OCQ), a measure that has been, and continues to be, used extensively by researchers. In 1979, Mowday, Steers and Porter outlined the conceptual foundation of commitment as they saw it, described the development of the measure and its psychometric properties, and summarized several studies in which the measure had been used. Thus, we know a considerable amount about this particular measure of organizational commitment and its correlates.

Unfortunately, few other commitment measures used in research during this period received this sort of careful scrutiny. Many of the measures that researchers used were created for one or two studies only and were rarely examined in light of existing measures. Typically, little detail was provided about how these scales were constructed. Almost no attention was paid to how commitment should be related to other conceptually similar (or dissimilar) variables, on what basis it should develop, or, with the notable exception of employee turnover, what specific implications it should have for employee behavior. Further, the commitment construct, as defined in a given study, did not always seem to correspond with the measure used to assess it. For example, following Becker's (1960) side-bet theory, several researchers (Alutto, Hrebiniak, & Alonso, 1973; Hrebiniak & Alutto, 1972; Ritzer & Trice, 1969) defined commitment in terms of the costs associated with leaving the organization. In the particular measure they used, however, respondents were asked the likelihood that they would leave the organization if given various attractive inducements to do so. Getting a high "commitment" score on this measure meant that the respondents were unwilling to leave even in the presence of attractive options. Rather than suggesting that costs associated with leaving were at stake here, this suggests that high scorers found their organization so desirable that little could lure them away. Conceptually (Stebbins, 1970), and empirically (Meyer & Allen, 1984), it does not appear that the measure assesses commitment at all as Becker conceptualized it. In sum, with one notable exception (Mowday et al., 1979), there is little evidence in the early literature that attention was given to the construct validity of organizational commitment measures.

Perhaps not surprisingly, then, the third feature of the early commitment research is the inconsistency of empirical findings that it produced. This was particularly noticeable, and, arguably, most disappointing when considering the behavioral "consequences" of commitment. Although most putative measures of commitment were correlated with turnover intention, results regarding other hypothesized consequences were mixed. In their meta-analysis of commitment research conducted during this period, Mathieu and Zajac (1990) noted that relations between commitment and various outcome measures (e.g., job performance) were moderated by the type of measure used. Beyond this, however, the commitment literature up until the mid-1980s provided little guidance as to how findings regarding the consequences of commitment might reasonably be interpreted.

We have suggested here that the early research on organizational commitment was characterized by three features: varying conceptual definitions, inadequate attention to measure development, and mixed empirical findings. Taken together, these three features made for a very confusing situation.

Organizational Commitment Research: Mid-1980s to the Present

During the 1980s, the organizational commitment literature underwent two important and related changes. First, although earlier work in the area was characterized by various, and often conflicting, uni-dimensional views of the construct, organizational commitment came to be recognized as a multidimensional work attitude (e.g., Mayer & Schoorman, 1992; Meyer & Allen, 1984, 1991; O'Reilly & Chatman, 1986).   For example, O'Reilly and his colleagues conceptualized organizational commitment as having three distinct bases. Specifically, they argued that the psychological bond between the employee and the organization is based, jointly, on the employee's interest in gaining rewards from the organization (compliance), pride in his/her relationship with the organization (identification) and congruence between the values of the employee and those of the organization (internalization). Although some studies support the distinctions between these three dimensions (e.g., Becker, Billings, Eveleth, & Gilbert, 1996), other researchers have encountered difficulties distinguishing between identification and internalization (e.g., Vandenberg, Self, & Seo, 1994). Furthermore, because compliance is positively, rather than negatively, associated with turnover, it is not clear in what sense the compliance measure assesses commitment to the organization. Despite these concerns, this work, and that of others who took a multidimensional view of commitment, prompted researchers to scrutinize some of the inconsistencies in the commitment literature.

A second, and perhaps more critical, change in the commitment literature was that greater attention was paid to the construct in question and to its measurement. Theoretical discussions by Morrow (1983), Reichers (1985), Scholl (1981) and others, likely contributed considerably to this change, as did the frustration that researchers felt with the confusing set of findings in the empirical literature. The growing awareness within organizational psychology of the construct approach and its value also played a role in stimulating this change.

Not surprisingly, some of the conceptual changes in the study of organizational commitment have been accompanied by efforts to refine and validate measures of the organizational commitment construct. One program of research in which explication of the organizational commitment construct and programmatic measurement work have gone hand in hand resulted in a three-component view of organizational commitment (Allen & Meyer, 1990a; Meyer & Allen, 1991, 1997). In the sections that follow, we outline the organizational commitment construct as conceptualized in the three-component model, describe the development of the measures of organizational commitment, and discuss evidence of relevance to the construct validity of the measures.

THE ORGANIZATIONAL COMMITMENT CONSTRUCT

It could be argued that the scientific study of commitment has been hampered somewhat by the fact that the word commitment is used so frequently in everyday language and, apparently, has been ascribed various meanings. Consequently, although commitment almost always refers to a psychological bond or tie between the employee and the organization that reduces the likelihood of voluntary turnover, the nature of the bond varies considerably. As indicated above, however, the various views of organizational commitment seem to reflect three general themes: affective attachment to the organization, perceived costs associated with leaving the organization, and feelings of obligation to the organization.

These three themes represent the bases of a three-component view of the organizational commitment construct that we forwarded several years ago (Allen & Meyer, 1990a; Meyer & Allen, 1991). Consistent with other researchers, we described organizational commitment as a psychological state, or "mind-set," that serves to link the employee to the organization. In contrast to earlier researchers who saw organizational commitment as a uni-dimensional construct, however, we argued that this psychological state could take three quite distinct forms and, therefore, that commitment was best seen as a multidimensional construct. To refer to these dimensions, or components, we used the terms affective, continuance, and normative commitment. Although each of these components serves to strengthen the likelihood that the employee will choose to remain with the organization, the nature of each of these psychological ties differs from the others. *Affective commitment* refers to the degree to which the employee identifies with, is involved in, and is emotionally attached to the organization. An affectively committed employee believes in the goals and values of the organization and enjoys being a member of it. Thus, employees with strong affective commitment remain with the organization because they *want to* do so. *Continuance commitment* refers to the degree to which the employee recognizes that costs associated with leaving the organization tie him/her to the organization. Those with strong continuance commitment are aware that the costs of discontinuing membership will be high. Thus, such employees remain with the organization because they *have to* do so. *Normative commitment* refers to the degree to which the employee feels an obligation to the organization. Normatively committed employees believe that continuing their membership in the organization is the "right and moral" thing to do. Thus, such employees remain with the organization because they feel they *ought to* do so.

Conceptual work on affective, continuance, and normative commitment did not develop in isolation from a consideration of other variables. Rather, the three components of organizational commitment are embedded in a model of organizational commitment from which several hypotheses can be derived. In essence, then, the model forms a "nomological network" (Cronbach & Meehl,

1955) that helps to elaborate the meaning of affective, continuance, and normative commitment and which provides a basis on which we can evaluate the construct validity of commitment measures.   An understanding of the organizational commitment construct as we have conceptualized it requires that we elaborate on several features of the model.

First, it is important to point out that affective, continuance, and normative commitment are considered to be components, rather than separate types, of organizational commitment.   We are not suggesting, for example, that a given employee's commitment to the organization can be described as either "affective," "continuance," or "normative."   Rather, each employee will feel affective, continuance, and normative commitment to his or her organization and, likely, will experience each of these to varying degrees.   Thus, just as an individual's personality can be described in terms of a profile consisting of several personality traits, the commitment an employee feels toward his/her organization can be described in terms of a profile made up of each of the three components.   Recently, Law, Wong and Mobley (1998) presented a taxonomy that can be used to understand various kinds of multidimensional constructs.   The distinction they draw between latent model constructs, aggregrate model constructs, and profile model constructs is based on the relations hypothesized between the construct and its various dimensions.   In particular, attention focuses on (a) whether or not the multidimensional construct exists at the same level as its dimensions and (b) whether or not empirical measures of the construct can be summed to represent the overall construct.   In the case of the three-component model, the answers to (a) and (b) are "yes" and "no", respectively.   Thus, the theoretical relations between the construct (commitment) and its three dimensions (affective, continuance, and normative commitment) suggest, following Law et al. (1998), that the three-component view of commitment should be classified as a profile model.

Second, the model specifies that the three components are conceptually distinguishable from each other and thus, that measures developed for each of the three are relatively uncorrelated with the other two. An employee's feeling of emotional attachment to, and desire to stay with, the organization is psychologically different from his or her sense of the need to stay (due to perceived costs associated with leaving) and different again from the feeling of obligation to stay with the organization.

Third, a critical feature of the model is that each of the three components is hypothesized to develop independently on the basis of different antecedent variables and via different processes (Meyer & Allen, 1991, 1997). Based on the construct as we defined it, and on the results of earlier studies that used conceptually comparable measures of commitment (e.g., the OCQ), we argued that affective commitment develops on the basis of work experiences that represented two central themes: (a) organizational supportiveness and fairness, and (b) personal importance and competence. Employees will feel affective commitment to the extent that they feel that the organization has treated them in a fair and just manner – particularly as this relates to principles of procedural justice. Affective commitment will also be stronger among employees who perceive that the organization values, is supportive of, and cares about them as people. In addition to fair and supportive treatment, we also hypothesized that affective commitment is stronger among employees who feel that they make important contributions to the organization – that their ideas are valued and trusted and that they are working in an environment that allows them to increase their sense of competence. Clearly, no single event can be isolated as the conduit of either of these themes; organizations communicate them through a myriad of policies, practices, and everyday dealings with employees. Moreover, in order for work experiences that convey these themes to impact upon affective commitment, it would seem important that they are attributed to the organization in question and not to other influences such as the law or cross-organizational norms (Meyer & Allen, 1995). In hypothesizing these general themes, we are suggesting that they are "universally rewarding;" they serve to make people feel good about themselves and will do so for most people. This does not rule out the possibility that "person-organization fit" processes will also be operative. Indeed, it seems quite likely that there will be particular organizational cultures that are more personally rewarding – and, thus, can invoke stronger affective commitment – in some people than in others.

The development of continuance commitment is, in one sense, simpler than affective commitment and, in another, more complex. Strong continuance commitment develops to the extent: (a) that there are conditions (e.g., "investments" the employee makes in the organization, an unfavorable job market) that make leaving costly *and* (b) that the employee recognizes that these costs exist. It is difficult to predict exactly the specific conditions that will invoke this recognition; likely, they are highly idiosyncratic. That is, whether a particular condition will be acknowledged as an important cost of leaving might depend on the employee' s own preferences and concerns and/or situational variables that serve to make the condition salient to the employee (Vandenberghe & Peiro, 1999). For whatever reasons, for one employee, a critically important cost associated with leaving the organization might be the prospect of having to relocate to another town. For another, relocation might matter little; instead, an important cost associated with leaving might be that the skills acquired in the organization would no longer be valuable and, hence, represent a "forfeited investment." Although we recognized that the *details* of the "antecedents" of continuance commitment would vary greatly (potentially playing havoc with operationalization!), we nonetheless predicted that commitment would develop on the basis of two general classes of variables: perceived investments and perceptions of employment alternatives. According to the model, therefore, employees who feel that they have invested a great deal in their current organization and have few alternatives will have stronger continuance commitment that those with few perceived investments and several alternatives.

We hypothesized that normative commitment develops primarily through the process of internalization during one's early life. Employees whose family and/or culture provides experiences that reinforce the importance of commitment to one's employer (e.g. parents who stress corporate loyalty; a culture that encourages lifetime employment) will likely have stronger normative commitment to an organization than one who is not exposed to such experiences. To the extent that these experiences exist, and are internalized, normative commitment develops. We also hypothesized that normative commitment can develop on the basis of experiences within the organization; in particular, normative commitment will become stronger to the extent that the organization makes the kind of investments in an employee that he or she would feel obliged to reciprocate (e.g., tuition payments made by the organization; interest-free loans).

Fourth, all three components of commitment have straightforward implications for staying with (or leaving) an organization. The stronger the commitment, the stronger the intention to stay and the likelihood of actually staying. Beyond that, however, it is expected that each of the three components of organizational commitment will have a different pattern of behavioral consequences. In describing the predictions that the model makes about potential behavioral consequences of affective, continuance, and normative commitment, we allude to some "profile effects" (i.e., the effect of one component of commitment will be influenced by the level of the other two). For the most part, however, hypotheses are presented, in the interests of simplicity, in terms of the "main effects" of each commitment component

Because an employee with strong affective commitment has an emotional attachment to the organization, it seems likely that he or she will be motivated to make a greater contribution to the organization than an employee with weak affective commitment. Thus, the model predicts that affective commitment will be positively related to attendance at work and various aspects of job performance. Included in the latter are behaviors that are required by the organization as well as discretionary extra-role behavior that benefits the organization. All else being equal, employees with strong continuance commitment will feel no particular need to contribute to the organization beyond what is needed to keep their jobs. Thus, we hypothesized that continuance commitment would be unrelated to attendance and job performance. Moreover, among employees for whom continuance commitment represents the primary tie that binds them to the organization (i.e., both affective and normative commitment are weak), continuance commitment might be negatively related to work behaviors. That is, in the absence of other reasons for staying, those with strong continuance commitment might feel particularly resentful of the situation in which they find themselves; potentially, this could lead to undesirable work behavior. Finally, we hypothesized that normative commitment is positively related to job performance; employees who feel an obligation to the organization will likely want to make positive contributions to it. However, because feelings of obligation do not carry with them the same feelings of enthusiasm and involvement as affective commitment, we hypothesized that these positive relations will be more modest in magnitude. In addition, normative commitment might affect the "tone" with which some aspects of work are carried out. Particularly among employees whose primary tie to the organization is normative commitment (i.e., affective and continuance commitment are weak), those with strong normative commitment might feel resentful of their sense of indebtedness to the organization. Possibly, this could affect how willingly – or grudgingly – they carry out particular duties.

Fifth, despite the confusion created by some of the earlier commitment literature, it should be noted that there is parallelism between some early measures and the components described in the model. Affective commitment, for example, is very similar to organizational commitment as conceptualized and measured using the Organizational Commitment Scale (Mowday et al.,1979). Similarly, a measure developed by Wiener (1982) is fairly close to normative commitment as conceptualized here. Thus, this parallelism means that we have been able to interpret some of the earlier research within the context of the model (see Meyer & Allen, 1991; 1997).

Development of the Organizational Commitment Measures

Two of the commitment measures developed on the basis of this model were first used in published research by Meyer and Allen (1984); the third, by Allen and Meyer (1990a). Since then, the measures, referred to as the Affective, Continuance, and Normative Commitment Scales (ACS, CCS, and NCS, respectively), have been administered in several studies and have been revised (Meyer, Allen, & Smith, 1993).

The development of the ACS, CCS, and NCS was based on the scale construction principles outlined by Jackson (1970). Although they are described in detail elsewhere (Allen & Meyer, 1990a), we provide a brief overview here of the procedures we followed. First, the definitions of the three commitment constructs were used to develop an initial pool of items. In this instance, our task during the item-writing process was somewhat different than that involved in developing personality measures. Rather than writing items that described behavioral exemplars of a construct – as might be the case in personality assessment – our task involved writing items that dealt with the way in which an employee with strong (or weak) affective, continuance, or normative commitment would perceive his/her relationship with the organization. As much as possible, we tried to avoid reference to particular behaviors that, rather than being part of the commitment construct per se, represented behavioral consequences of it.   A similar effort was made to exclude reference to hypothesized antecedents.   On the basis of the definitions, a pool of 51 items were generated; each item corresponded to one of the three components of commitment.   Second, this item pool was administered to an organizationally and occupationally heterogenous sample with a fairly balanced gender representation (over 250 full-time employees from three organizations; 57% were female).   Third, as stipulated by Jackson (1970), items were selected for inclusion in the scales on the basis of a series of decision rules that took into account the endorsement proportions associated with each item, item-scale correlations, content redundancy, and the desire to include both positively and negatively keyed items.   Each of the three scales resulting from this process is made up of 8 items.   Respondents indicate their degree of agreement or disagreement with each item and scale scores are calculated by averaging across item responses.   A similar process was undertaken a few years later when the scales were revised and shortened to 6 items (Meyer et al., 1993). Sample items from the original version of the ACS, CCS, and NCS are shown below.

Affective Commitment Scale
> I really feel as if this organization's problems are my own.
> I do not feel "emotionally attached" to this organization. (Reverse keyed)

Continuance Commitment Scale
> Too much of my life would be disrupted if I decided I wanted to leave my organization right now.
> I believe that I have too few options to consider leaving this organization.

Normative Commitment Scale
> If I got an offer for a better job elsewhere, I would not feel it was right to leave my organization.
> I do not believe a person must always be loyal to his or her organization. (Reverse keyed)

Evaluating the Organizational Commitment Measures

Several quite different kinds of evidence can be used to evaluate the construct validity of self-report measures such as these.   Since the commitment measures were developed they have been administered to a wide variety of samples in several dozen studies.   A few years ago, we reviewed over 40 studies (involving 16,000 employees from a wide variety of organizations) that had examined one or more of the three commitment measures (Allen & Meyer, 1996).   Since then, some of the relations forwarded in the model have been examined meta-analytically with over 80 samples (Stanley, Meyer, Topolnytsky & Herscovitch, 1999). Consequently, there now exists a considerable body of evidence regarding the psychometric properties of the measures and their relations with other variables.   Our intention in what follows is to provide an overview, rather than detailed information, about what we have learned about the construct validity of the three commitment measures and, in doing so, to highlight areas where more remains to be done.

The reliabilities of the measures have been assessed in virtually all studies in which they have been used. In their recent meta-analysis, Stanley et al. (1999) reported the following mean reliabilities: ACS (.82), CCS (.76) and NCS (.75). Although the vast majority of studies using the meaures have been cross-sectional, a few researchers have used them in longitudinal studies, thus allowing us to also examine test-retest reliabilities. In all cases, reliabilities have been within acceptable range and comparable to those found in other commitment measures. With one exception (Blau, Paul & St. John, 1993), however, longitudinal data have been collected from organizational newcomers, typically those in the first several months of their tenure with the organization. This raises a question about the "time course" of developing commitment and when, in fact, it might be appropriate to begin collecting such data from new employees. One argument that could be advanced is that, because would-be employees engage in "anticipatory socialization" with respect to an organization as soon as they start to consider it as a potential employer (Feldman, 1976), commitment can be meaningfully assessed very soon after organizational entry. Another is that employees can only meaningfully reflect on their commitment to an organization after they have had some experience working in it. Particularly interesting, with respect to this, are the reliabilities reported in the longitudinal study conducted by Vandenberg and Self (1993). They administered the ACS and CCS on employees' first *day* at the organization and at both 3 months and 6 months post entry. The test-retest reliabilities involving Day 1 data were particularly low for both the ACS (.48 for Day 1- 3 months; .38 for Day 1 - 6 months) and the CCS (.44 for both lags) and were in contrast to those involving the 3 - 6 month lag (ACS:.77; CCS:.63) and to other studies that involved employees who had been employed for a least one month before commitment was first assessed (Blau et al., 1993; Meyer, Bobocel, & Allen, 1991, Meyer et al., 1993). This pattern is consistent with that found with other measures of organizational attitudes (Vandenberg & Self, 1993); thus, it may well reflect something about the stabilization of attitude that occurs as newcomers gain experience with their organizations.

Meta-analytic examination (Stanley et al., 1999) reveals that, as expected, the ACS and CCS are only modestly related (r=.07), as are the CCS and the NCS (r=.18). The relation between the ACS and the NCS (r=.64), however, is substantial. Despite this, results of both exploratory (e.g., Reilly & Orsak, 1991) and confirmatory (e.g., Dunham, Grube, & Castaneda, 1994; Hackett, Bycio, & Hausdorf, 1994; Meyer et al., 1993) factor analyses suggest that items making up the three commitment measures load separately on the appropriate factors. Further, in factor analytic studies that included other work attitude measures, the pattern of findings is as would be expected. For example, the ACS items loaded on a factor separate from those measures that assessed career, job, and work value constructs (Blau et al., 1993). Shore and Tetrick (1991) reported evidence supporting the distinction between the ACS, the CCS, job satisfaction and perceived organizational support. As expected, however, ACS and OCQ items loaded on the same factor. Similarly, Dunham et al. (1994) showed that the OCQ converged with the ACS but, as hypothesized, was distinct from the CCS and NCS.

One issue that has arisen from some of the factor analytic work has to do with the uni-dimensionality of the CCS. Several years ago, on the basis of results of exploratory factor analyses, McGee and Ford (1987) suggested that the CCS is better represented as two dimensions, one dealing with the employee's perceptions of alternatives and the other on perceptions of personal sacrifices associated with leaving the organization.. Since then, the CCS has received considerable scrutiny using confirmatory factor analysis (e.g., Dunham et al., 1994; Meyer, Allen, & Gellatly, 1990; Somers, 1993). Although the superiority is modest, a model hypothesizing a two-dimensional structure for the CCS generally provides a better fit to the data than does a uni-dimensional model. One dimension includes items that assess the employee's recognition that investments made in the organization would be sacrificed upon leaving it (High Sacrifice); the other includes items that refer to the employees' recognition that alternatives are few (Low Alternatives). One way to interpret this pattern of findings is to suggest that organizational commitment is best conceptualized as a four-, rather than three-component construct. There is reason to suggest, however, that this might not be the best approach. As has been noted in some studies (e.g., Hackett et al., 1994, Jaros, 1997), and reinforced in a recent meta-analysis (Stanley et al., 1999), turnover intention is correlated with the High Sacrifices subscale ($r = -.17$), but not the Low Alternatives subscale ($r = -.01$), suggesting that the items making up the latter do not well represent commitment to the organization. Neither is it the case, conceptually, that perceptions of low alternatives, per se, represent commitment. Recall that continuance commitment is defined as a psychological tie to the organization that is based on the employee's recognition that leaving would be costly.   In our elaboration of the construct above, we noted that various events, some idiosyncratic to the employee, could serve as the basis for these perceived costs.   Although one of these *antecedents* might be the perception of viable alternatives (with low alternatives making the perceived costs / sacrifices associated with leaving higher), it need not be integral to the definition of continuance commitment itself.   In retrospect, then, it might be wise to exclude "low alternatives" type items from subsequent refinements of the CCS.   This approach would seem more appropriate than the addition of a fourth and, arguably, conceptually murky component of commitment.

Several studies have examined the relations between the components of commitment and variables that would be expected to contribute to their development.   As hypothesized, the ACS was positively related to various indicators of organizational/supervisory support (e.g., Allen & Meyer, 1990a,b; Shore & Wayne, 1993; Withey, 1988) and several aspects of workplace justice (e.g., Gellatly, 1995; Konovsky & Cropanzano, 1991; Moorman, Niehoff, & Organ, 1993). In addition, the ACS was related to other variables that convey concern for employees such as role clarity (Allen & Meyer, 1990a) and transformational leadership (Bycio, Hackett, & Allen, 1995). For the most part, and consistent with theoretical predictions, these variables were uncorrelated with the CCS and were either uncorrelated, or only weakly correlated, with the NCS (Allen & Meyer, 1996).

Continuance commitment has been shown to be related to a number of variables that "tie" the employee to his or her organization such as perceptions about the transferability of skills (Allen & Meyer, 1990a; Lee, 1992) and transferability of education (Lee, 1992). Stronger continuance commitment was expressed by employees who thought their education or training was less easily transferred elsewhere. As would be expected, CCS scores also related to perceptions of acceptable alternative employment (Allen & Meyer, 1990a; Lee, 1992; Meyer et al., 1991) and the attractiveness of alternatives (Whitener & Walz, 1993). Whitener and Walz also used regional unemployment rates as a more objective measure of alternatives. Although the attractiveness variable was correlated with CCS scores, unemployment rates were not. Possibly, the latter were not seen as personally relevant, something that might be necessary in order for a potential antecedent to influence an individual's feelings of perceived costs.

Thus far, very little research has examined the hypothesized antecedents of normative commitment. Although there have been calls for studies that directly examine the role of early familial socialization on normative commitment (e.g., Dunham et al., 1994: Meyer & Allen, 1991; 1997), to our knowledge these have not been done. In addition, we need to understand better the role of culture in the development of normative commitment, a point we return to in some detail later. There is evidence, however, that normative commitment and continuance commitment (but not affective commitment) are related to a generalized belief in, and need to fulfill, one's obligations (Meyer et al., 1993). To the extent that such beliefs are the product of early socialization, this suggests a possible link between socialization and feelings of obligation to the organization. Finally, we noted earlier that, although affective and normative items load on separate factors, the ACS and NCS (both versions) are highly correlated. To this point, it is not clear whether this is "simply" a measurement problem or whether it represents evidence suggesting that the two constructs share some antecedents (cf. Allen & Meyer, 1990b; Ashforth & Saks, 1996) and/or are, themselves, causally related.

Variables that have been hypothesized to be "consequences" of organizational commitment have also received considerable research attention and recently some of these relations have been examined meta-analytically (Stanley et al., 1999).

Quite reasonably, a great deal of research has focussed on turnover variables. Stanley et al. (1999) provide evidence that affective commitment, continuance, and normative commitment are negatively related to both actual turnover (ACS:-.23; CCS: -.07; NCS: -.16) and turnover intention (ACS: -.43; CCS: -.18; NCS: -.23). Results of this study also show, as hypothesized, that affective commitment is negatively related to absenteeism. Neither continuance commitment nor normative commitment, however, are related to absenteeism. Also as hypothesized, relations with required aspects of job performance are positive, both for affective commitment (r =.16) and, albeit quite weakly, for normative commitment (r = .05). In contrast, there is a small negative correlation between continuance commitment and job performance (r =-.06). Finally, both affective commitment (r = .29) and normative commitment (r = .19) were shown to be positively related to organizational citizenship behavior; continuance commitment and citizenship behavior were unrelated.

The Model to Date

Taken together, the findings seem to provide considerable evidence in support of the three-component model and, hence, the nomological network surrounding the affective, continuance, and normative commitment constructs. Although some fine-tuning of the measures might be warranted, there appears to be much value in conceptualizing organizational commitment in this manner and in measuring it as we have done. At this point, perhaps the most interesting questions one might ask about this three-component construct have to do with the extent to which it has applicability to other foci (or domains) to which people are committed and to cultures beyond North America. We turn now to a consideration of these issues.

CONSTRUCT RELEVANCE AND OTHER FOCI

The three-component commitment model was developed in order to facilitate our understanding of commitment to the work organization. There are, of course, numerous foci, or domains, to which people can feel committed in both work (e.g., occupation, project, union) and non-work (e.g., family, hobbies) aspects of life. Moreover, although the organization remains the most extensively studied focus of the commitment literature, considerable attention has been given to commitment to some of these other specific work foci including unions (e.g., Fullagar & Barling, 1989; Gordon, Philpot, Burt, Thompson, & Spiller, 1980), occupations (e.g., Morrow & Wirth, 1989; Wallace, 1988), and work/employment (e.g., Blau et al., 1993; Jackson, Stafford, Banks, & Warr, 1983). As with most of the early organizational commitment research, however, these investigators have typically taken a uni-dimensional view of the commitment construct. In addition, most of this research tends to examine commitment only to the focus of particular interest (e.g., union, occupation, etc.) and not "across foci" (see Wallace, 1988 for an exception). Indeed, although theoretical discussions of "multiple commitments" at work have been part of the organizational behavior literature for several years (e.g., Morrow, 1983, 1993; Reichers, 1985), empirical work examining interrelationships between various forms of commitment to various foci has only begun relatively recently (e.g., Becker, 1992; Becker & Billings, 1993; Becker et al., 1996; Meyer et al., 1993).

It seems reasonable to suggest that the "want to," "have to," and "ought to" notions that embody affective, continuance, and normative commitment might have relevance to other foci within the organization as well as to those beyond the organization. Meyer and Allen (1997) proposed a framework within which commitment can be considered multidimensional both in terms of its (three-component) psychological nature *and* its focus. More recently, a general model of workplace commitment has been proposed that extends this thinking considerably (Meyer & Herscovitch, in press). In order to evaluate relations within an integrated framework, however, it is first necessary to determine whether or not the affective, continuance, and normative commitment notions have relevance to these domains.

Thus far, empirical work examining the generalizability, or extension, of the three-component model to other foci has been relatively limited although promising. Meyer et al. (1993) examined this issue with respect to commitment to the occupation using participants from a single occupation, nursing. In the first study, a pool of occupational commitment items, each written to correspond to one of the three conceptual definitions of commitment, was administered to a sample of student nurses from all four years of a university nursing program. Following item analysis procedures similar to those used in the development of the ACS, CCS, and NCS (Allen & Meyer, 1990a), Meyer et al. selected items from the pool and developed parallel measures of affective, continuance, and normative commitment to the occupation. These measures, along with several other conceptually relevant variables, were administered to a second sample consisting of registered nurses. Results of this research provide support for a three-component conceptualization of occupational commitment and validity data for the newly developed measures. Specifically, Meyer et al (1993) found that: (a) confirmatory factor analyses based on the registered nurse data showed that a 6-factor solution (three occupational and three organizational commitment components) provided the best fit to the data, (b) correlations between the occupational commitment scales and several antecedent variables were as hypothesized, and (c) the occupational commitment scales correlated as expected with intention to leave nursing, as well as some other outcome variables (e.g., voluntary absenteeism, reactions to dissatisfying experiences, citizenship behavior). In addition, the occupational commitment measures contributed to the prediction of some of these outcomes over and above the contribution made by organizational commitment.

This is a particularly important finding, conceptually, in light of concerns about construct redundancy (Morrow, 1983, 1993) within the commitment literature. Since the development of the occupational commitment scales, they have been used in samples of accountants (Gross & Fullagar, 1996), students in the rehabilitation field (Speechley, Noh, & Beggs, 1993) and government employees representing several occupations (Irving, Coleman, & Cooper, 1997). All three studies provided factor analytic evidence supporting the three hypothesized components of occupational commitment. In addition, the Irving et al. (1997) study examined correlations between the three occupational commitment measures and several other variables; results were generally as predicted. Overall, although research is still in a fairly preliminary stage, it appears that the three-component conceptualization of commitment has merit as a way of thinking about the psychological bond that people have to their occupations. Further, this work suggests that the three-component model is not limited to the organization and might be fruitfully explored with respect to other foci.

Recently, Meyer and Herscovitch (in press) have argued that, "commitment should have a 'core essence' regardless of the context in which it is studied" and, therefore, that the development of a general model of workplace commitment should be possible. As we move across foci, in an attempt to assess this possibility, it seems reasonable to take the general approach that was taken in examining occupational commitment. Critical to this approach, of course, are clear conceptual definitions of affective, continuance, and normative commitment to the focal domain in question. To do this, researchers require a good sense of what that focal domain is (e.g., an entity, such as the organization, or something more abstract such as a set of principles), the bases on which the "multiple mind sets" of commitment (Meyer & Herscovitch, in press) will develop, and how this commitment will be expressed.

Perhaps because of the tradition from which it evolved – one that emphasized staying/leaving as the critical consequence of commitment – it is more common to envisage "commitment" to foci in which staying / leaving is a salient consequence. Clearly, people can choose to leave their organization. Similarly, they can also choose to leave an occupation (e.g., discontinue membership in an occupational association; accept a job in a different line of work). Leaving is also a salient behavioral marker of various relationships, both personal and work-related (e.g., selling a franchise, divorcing a spouse, dissolving a business partnership). For some foci, however, the most salient behavioral consequence – or focal behavior – might be something other than staying/leaving. Consider, for example, commitment to less tangible foci such as a goal or change initiative. Commitment with regard to these foci might involve a sense of being bound (out of desire, cost, or obligation), not to staying or leaving, but to attainment of the goal or to changing one's behavior to be compatible with the initiative. As was the case with organizational commitment, commitment of any form should be sufficient to insure the focal behavior. The impact of different forms of commitment will most likely be detected in "discretionary" behaviors associated with the focal behavior. For example, employees whose commitment to attain an assigned goal is due primarily to perceived costs of failure to do so are less likely to persist when faced with obstacles that would alleviate their responsibility for failure than are those employees who are committed primarily out of a belief in the value of the goal. Similarly, those who are committed to a change initiative primarily out of concern for the consequences of failure to change are less likely than those who are committed due to a belief in the objectives of the change to go out of their way to insure that the change achieves its intended objectives.

In sum, there is good reason to believe that the different forms of commitment identified in the three-component model of organizational commitment are equally meaningful in the study of commitment to other aspects of the workplace. Commitment binds an individual to a course of action that is of relevance to a particular entity. The nature of that behavior, particularly the discretionary aspects of its enactment, however, will be influenced by the nature of the mind set characterizing that commitment (i.e., want to, have to, ought to). Thus far, it appears that a three-component commitment construct has relevance for the occupation. Further research is needed to evaluate the ideas presented here and to demonstrate, empirically, construct relevance to other workplace foci.

CONSTRUCT RELEVANCE AND MEASUREMENT ACROSS CULTURES

At the time that Allen and Meyer (1996) conducted their review of the research using the ACS, CCS and NCS, they found only one study that had been conducted in organizations outside North America (i.e., Lee, 1992). Since then, one or more of these scales has been used in research conducted in several countries around the world, including Australia (Griffin, 1996; Travaglione, 1998), Belgium (Vandenberghe, 1996, 1998; Vandenberghe, Bonami & Jacquemyns, 1998; Vandenberghe & Peiro, 1999; Vandenberghe, Stinglhamber, Bentein & Delhaise, 1999); Germany (Freund, 1995; Lubich, 1997), Japan (Takao, 1995; Takahashi, 1997; Takahashi, Noguchi & Watanabe, 1998), Korea (Chang, 1997; Hahn, Hwang & Pak, 1997; Ko, Price & Mueller, 1997; Lee, Allen, Meyer & Rhee, 1999), The Netherlands (Allen & de Gilder, 1997; den Hartog, 1997; Ellemers, de Gilder & van den Heuvel, 1998), Spain (González & Antón, 1995), Sweden (Sverke & Sjoberg, 1994) and Turkey (Wasti, 1999). Interest in the study of commitment outside of North America provides additional challenges in the construct validation process. In this section, we provide a summary of some of the key issues of relevance to researchers as they begin to study commitment more globally. We also examine the strategies that are being used in this research, summarize the findings, and identify limitations. Finally, we outline a strategy for the conduct of future research to assess the cross-cultural generalizability of the three-component model, and of the measures of the three components.

To begin our discussion, let us consider four questions that might be of interest in cross-cultural research: (a) Are affective, continuance, and normative commitment to the organization meaningful in other cultures (i.e., do the constructs generalize)? (b) Do the ACS, CCS, and NCS (translated when necessary) measure the same constructs in different cultures? (c) Are the antecedents, consequences and correlates of affective, continuance and normative commitment the same across cultures? and (d) Are mean levels of the three components of commitment the same or different across cultures? The answers to these questions are not independent (Hui & Triandis, 1985). For example, the questions concerning equivalence of measures, equivalence of relations, and equivalence of means only become relevant if it can be demonstrated that the constructs themselves generalize across cultures. Of course, if evidence for equivalence of measures, relations, and means is found, it would follow that the constructs themselves generalize. As we discuss later, however, failure to provide evidence of equivalence does not necessarily imply that the constructs do not generalize. For this reason, we believe it is important to seek answers to the more abstract question concerning construct equivalence before attempting to answer the more concrete questions concerning equivalence of measurement, relations, and means. For the most part, however, this has not been the case.

Much of the research conducted to date has been directed at determining whether the factor structure of the commitment measures generalizes across countries/cultures (e.g., González & Antón, 1995; Lubich, 1997; Ko et al., 1997; Travaglione, 1998; Vandenberghe, 1996), and whether commitment relates to other variables (e.g., leadership; turnover intention; organizational citizenship behavior) in other countries/cultures in the same way it does in North America (e.g., Griffin, 1996; Ko et al., 1997; Lubich, 1997). Other cross-cultural researchers have used the measures in research whose primary focus was something other than the generalizability of the commitment model or measures (e.g., den Hartog, 1997; Ellemers et al., 1998; Sverke & Sjoberg, 1994). In one study that we are aware of, an attempt was made to compare mean levels of the three components of commitment across cultures (Vandenberghe et al., 1999).

Research to assess the generalizability of the factor structure of the three commitment measures has typically been conducted within a single country, with the results being compared to those obtained in North America. In general, these studies have found strong evidence for the existence of three oblique factors corresponding to affective, continuance and normative commitment (e.g., Lubich, 1997; Ko et al., 1997; Vandenberghe, 1996). In some cases, however, it was necessary for investigators to eliminate items before a clear and well-fitting factor structure emerged (e.g., den Hartog, 1997; Travaglione, 1998; Vandenberghe,

1998). Studies that used confirmatory factor analysis to compare the relative fit of three- and four-factor (i.e., including two continuance commitment factors) models provided mixed results, with González and Antón (1995), Ko et al. (1997) and Vandenberghe (1996) finding stronger support for a three-factor model, and Lee et al. (1999) and Lubich (1997) finding evidence for the superiority of a four-factor solution. Another popular research strategy has been to examine the relations between the components of commitment and theoretically related variables across cultures (e.g., Freund, 1995; Griffin, 1996; Lubich, 1997; Ko et al., 1997), and to compare the findings to those obtained in North America. To the extent that patterns of relations are the same as those reported in North America (i.e., the nomological network is the same), evidence is provided for the construct validity of the measures outside North America.   Failure to find such evidence, however, cannot be interpreted unequivocally. It is possible that the difference in relations reflects lack of equivalence of the measures, unique features of the sample or contextual characteristics, or other methodological problems (see Paunonen, this volume). Therefore, to draw conclusions concerning cross-cultural differences, it is necessary to rule out alternative explanations. Campbell (1964) has noted that, to find cross- cultural differences, it is first necessary to identify similarities (i.e., to demonstrate that the constructs are indeed meaningful across cultures). Consequently, demonstrating the existence of cross-cultural differences will inevitably require the conduct of multiple studies, ideally using different research methods (cf. van de Vijver & Leung, 1997).

As noted earlier, almost all of the studies described above involved the collection of data in a single country/culture. Comparisons were made, implicitly or explicitly, to findings obtained previously in North America, but data were not collected simultaneously in the two cultures and no effort was made to ensure comparability of organization or sample characteristics. Moreover, research has not yet been conducted to examine systematically the implications of culture on commitment (i.e., its structure, level, or relations with other variables).   A systematic investigation of cultural influences requires the measurement of commitment (and possibly related variables) in several cultures varying on one or more relevant dimensions (e.g., Hofstede's [1980, 1991] four value-based dimensions). The only studies to date that have directly considered the potential influence of culture on commitment are those of Vandenberghe et al. (1999) and Wasti (1999).

Vandenberghe et al. (1999) collected data from a large sample of employees from different countries/cultures working for the same organization (the European Commission) and in a single location (i.e., Brussels).   Moreover, because participants were translators working for the European Commission, they were all fluent in either English or French, thereby restricting the translation to a single "foreign" language. Although this strategy has the advantage of controlling for, or minimizing, problems associated with sample characteristics, organizational context, and translation, the sample is unique in that all participants were well educated and were largely expatriates with experience working in a common culture/country (i.e., Belgium).

The primary focus of Vandenberghe et al.'s research was on testing the hypotheses that (a) it is possible to distinguish among multiple bases (affective, continuance, normative) and multiple foci (e.g., organization, occupation, work group) of commitment, and (b) prediction of intention to leave the organization can be improved by including commitment to foci other than the organization itself.   They further hypothesized that the factor structure underlying their multidimensional commitment model, and the relations between the multiple commitments and turnover intentions, would be invariant across subgroups created on the basis of Hofstede's (1980, 1991) dimensions (i.e., individualism/collectivism, uncertainty avoidance, masculinity/ femininity, and power distance).   Their hypotheses concerning the cultural invariance of factor structure and relations with turnover intention were generally supported. Only in the comparison of subgroups differing on the masculinity/femininity dimension was a statistical difference in the structural model (predicting turnover intention) found. Because the same model fitted the data well for both subgroups, however, the authors concluded that this difference was not practically significant. Finally, Vandenberghe et al. conducted exploratory analyses to determine whether mean levels of commitment varied across these same subgroups. Only a few significant differences were observed. For example, they found that employees from individualistic countries had higher levels of continuance commitment to their organization.

Wasti (1999) took a somewhat different approach in testing for cultural differences. Specifically, she measured culture as an individual difference variable. She was particularly interested in the implications of the individualism/collectivism dimension on the relative strength of relations between the commitment components and turnover intention.   Following Triandis (e.g., Triandis, Leung, Villareal & Clack, 1985), she argued that there is considerable variation in the extent to which individuals within a particular culture take an individualist or collectivist perspective.   When measured as an individual difference, the internalization of an individualist perspective is referred to as *idiocentrism* whereas the internalization of a collectivist perspective is referred to *allocentrism*. Using a large sample of employees from Turkey, Wasti found that affective commitment was a strong predictor of turnover intention for both idiocentrics and allocentrics, but that normative commitment was a stronger predictor for allocentrics than for idiocentrics. This finding is consistent with Meyer and Allen's (1997) suggestion that normative commitment might be a better predictor of turnover intentions in collectivist cultures than has been the case in the North America with its strong individualistic orientation. It is important, however, that this findings be replicated in between- rather than within-culture comparisons before firm conclusions are drawn.

The findings reported by Vandenberghe et al. (1999) and Wasti (1999) are interesting in that they provide some evidence for generalizability of the three-component model, as well as for the possibility of cross-cultural differences in mean levels of commitment and the relations between the commitment components and turnover intention. Nevertheless, there is much more to be learned about the cross-cultural generalizability of the commitment model. As we noted earlier, validation of the model and measures within cultures is a complex process. In the following section, we provide a general framework for future research to examine the cross-cultural generalizability of the three-component model of commitment. This strategy is based largely on the emic-etic approach developed by Triandis (1972, 1992). Detailed discussion of research methods and their strengths and limitations – that is, the use of emic (culturally tailored) measures to assess etic (presumably universal) constructs – is beyond the scope of this chapter. Interested readers should consult van de Vijver and Leung (1997) for a more detailed review.

A Plan for the Future

Triandis (1992) recently outlined a multi-stage strategy for conducting cross-cultural research that might serve as a valuable guide in the conduct of research to assess the cross-cultural generalizability of the three-component model of commitment. This strategy is intended to assess the meaningfulness of etic constructs across cultures by developing emic measures designed to assess more appropriately those constructs in different cultures. Following this strategy, it should be possible to address each of the basic questions raised earlier in this section.

The first stage of research in the emic-etic strategy is to involve "experts" within the target culture in the evaluation of the etic construct(s). As noted earlier, the question concerning the generalizability of the core constructs is the most fundamental question in the cross-cultural evaluation of the three-component model. It is important to determine whether employees in other cultures experience the same psychological states of "want to," "need to," and "ought to" in defining their relationship with their employer as has been observed among employees in North America. Only if this is the case does it make sense to ask questions pertaining to the generalizability of the measures, nomological network of relations with antecedent, correlate, and consequence measures, and differences in levels of commitment.

A starting point for the investigation of the generalizability of the commitment constructs, therefore, would involve having individuals who are knowledgeable about both the commitment model and the target culture make an assessment of the meaningfulness of the construct definitions in the new culture(s). This analysis might also include an assessment of whether the three components identified in the model are "exhaustive" within other cultures, or whether additional components are required to fully account for commitment-relevant behavior. Care must be taken in this assessment to ensure that any additional components truly reflect a form of "commitment to the organization" rather than related constructs that might have implications for similar forms of behavior (see Meyer & Herscovitch, in press). For example, employees might remain in the organization because of a strong sense of attachment to a supervisor or work group. Although the consequences of this attachment are the same as the consequences of organizational commitment, attachment to co-workers should not be considered a separate *form* of organizational commitment.

In most cases, studies conducted outside North America have been conducted by individuals who are knowledgeable about the target cultures. Consequently, implicit in their efforts to assess the cross-cultural generalizability of the ACS, CCS and NCS is the belief that the underlying constructs are potentially meaningful in the target culture. Research therefore begins with an attempt to determine whether the factor structure of translated measures is consistent with that predicted by the model. Thus, tests of the generalizability of the model are confounded with tests of the generalizability of the measures. Finding evidence to support the generalizability of the measures implies that the constructs themselves are relevant. As noted earlier, however, caution must be exercised in the interpretation of negative findings. Failure to provide partial or complete support for the generalizability of the measures does not necessarily imply that the constructs are not meaningful (see Hui & Triandis, 1985; Paunonen, this volume). The problem might lie, for example, in the way in which the constructs were operationalized. Consequently, a second important stage in emic-etic approach to cross-cultural research involves the development and validation of measures for each culture of interest.

Research conducted in non-English speaking countries outside North America requires that the commitment measures be translated into the host language. To date, the most common strategy has been to use translation and back-translation of the original English items (e.g., den Hartog, 1997; Lubich, 1997; Vandenberghe, 1996). Although it can be effective, this strategy alone does not ensure measure equivalence and can, in fact, result in the development of items that are awkwardly worded and do not truly reflect the intended construct (Brislin, 1980, 1986). Using the emic-etic approach, an etic construct is measured using emic items. These items are written by experts who are knowledgeable about both the culture and the etic constructs. Of course, the use of emic items means that the constructs will be operationalized differently in different cultures, which can create difficulties for cross-cultural comparisons. These difficulties can be minimized by following procedures for item development and evaluation outlined by Triandis (1992). For example, to ensure that the items reflect the underlying construct to the same degree across cultures, a sample of knowledgeable individuals within each culture can sort items into categories representing different levels of commitment, and items can then be selected to ensure comparability of level across cultures. Consequently, even though the item content is different, researchers can be reasonably confident that the items are at comparable levels of "difficulty" (i.e., the level of commitment required for an individual to agree with items in the different cultures is roughly the same). To determine whether item equivalence has been achieved, researchers can use item response theory procedures (see Hulin, Drasgow & Komocar, 1982). Confirmatory factor analyses can be used to ensure that the factor structure of the measures is consistent across cultures, and that the structure suggested by the three-component model fits the data well.

Once measurement equivalence has been established, a next step in cross-cultural research would be to assess the generalizability of the proposed relations between commitment and various antecedent (e.g., leadership; person-organization fit; employment opportunities), correlate (e.g., job satisfaction, occupational commitment), and consequence (e.g., turnover, performance, organizational citizenship behavior) variables. (Note that measurement equivalence for these other constructs must also be assessed). As noted earlier, these hypothesized relations represent the nomological network used to assess the validity of the model within North America. They can serve the same purpose in cross-cultural research (Hui & Triandis, 1985; van de Vijver & Leung, 1997). Of course, it is possible that some of these relations *should* be different across cultures. Consequently, finding differences in the strength or direction of correlations across cultures does not necessarily invalidate the model. These differences must be interpreted in context. First, if there are a number of similarities in relations across cultures, it is more likely that observed differences are meaningful and not simply a function of sampling or measurement problems (cf. Campbell, 1964). Second, the differences are more likely to be meaningful if they can be explained by existing theory (e.g., Hofstede, 1980, 1991). For example, if the strength of the relation between a particular antecedent variable (e.g., leadership style) and commitment differs in a predictable manner between cultures varying along a known dimension (e.g., individualism/collectivism), we can be reasonably confident that this difference is meaningful. For this reason, a systematic investigation of the cross-cultural generalizability of the three-component model would ideally involve representative sampling of cultures reflecting differences on one or more well-established cultural dimensions. Representative sampling (e.g., employees, occupations, organizations) *within* cultures is also important (van de Vijver & Leung, 1997).

As noted earlier, some investigators might be interested in comparing levels of commitment across cultures. Such comparison requires prior demonstration of measurement and scalar equivalence (cf. Riordan & Vandenberg, 1994; Ryan,

Chan, Ployhart & Slade, 1999).   If these assumptions are met, tests for mean differences in the raw or latent variables across cultures are meaningful.   Although such comparisons are simpler if the same (etic) items are used across cultures, Triandis (personal communication, May 1999) notes that such comparisons can be meaningful even with combinations of etic and emic items (assuming appropriate consideration is given to item equivalence in the scale development phase described above).

To our knowledge, the combined emic-etic approach has been applied only once to assess the cross-cultural generalizability of the three component model of organizational commitment.   Wasti (1999) conducted semi-standardized interviews with Turkish employees to assess the content relevance of items from Meyer et al.'s (1993) commitment scales, and to develop additional (emic) items of relevance to the constructs within the Turkish culture.   The results of her study were summarized briefly above.   We believe that this strategy has great promise and should guide future cross-cultural tests of the model.   Although its use has perhaps most obvious advantage for conducting research in non-English speaking countries, it might be useful as well in English-speaking countries outside of North America.   Investigators in Australia, for example, found that several of the items on the ACS, CCS and NCS did not define the intended factors and had to be dropped (Griffin, 1996; Travaglione, 1998).   Some expressions used in North America might not be interpreted the same by Australian employees. Consequently, it might be necessary to develop emic items to ensure appropriate domain coverage in English-speaking countries outside North America as well.

Finally, it is important to recognize that commitment theory and research as it exists in North America might benefit from the findings of cross-cultural research. For example, collaborative work with researchers in other cultures to develop equivalent measures might provide suggestions for improvement in the commitment scales.   Indeed, to facilitate cross-cultural research involving employees from North America, it might be helpful to modify existing items to make them more similar to those used elsewhere. This process is referred to as decentering (i.e., item generation becomes less dependent on operationalization within the culture of origin; cf. van de Vijver & Leung, 1997).   Similarly, it might become apparent that the constructs themselves (i.e., the three components) require modification, or that additional components need to be added.   Again, we caution that, if this is the case, care be taken to ensure that revisions or additions be based on a core definition of commitment, and that the construct not be misused or overgeneralized (see Meyer & Herscovitch, in press).

CONCLUSIONS

We began this chapter with the observation that organizational psychology has paid less-than-optimal attention to construct validation issues and, using the case of organizational commitment, illustrated some of the interpretive problems this can create.   Consistent with the arguments that Douglas Jackson made so effectively over two decades ago, it appears that more careful attention to the construct and an examination of various aspects of its nomological network has ameliorated some of these problems associated with early commitment research. Further, the evidence suggests that the three-component conceptualization of commitment has merit.   Nonetheless, construct validation is an ongoing process and there are issues associated with the three-component model and its measures that can use further exploration.   Some of these require that we take the model "further afield".   Indeed, as we have indicated, much remains to be done in evaluating its applicability to other foci and to cultures outside of North America. We look forward to this and other construct-driven commitment research and, more generally, to an increasing appreciation of the construct approach within the study of organizational behavior.

REFERENCES

Allen, N. J., & de Gilder, D.   (1997, June). *An examination of dispositional affect, organizational commitment, and turnover intention.* Presented at the annual meeting of the Canadian Psychological Association, Toronto.

Allen, N. J., & Meyer, J. P. (1990a).   The measurement and antecedents of affective, continuance, and normative commitment to the organization. *Journal of Occupational Psychology, 63*, 1-18.

Allen, N. J., & Meyer, J. P. (1990b). Organization socialization tactics: A longitudinal analysis of links to newcomers' commitment and role orientation. *Academy of Management Journal, 33*, 847-858.

Allen, N. J., & Meyer, J. P. (1996). Affective, continuance, and normative commitment to the organization: An examination of construct validity. *Journal of Vocational Behavior, 49*, 252-276.

Alutto, J. A., Hrebiniak, L. G., & Alonso, R. C. (1973). On operationalizing the concept of commitment. *Social Forces, 51*, 448-454.

Ashforth, B. E., & Saks, A. M. (1996). Socialization tactics: Longitudinal effects on newcomer adjustment. *Academy of Management Journal, 39*, 149-178.

Becker, H. S. (1960). Notes on the concept of commitment. *American Journal of Sociology, 66*, 32-42.

Becker, T.E. (1992). Foci and bases of commitment: Are they distinctions worth making? *Academy of Management Journal, 35*, 232-244.

Becker, T.E., & Billings, R. S. (1993). Profiles of commitment: An empirical test. *Journal of Organizational Behavior, 14*, 177-190.

Becker, T. E., Billings, R. S., Eveleth, D. M., & Gilbert, N. L. (1996). Foci and bases of employee commitment: Implications for job performance. *Academy of Management Journal, 39*, 464-482.

Blau, G., Paul, A., & St. John, N. (1993). On developing a general index of work commitment. *Journal of Vocational Behavior, 42*, 298-314.

Brislin, R. W. (1980). Translation and content analysis of oral and written material. In H. C. Triandis & J. W. Berry (Eds.). *Handbook of cross-cultural psychology* (pp. 389-444). Boston: Allyn & Bacon.

Brislin, R. W. (1986). The wording and translation of research instruments. In W. J. Lonner & J. W. Berry (Eds.). *Field methods in cross-cultural research* (pp. 137-164). Newbury Park, CA: Sage.

Buchanan, B. (1974). Building organizational commitment: The socialization of managers in work organizations. *Administrative Science Quarterly, 19*, 533-546.

Bycio, P., Hackett, R. D., & Allen, J. S. (1995). Further assessment of Bass's (1985) conceptualization of transactional and transformational leadership. *Journal of Applied Psychology*, **80**, 468-478.

Campbell, D. T. (1964). Distinguishing differences of perception from failures of communication in cross-cultural studies. In F. S. C. Northrop & H. H. Livingston (Eds.), *Cross-cultural understanding: Epistomology in anthropology* (pp. 308-336). New York: Harper & Row.

Chang, E. (1997). Career commitment as a complex moderator of organizational commitment and turnover intention. *Korean Journal of Management*, **5**, 217-253.

Cronbach, L. J., & Meehl, P. E. (1955). Construct validity in psychological tests. *Psychological Bulletin*, **52**, 281-302.

den Hartog, D. N. (1997). *Inspirational leadership*. Unpublished doctoral dissertation, Free University, Amsterdam, The Netherlands.

Dunham, R. B., Grube, J. A., & Castaneda, M. B. (1994). Organizational commitment: The utility of an integrative definition. *Journal of Applied Psychology*, **79**, 370-380.

Ellemers, N., de Gilder, D., & van den Heuvel, H. (1998). Career-oriented versus team-oriented commitment and behavior at work. *Journal of Applied Psychology*, **83**, 717-730.

Feldman, J.C. (1976). A contingency theory of socialization. *Administrative Science Quarterly*, **21**, 433-452.

Freund, C. G. (1995). *The dual impact of leadership behavior and leader-follower tolerance of ambiguity congruence of organizational commitment*. Unpublished doctoral dissertation, United States International University, San Diego, CA.

Fullager, C., & Barling, J. (1989). A Longitudinal test of a model of antecedents and consequences of union loyalty. *Journal of Applied Psychology*, **74**, 213-227.

Gellatly, I. R. (1995). Individual and group determinants of employee absenteeism: Test of a causal model. *Journal of Organizational Behavior*, **16**, 469-485.

González, L., & Antón, C. (1995). Dimensiones del compromiso organizacional. In L. González, A. De La Torre & J. De Elena (Eds.). *Psicología del trabajo y de las organizaciones, Gestión de recursos humanos y nuevas tecnologías*, Salamanca, Spain: Eudema.

Gordon, M. E., Philpot, J. W., Burt, R. E., Thompson, C. A., & Spiller, W. E. (1980). Commitment to the union: Development of a measure and an examination of its correlates [Monograph]. *Journal of Applied Psychology*, **65**, 479-499.

Griffin, R. W., & Bateman, T. S. (1986). Job satisfaction and organizational commitment. In C.L. Cooper & I. T. Robertson (Eds.) *International review of industrial and oganizational psychology*. Chichester: Wiley.

Griffin, M. A. (1996, April). *Organizational commitment and extra-role behavior*. Presented at the annual meeting of the Society for Industrial and Organizational Psychology, San Diego, CA.

Gross, A.B., & Fullagar, C. (1996, April). *Professional association participation: An application and extension of labor union models*. Presented at the annual meeting of the Society of Industrial and Organizational Psychology, San Diego, CA.

Hackett, R. D., Bycio, P., & Hausdorf, P. A. (1994). Further assessments of Meyer and Allen's (1991) three-component model of organizational commitment. *Journal of Applied Psychology*, **79**, 15-23.

Hahn, J., Hwang, W., & Pak, S. (1997). The impact of the characteristics of organizational culture on the bases for organizational commitment. *Korean Journal of Management*, **5(2)**, 95-134.

Hinkin, T. R. (1995). A review of scale development practices in the study of organization. *Journal of Management*, **21**, 967-988.

Hinkin, T.R. (1998). A brief tutorial on the development of measures for use in survey questionnaires. *Organizational Research Methods*, **1**, 104-121.

Hofstede, G. (1980). *Culture's consequences: International differences in work-related values*. Beverly Hills, CA: Sage.

Hofstede, G. (1991). *Cultures and organizations: Software of the mind*. New York: McGraw-Hill.

Hrebiniak, L. G., & Alutto, J. A. (1972). Personal and role-related factors in the development of organizational commitment. *Administrative Science Quarterly*, **17**, 555-573.

Hui, C. H., & Triandis, H. C. (1985). Measurement in cross-cultural psychology: A review and comparison strategies. *Journal of Cross-Cultural Psychology*, **16**, 131-152.

Hulin, C. L., Drasgow, F., & Komocar, J. (1982). Applications of item response theory to analysis of attitude scale translation. *Journal of Applied Psychology*, **67**, 818-825.

Irving, P. G., Coleman, D. F., & Cooper, C. L (1997). Further assessments of a three-component model of occupational commitment: Generalizability and differences across occupations. *Journal of Applied Psychology*, **82**, 444-452.

Jackson, D. N. (1970). A sequential system for personality scale development. In C. D. Spielberger (Ed.), *Current topics in clinical and community psychology* (Vol.2, pp. 61-96). San Diego, CA: Academic Press.

Jackson, D. N. (1979). Construct validity and personality assessment. In *Construct validity in psychological measurement*. Proceedings of colloquium on theory and application in education and a employment. Educational Testing Service: Princeton, NJ.

Jackson, P. R., Stafford, E. M., Banks, M. H., & Warr, P. B. (1983). Unemployment and psychological distress in young people: The moderating role of employee commitment. *Journal of Applied Psychology*, **68**, 525-535.

Jaros, S.J. (1997). An assessment of Meyer and Allen's (1991) three-component model of organizational commitment and turnover intentions. *Journal of Vocational Behavior*, **51**, 319-337.

Kanter, R. M. (1968). Commitment and social organization: A study of commitment mechanisms in utopian communities. *American Sociological Review*, **33**, 499-517.

Ko, J-W., Price, J. L., & Mueller, C. W. (1997). Assessment of Meyer and Allen's three-component model of organizational commitment in South Korea. *Journal of Applied Psychology*, **82**, 961-973.

Konovsky, M. A., & Cropanzano, R. (1991) Perceived fairness of employee drug testing as a predictor of employee attitudes and job performance. *Journal of Applied Psychology*, **76**, 698-707.

Law, K. S., Wong, C-S., & Mobley, W. H. (1998). Toward a taxonomy of multi-dimensional constructs. *Academy of Management Review*, **23**, 741-755.

Lee, K. (1992). *A study of affective, continuance, and normative commitment to the organization.* Unpublished master's thesis, Sungkyunkwan University, Seoul, Korea.

Lee, K., Allen, N. J., Meyer, J. P., & Rhee, K-Y. (1999, May). *Cross-cultural generalizability of the three-component model of organizational commitment.* Presented at the annual meeting of the Society for Industrial and Organizational Psychology, Atlanta, GA.

Lubich, R.D. (1997). *Organizational commitment: An examination of its linkages to turnover intention.* Unpublished doctoral dissertation. Nova Southeastern University, Fort Lauderdale, FL.

Marsh, R. M., & Mannari, H. (1977). Organizational commitment and turnover: A predictive study. *Administrative Science Quarterly*, **22**, 57-75.

Mathieu, J. E., & Zajac, D. (1990). A review and meta-analysis of the antecedents, correlates, and consequences of organizational commitment. *Psychological Bulletin*, **108**, 171-194.

Mayer, R. C., & Schoorman, F. D. (1992). Predicting participation and production outcomes through a two-dimensional model of organizational commitment. *Academy of Management Journal*, **35**, 671-684.

McGee, G. W., & Ford, R. C. (1987). Two (or more) dimensions of organizational commitment: Reexamination of the Affective and Continuance Commitment Scales. *Journal of Applied Psychology*, **72**, 638-642.

Meyer, J. P., & Allen, N. J. (1984). Testing the "side-bet theory" of organizational commitment: Some methodological considerations. *Journal of Applied Psychology*, **69**, 372-378.

Meyer, J. P., & Allen, N. J. (1991). A three-component conceptualization of organizational commitment. *Human Resource Management Review*, **1**, 61-89.

Meyer, J. P., & Allen, N. J. (1995, May). *Work characteristics and work attitude relations: Moderating effect of attributions.* Presented at the annual meeting of the Society for Industrial and Organizational Psychology, Orlando, FL.

Meyer, J. P., & Allen, N. J. (1997). *Commitment in the workplace: Theory, research, and application.* Thousand Oaks, CA: Sage Publications.

Meyer, J. P., Allen, N. J., & Gellatly, I. R. (1990). Affective and continuance commitment to the organization: Evaluation of measures and analysis of concurrent and time-lagged relations. *Journal of Applied Psychology*, **75**, 710-720.

Meyer, J. P., Allen, N. J., & Smith, C. A. (1993). Commitment to the organization and occupations: Extension and test of a three-component conceptualization. *Journal of Applied Psychology*, **78**, 538-551.

Meyer, J. P., Bobocel, D. R., & Allen, N. J. (1991). Development of organizational commitment during the first year of employment: A longitudinal study of pre- and post-entry influences. *Journal of Management*, **17**, 717-733.

Meyer, J. P., & Herscovitch, L. (in press). Commitment in the workplace: Toward a general model. *Human Resource Management Review.*

Moorman, R. H., Niehoff, B. P., & Organ, D. W. (1993). Treating employees fairly and organizational citizenship behavior: Sorting the effects of job satisfaction, organizational commitment, and procedural justice. *Employee Responsibilities and Rights Journal, 6,* 209-225.

Morrow, P. C. (1983). Concept redundancy in organizational research: The case of work commitment. *Academy of Management Review, 8,* 486-500.

Morrow, P.C. (1993). *The theory and measurement of work commitment.* Greenwich, CT: JAI Press.

Morrow, P. C., & Wirth, R. E. (1989). Work commitment among salaried professionals. *Journal of Vocational Behavior, 34,* 40-56.

Mowday, R. T., Porter, L. W., & Steers, R. M. (1982). *Organizational linkages: The psychology of commitment, absenteeism, and turnover.* San Diego, CA: Academic Press.

Mowday, R. T., Steers, R. M., & Porter, L. W. (1979). The measurement of organizational commitment. *Journal of Vocational Behavior, 14,* 224-247.

O'Reilly, C. A., & Chatman, J. (1986). Organizational commitment and psychological attachment: The effects of compliance, identification, and internalization on prosocial behavior. *Journal of Applied Psychology, 71,* 492-499.

Paunonen, S. V. (2000). Construct validity and the search for cross-cultural consistencies in personality. In R. Goffin and E. Helmes (Eds.). *Problems and solutions in human assessment: Honoring Douglas N. Jackson at seventy* (pp. 121-138).

Reichers, A. E. (1985). A review and reconceptualization of organizational commitment. *Academy of Management Review, 10,* 465-476..

Reilly, N. P., & Orsak, C. L. (1991). A career stage analysis of career and organizational commitment in nursing. *Journal of Vocational Behavior, 39,* 311-330.

Riordan, C. M., & Vandenberg, R. J. (1994). A central question in cross-cultural research: Do employees of different cultures interpret work-related measures in an equivalent manner? *Journal of Management, 20,* 643-671.

Ritzer, G., & Trice, H. M. (1969). An empirical study of Howard Becker's side-bet theory. *Social Forces, 47,* 475-479.

Ryan, A. M., Chan, D., Ployhart, R. E., & Slade, L. A. (1999). Employee attitude surveys in a multinational organization: Considering language and culture in assessing measurement equivalence. *Personnel Psychology, 52,* 37-58.

Scholl, R. W. (1981). Differentiating commitment from expectancy as a motivating force. *Academy of Management Review, 6,* 589-599.

Schwab, D. P. (1980). Construct validity in organizational behavior. *Research in Organizational Behavior, 2,* 3-43.

Shore, L.M., & Tetrick, L. E. (1991). A construct validity study of the Survey of Perceived Organizational Support. *Journal of Applied Psychology, 76,* 637-643.

Shore, L. M., & Wayne, S. J. (1993). Commitment and employee behavior: Comparison of affective and continuance commitment with perceived organizational support. *Journal of Applied Psychology, 78,* 774-780.

Somers, M. J. (1993). A test of the relationship between affective and continuance commitment using non-recursive models. *Journal of Occupational and Organizational Psychology, 66,* 185-192.

Speechley, M. J., Noh, S., & Beggs, C. (1993). Examining the psychometric properties of a scale on a smallish sample: An example using an occupational commitment scale. *Canadian Journal of Rehabilitation, 7,* 90-93.

Stanley, D., Meyer, J. P., Topolnytsky, L., & Herscovitch, L. (1999). *Affective, continuance, and normative commitment: Meta-analyses of interrelations and outcomes.* Presented at the annual meeting of the Society for Industrial and Organizational Psychology, Atlanta, GA.

Stebbins, R.A. (1970). On misunderstanding the concept of commitment: A theoretical clarification. *Social Forces, 48,* 526-529.

Sverke, M., & Sjoberg, A. (1994). Dual commitment to company and union in Sweden: An examination of predictors and taxonomic split methods. *Economic and Industrial Democracy, 15,* 531-564.

Takahashi, K. (1997). Item characteristics of an organizational commitment scale and its application: Based on the Allen and Meyer three-dimensional commitment scale. *Japanese Journal of Administrative Behavior, 11,* 123-136.

Takahashi, K., Noguchi, H., & Watanabe, N. (1998, March). *Development of Allen and Meyer Commitment Scale Japanese Version Based on Item Response Theory.* Paper presented at the first workshop of the Japanese Association of Administrative Science. Nanzan University, Nagoya, Japan.

Takao, S. (1995). *The multidimensionality of organizational commitment: An analysis of its antecedents and consequences among Japanese systems engineers.* Unpublished doctoral dissertation, Cornell University, Ithaca, NY.

Travaglione, A. (1998). *The determinants and outcomes of organizational commitment.* Unpublished doctoral dissertation, Curtin Graduate School of Management, Perth, Australia.

Triandis, H. C. (1972). *The analysis of subjective culture.* New York: Wiley.

Triandis, H. C. (1992). Cross-cultural research in social psychology. In D. Granberg & G. Sarup (Eds.), *Social judgment and intergroup relations: Essays in honor of Musafer Sherif* (pp. 229-243). New York: Springer-Verlag.

Triandis, H. C., Leung, K., Villareal, M., & Clack, F. L. (1985). Allocentric vs. idiocentric tendencies: Convergent and discriminant validation. *Journal of Research in Personality*, **19**, 395-415.

van de Vijver, F., & Leung, K. (1997). *Methods and data analysis for cross-cultural research.* Thousand Oaks, CA: Sage

Vandenberg, R. J., & Self, R. M. (1993). Assessing newcomers' changing commitments to the organization during the first 6 months of work. *Journal of Applied Psychology*, **78**, 557-568.

Vandenberg, R. J., Self, R. M., & Seo, J. H. (1994). A critical examination of the internalization, identification, and compliance commitment measures. *Journal of Management*, **20**, 123-140.

Vandenberghe, C. (1996). Assessing organizational commitment in a Belgian context: Evidence for the three-dimensional model. *Applied Psychology: An International Review*, **45(4)**, 371-386.

Vandenberghe, C. (1998). *An examination of the attitudinal consequences of person-culture fit in the health care industry.* Unpublished manuscript, Catholic University of Louvain, Belgium.

Vandenberghe, C., Bonami, M., & Jacquemyns, B. (1998). *Perceived support, organizational commitment, and job satisfaction as correlates of citizenship behaviors: A test in retail stores.* Unpublished manuscript, Catholic University of Louvain, Belgium.

Vandenberghe, C., & Peiro, J. M. (1999). *Organizational and individual values: Their main and combined effects on work attitudes and perceptions.* Unpublished manuscript, Catholic University of Louvain, Belgium.

Vandenberghe, C., Stinglhamber, F., Bentein, K., & Delhaise, T. (1999). *An examination of the cross-cultural validity of a multidimensional model of commitment in the European Community.* Unpublished manuscript, Catholic University of Louvain, Belgium.

Wallace, J.E. (1988). Professional and organizational commitment: Compatible or incompatible? *Journal of Vocational Behavior*, **42**, 333-349.

Wasti, S. A. (1999, August). *A cultural analysis of organizational commitment and turnover intentions in a collectivist society.* Presented at the annual meeting of the Academy of Management, Chicago, IL.

Whitener, E.M. & Walz, P.M. (1993). Exchange theory determinants of affective and continuance commitment. *Journal of Applied Psychology*, **42**, 265-281.

Wiener, Y. (1982). Commitment in organizations: A normative view. *Academy of Management Review*, **7**, 418-428.

Wiener, Y., & Vardi, Y. (1980). Relationships between job, organization, and career commitments and work outcomes: An integrative approach. *Organizational Behavior and Human Performance*, **26**, 81-96.

Withey, M. (1988). Antecedents of value based and economic organizational commitment. *Proceedings of the Administrative Sciences Association of Canada-Organizational Behavior Division*, **9**, 124-133.

14 THE CONSTRUCT OF GOAL COMMITMENT: MEASUREMENT AND RELATIONSHIPS WITH TASK PERFORMANCE

Gerard H. Seijts
Gary P. Latham

INTRODUCTION

Among the most robust findings in the behavioral science literature is that setting a specific, difficult goal leads to higher performance than urging individuals to "do their best" (Latham & Locke, 1991; Locke & Latham, 1984; 1990). Moreover, research has repeatedly shown that the higher the specific goal, the higher the individual's performance. Only when individuals reach the limits of their abilities does the linear relationship between goal difficulty and performance level off (Garland, 1982; Locke, 1982; Seijts, Meertens, & Kok, 1997).

Latham and Lee (1986) found that the positive effect of goal setting on performance generalizes across laboratory and field studies, soft and hard criteria, individual and group goals, and goals that are set by an individual (self-set), assigned by an authority figure (e.g., supervisor, and experimenter) or set participatively. In short, the beneficial effect of goal setting on performance has been replicated across a wide variety of participants, tasks, criterion measures, settings, and countries using a multitude of research designs (Bandura, 1997; Locke & Latham, 1990). Thus, it is not surprising that numerous authors have concluded that goal setting theory is among the most valid and practical theories of motivation (Lee & Earley, 1992; Miner, 1984; Pinder, 1998).

It is virtually axiomatic that a goal that a person is not really trying for is not truly a goal and therefore has little or no effect on subsequent performance (Bargh

& Chartrand, 1999; Gollwitzer, 1999; Locke, 1968; Locke & Latham, 1990; Locke, Latham, & Erez, 1988). Goal commitment is related to performance in two ways.First, empirical studies, including a meta-analysis, have shown that goal commitment moderates the relationship between goal difficulty and performance (Erez & Zidon, 1984; Hollenbeck, Williams & Klein, 1989a; Klein, Wesson, Hollenbeck, & Alge, 1999a; Tubbs, 1993). The correlation between goal difficulty and performance is higher among individuals with high goal commitment than among those with low goal commitment.

Second, the level of goal commitment can have a main effect on performance (Hollenbeck & Klein, 1987; Klein et al., 1999a; Locke & Latham, 1990). Individuals who are highly committed to a difficult goal perform at significantly higher levels than individuals who are not committed to the same goal (Hollenbeck, Klein, O'Leary-Kelly, & Wright, 1989b; Klein et al., 1999a; Locke & Shaw, 1984; Seijts & Latham, 1999a). This is because highly committed individuals exert more effort, and are more persistent toward goal attainment, than individuals who are less committed to the goal. However, when an assigned goal is easy or moderately difficult, high commitment may lead to poorer performance than low commitment to the same goal (Locke & Latham, 1990). Individuals with low commitment to the assigned goal may set a higher personal goal that, in turn, may lead to higher performance.

Given the critical role of goal commitment in goal setting theory, one would expect that the assessment of this construct has played a prominent role in goal setting research. However, in a review of the goal setting literature through the mid 1980s, Hollenbeck and Klein (1987) found that in the majority (61 percent) of goal setting studies they reviewed (66 of 109), no mention was made of goal commitment. In 12 percent of the studies, goal commitment was mentioned but not empirically assessed. In none of the studies did the authors attempt to establish the construct validity of their measure of goal commitment. In addition, Hollenbeck and Klein (1987) found that many goal setting researchers used a single-item measure (e.g., "How committed are you to attaining the goal set?"). Hence the reliability of the measure of goal commitment was not known.

Hollenbeck and Klein's (1987) findings were troubling for at least two reasons. First, they found that the critical role of goal commitment to goal setting theory had been largely ignored. Second, they reported that unmeasured goal commitment effects were often used as post hoc explanations for non-significant goal setting effects. That is, even when goal commitment was not assessed, the varying effect-sizes for goal setting, as well as inconsistent results with moderating variables (e.g., participation, feedback, and rewards) were often attributed to unmeasured goal commitment effects. Hollenbeck and Klein concluded that, given the central role of goal commitment in goal setting theory, subsequent research must assess goal commitment.

Within the past decade, effort has been directed to defining goal commitment, suggesting ways of measuring it, and assessing the construct validity of the respective measures (DeShon & Landis, 1997; Hollenbeck et al., 1989a; Klein, Wesson, Hollenbeck, Wright, & DeShon, 1999b; Tubbs, 1993; Wright, O'Leary-Kelly, Cortina, Klein, & Hollenbeck, 1994). Instrumental to the development of a psychometrically sound goal commitment measure has been the willingness on the part of researchers to be guided by empirical data, and to correct their conceptions and misconceptions on the basis of empirical findings.

The purpose of this chapter is four-fold. First, consistent with Jackson's recommendation for scale development and construct validation strategies, the construct of goal commitment is defined conceptually. Second, the methods used to assess this construct are reviewed and critiqued. Third, theoretical, empirical, and practical concerns of the goal commitment scale developed by Hollenbeck and his colleagues are addressed (Hollenbeck et al., 1989a; Hollenbeck et al., 1989b). Fourth, consistent with the theme of this book, measurement opportunities regarding the goal commitment construct are explored.

CONCEPTUAL DEFINITION OF GOAL COMMITMENT

Construct validation is a multi-step process. Jackson (1970; 1971; 1979) argued that an initial step is to define the theoretical construct and its dimensions under investigation in precise terms. Specification of a content domain allows the researcher to develop a pool of measurement items that represent the content domain. This is the second step in designing and validating a measurement scale. The important role played by construct definition in scale construction is shown in Jackson's work. His research suggested that when construct definitions are made explicit, average undergraduate psychology students can, in a matter of hours, generate multi-item scales with validities and reliabilities comparable to those of popular empirically-derived scales that took months or years to develop (Jackson, 1975; 1979; see Chapter 11 of this volume by Goffin, Rothstein, & Johnston for a discussion of the empirical scale development strategy).

Theory facilitates scale construction in that it explains how the focal construct can be differentiated from other constructs. This is because theory and construct definition suggest a basis for obtaining evidence for discriminant validity (Campbell & Fiske, 1967; Jackson, 1970).

A plethora of conceptual definitions of goal commitment have been proposed (see Tubbs & Dahl, 1991 for a review). For example, Locke et al. (1988) described goal commitment as one's attachment to or determination to reach a goal, regardless of the goal's origin. Similarly, Kernan and Lord (1988) defined goal commitment as an unwillingness to lower goals when confronted with feedback that the goals have not yet been reached. Naylor and Ilgen (1984) defined goal commitment as the degree to which an individual commits resources such as time and effort toward accomplishing a goal. Most recently, DeShon and Landis (1997) defined this construct as "the degree to which the individual considers the goal to be important, is determined to reach it by expending effort over time, and is unwilling to abandon or lower the goal when confronted with setbacks and negative feedback" (p. 106).

Common to these definitions is the content domain of choice, effort, and persistence to attain a specific goal regardless of obstacles or initial failures to do so (Hollenbeck et al., 1989b; Klein et al., 1999b; Wright et al., 1994). Once the content domain of a construct is specified, researchers can shift their attention to the development of scale items to sample representatively processes related to content (Jackson, 1979).

The definitions of goal commitment suggest that it can be measured attitudinally or behaviorally. Indeed, Locke and Latham (1990) suggest that either approach is satisfactory. Employing both strategies can provide evidence for convergent validity of the measure of goal commitment.

OPERATIONALIZATION OF GOAL COMMITMENT

Measures of goal commitment that have been proposed in the literature include attitudinal self-report measures, goal discrepancy measures, subsequent goal change, and observable behavior. These alternate ways are complementary for increasing understanding of goal commitment, and how goal commitment affects subsequent performance. The advantages and limitations of each method are discussed below. In addition, consistent with Jackson's (1971; 1979; 1984) recommendations, strategies for item selection are discussed.

Attitudinal Self-Report Measures

Among the most widely used measure of goal commitment is a scale developed by Hollenbeck and his colleagues (Hollenbeck et al., 1989a; Hollenbeck et al., 1989b) (see Table 1). This measure operationalizes goal commitment as a self-report of an attitudinal reaction to a goal. Consistent with the literature on attitudes (Fishbein & Ajzen, 1975; Gollwitzer & Bargh, 1996), the scale items reflect the cognitive (e.g., "I think this goal is a good goal to shoot for"), affective (e.g., "Quite frankly, I don't care if I achieve this goal or not"), and behavioral (e.g., "It wouldn't take much to make me abandon this goal") components of an attitude.

To establish the adequacy of item sampling and the construct validity of their goal commitment measure, Hollenbeck et al. (1989a) collected data on self-set academic performance goals, commitment to those goals, and the academic performance of 190 undergraduate students enrolled in a management course. A principal-axis factor analysis on the original nine items indicated that 49.7 percent of the variance could be accounted for by a single factor. Seven items (items 1 thru 7 in Table 1) loaded on this factor with factor loadings greater than .61. A second factor (items 8 and 9 in Table 1) explained additional variance of 17 percent; because these two items seemed to load on this separate factor, they were deleted from the original nine-item scale. The remaining seven items were thus treated as a uni-dimensional measure of goal commitment. Cronbach's alpha of this measure was .88. The correlation between commitment to the self-set goal and academic performance was positive and significant ($r = .36, p < .05$).

Table 1. Hollenbeck, Williams and Klein's (1989) Goal Commitment Items.

1. It is hard to take this goal seriously. (R)

2. It is unrealistic for me to expect to reach this goal. (R)

3. It is quite likely that this goal may need to be revised, depending on how things go. (R)

4. Quite frankly, I don't care if I achieve this goal or not. (R)

5. I am strongly committed to pursuing this goal.

6. It would not take much to make me abandon this goal. (R)

7. I think this goal is a good goal to shoot for.

8. I am willing to put forth a great deal of effort beyond what I would normally do to achieve this goal.

9. There is not much to be gained by trying to achieve this goal. (R)

Note. Items followed by (R) indicate that the item was reverse-scored.

In a follow-up study, Hollenbeck et al. (1989b) reanalyzed the data (total $N = 752$ participants) from three separate studies (Hollenbeck et al., 1989a; Klein, 1987; Wright, 1987) that shared the same pool of goal commitment items. This was done in order to develop "an efficient, construct valid measure of goal commitment." Consistent with Jackson's (1971; 1979; 1984) recommendations, the construct validity analysis consisted of four empirical tests. First, a principal components factor analysis on the nine original goal commitment items was conducted. The results showed that all nine items exhibited factor loadings in excess of .50, with an average of .63. The nine-item pool revealed one major underlying factor that accounted for 40 percent of the variance. A second factor was extracted which accounted for 12 percent additional variance. Deleting this factor from the analysis resulted in a seven-item goal commitment scale (items 1 thru 7 in Table 1; see also Hollenbeck et al. (1989a)). The Cronbach's alpha of this seven-item version of the goal commitment scale was .80.

Second, evidence of convergent validity was obtained. Hollenbeck et al. (1989b) found that their self-report measure of goal commitment correlated negatively and significantly with an alternative measure of goal commitment, namely, the self-set - assigned goal discrepancy ($r = -.54$, $p < .05$). Self-reported goal commitment decreased as the absolute value of the self-set - assigned goal discrepancy increased. The correlation between the self-report measure of goal commitment and actual goal change, however, was not significant ($r = -.11$, $p > .05$). Collectively, these two findings provide modest evidence of convergent validity. Although convergent validity is a necessary condition for construct validation, it is not sufficient (Campbell & Fiske, 1967; Jackson, 1979; 1984; 1990).

A third step in construct validation is to specify, a priori, theoretical linkages between separate constructs that lie within the nomological net of the focal construct (Cronbach & Meehl, 1967; Jackson, 1979). Nomological validity refers to the network of theoretical expectations regarding the links in different combinations between particular independent, intervening, and dependent variables. The results obtained by Hollenbeck and his colleagues (1989b) showed that self-report commitment to difficult goals was consistently related to academic performance as well as performance on a computer card sorting task. Furthermore, consistent with their hypotheses, positive and significant correlations were obtained between the self-report measure of goal commitment and both situational (e.g., public evaluation of performance) and personal antecedents (e.g., need for achievement, and task involvement) of the construct.

Finally, evidence for discriminant validity was obtained. Specifically, Hollenbeck et al. (1989b) showed that their self-report measure of goal commitment was relatively independent from measures that are conceptually different from goal commitment. Various demographic variables and generalized intelligence (SAT score measures) did not correlate with goal commitment. These non-significant relationships provide some limited support for the discriminant validity requirement of construct validation.

Hollenbeck's scale appears to be a general, flexible measure in that it can be used to assess goal commitment regardless of goal origin or timing. It has been used by researchers to assess commitment to self-set, assigned, and participatively-set goals, and to assess initial goal commitment as well as ongoing commitment when striving to attain the goal. Moreover, this self-report scale of commitment has been used both at the individual and group level of analysis (Seijts & Latham, 1999b; Weingart, 1992; Weingart & Weldon, 1991).

A limitation of this scale is that it does not inform the researcher of the actual goal the individual is trying to attain when the goal is assigned or set participatively. An attitudinal self-report measure of goal commitment may not accurately reflect the discrepancy between assigned or participatively-set goals and the individual's personal goals. Locke and Latham (1990) thus recommended that self-set goals be measured. This is because assigned or participatively-set goals may be rejected, and self-set goals may change over time when a task includes multiple trials, and feedback suggests that the goal that was assigned or set participatively is too hard or too easy.

Self-set Goal - Assigned Goal Discrepancies

Several goal setting researchers have suggested that an indirect self-report measure of goal commitment is the discrepancy between an assigned or participatively-set goal and the individual's personal goal (Campion & Lord, 1982; Locke et al., 1988; Tubbs & Dahl, 1991). A large absolute discrepancy, that is, self-set goals either much higher or much lower than the assigned or participatively-set goal, suggests low commitment to the assigned or participatively-set goal.

The sign of the correlation between the discrepancy measure of goal commitment and actual task performance varies depending on the level of the self-set goal. If the assigned or participatively-set goal exceeds the individual's self-set personal goal, a large absolute discrepancy indicates relatively low personal goals. Thus, the discrepancy, that is, the indicator of goal commitment, will be negatively related to performance. In contrast, when participants set personal goals that are much higher than the assigned or participatively-set goal, the discrepancy will correlate positively with performance.

This operationalization of goal commitment is advocated by Tubbs and his colleagues (Tubbs, 1993; 1994; Tubbs & Dahl, 1991; Tubbs & Ekeberg, 1991). Their results showed that a direct calculation of the absolute discrepancy between assigned and self-set personal goals consistently moderated the relationship between assigned goals and performance. Nevertheless, there are several theoretical, empirical, and practical shortcomings to using this measure.

Theoretical Shortcomings

Wright and his colleagues (1994) criticized Tubbs' measure on the basis of four theoretical issues. First, they argued that even though the discrepancy measure of goal commitment correlated strongly with performance, effect size is not a basis for advocating the use of difference scores in goal setting research. This is because large effect sizes can be observed for reasons (e.g., sampling error) that have little or nothing to do with construct validity.

Second, the items in the attitudinal self-report measure of goal commitment (Hollenbeck et al., 1989a; Hollenbeck et al., 1989b) were developed to reflect the conceptual definition of goal commitment, namely, an attitude about a goal and the maintenance of the determination to achieve it. Thus, the self-report items displayed conceptual fidelity with the definition of goal commitment. This is important because item scales stand a greater chance of being construct valid if they are firmly grounded in theory (Jackson, 1970; 1971; 1979). In contrast, no theoretical rationale substantiates the claim that discrepancy scores in themselves capture the construct reflected in the label attached to them (Johns, 1981). Evidence of construct validity is not met by assuring that differences are calculated from components, namely, assigned or participatively-set goals and self-set personal goals, which are themselves construct valid.

Third, discrepancy measures are systematically related to their components. Therefore, in many situations, a discrepancy measure provides little incremental utility beyond simply examining one's personal or self-set goal. For example, in experimental conditions where there is no variance in assigned goals, there is a perfect correlation between the personal goal and the discrepancy between the assigned or participatively-set goal and the self-set goal.

A critical requirement in the construct validation of measures is the demonstration that the construct measured by a difference score is discriminable from the variables measured by its components (Jackson, 1971; 1979; 1984). The use of difference scores implies that they should do something "better" than other measures, especially their own components, which are already available and more likely to be grounded in theory (Johns, 1981). Such evidence, however, has not been found in the goal setting literature.

Fourth, the use of absolute differences between assigned or participatively-set goals and self-set goals assumes that the direction of this discrepancy is theoretically inconsequential. For example, the use of difference scores suggest that a person's reaction to an assigned goal that is higher than one's personal goal is equivalent to the reaction to an assigned goal that is lower than the personal goal. This assumption is tenuous. As Wright and his colleagues (1994) argued, individuals are likely to react more negatively to an assigned goal that exceeds their personal goal relative to an assigned goal that is lower than their personal goal. Thus, the direction of the difference between the components may suggest important information about the focal construct measured (e.g., moderating the relationship between the difference score and another variable).

Empirical Shortcomings

To the extent that ability is a strong determinant of one's personal goals and one's performance (Locke, 1998; Locke & Latham, 1990), the observed relationship between the discrepancy measure and performance will be spurious. To examine the relationship between a discrepancy measure of goal commitment and performance, one must thus partial out ability. Wright and his colleagues (1994) reanalyzed Tubbs' (1993) data and found that, after ability was partialled out, the correlation between the discrepancy measure of goal commitment and performance was reduced significantly.

Practical Shortcomings

There are at least four practical reasons for not using a discrepancy measure of goal commitment. First, it can only be used to measure goal commitment to assigned or participatively-set goals. To ask individuals to set their own goals and then to indicate their personal goals is redundant (Locke & Latham, 1990).

Second, the timing of measurement of goal commitment is problematic. If a goal is assigned or participatively-set and then a self-set goal is measured, the resulting self-set goals may be anchored to the assigned or participatively-set goal (Hinsz, Kalnbach, & Lorentz, 1997; Seijts & Latham, 1999b; Wright et al., 1994). Furthermore, if the individual is first assigned a goal, and then subsequently asked to self-set a personal goal, rejection of the assigned goal is implicitly if not explicitly encouraged (Locke et al., 1988). Alternatively, if individuals are first asked about their self-set personal goals and are then assigned a goal, the discrepancy measure is not likely to be reflective of the individual's subjective reaction to this assigned or participatively-set goal. In contrast, Hollenbeck et al. (1989a) demonstrated that the self-report attitudinal measure of goal commitment is relatively unaffected by the timing of measurement.

A third practical problem with discrepancy measures involves the potential lack of statistical power in significance testing (Wright et al., 1994). Large sample sizes are required as discrepancy measures should be studied within rather than across conditions. The rationale is that commitment is expected to be related to performance within goal conditions. Put differently, within a goal condition, the assigned goal is a constant, meaning that the discrepancy measure is an indirect reflection of one's personal goal.

Finally, discrepancy measures of goal commitment lack both parsimony and efficiency. The researcher is required to measure two variables directly (assigned or participatively-set goals, and self-set goals) and calculate a third variable, that is, the discrepancy score, to do what a single measure, namely the self-set goal might have done alone (Johns, 1981).

Subsequent Goal Change

The conceptual definition of goal commitment includes an unwillingness to change or abandon a goal over time. Therefore, another measure of goal commitment is whether individuals report a change in goals over time (Hollenbeck et al., 1989b; Locke & Latham, 1990; Yukl & Latham, 1978). Locke and Latham (1990) recommended that self-set goals should be measured to monitor a possible change in goals. For example, measuring self-set personal goals may provide additional insight why an assigned or participatively-set goal did or did not have an effect on performance. This measure of goal commitment, however, requires a repeated-measures design involving multiple trials during which participants are asked to report their self-set proximal or distal personal goals.

Performance

The degree of goal commitment may also be inferred from performance itself. For example, Salancik (1977) argued that action is the ultimate proof of commitment, and thus, by implication, the most accurate measure of it. Attitudes, in contrast, are an attempt to predict action before the fact. Salancik argued that commitment is grounded in behavior. Specifically, he stated that:

> "To act is to commit oneself ... An adulterer may proclaim unrelenting devotion to a lover, but to give up children, home, and joint bank accounts is to put meaning into the proclamation ... Thus, at a minimum, a concept of commitment implies that behavior, or action, be a central focus" (Salancik, 1977, p. 4).

Empirically, inferring commitment from performance seems justified if ability, self-efficacy, and so forth were (or can be assumed to have been) controlled or randomized across conditions. However, as stated earlier, performance should not be the sole measure of commitment; factors other than commitment affect performance including situational constraints. Consequently, it is useful to measure commitment attitudinally before action takes place.

Conclusion

There are three different ways for assessing goal commitment, namely, the attitudinal self-report measure developed by Hollenbeck and his colleagues, the measurement of self-set personal goals, and behavior (e.g., choice, effort, and persistence). Goal commitment should be assessed across time to examine the dynamic interplay between goals, commitment to these goals, and performance. Discrepancy measures should be avoided for theoretical, empirical, and practical reasons.

HOLLENBECK ET AL.'S REVISED GOAL COMMITMENT SCALE

As noted earlier in this chapter, a meta-analysis revealed that goal commitment moderates the relationship between goal difficulty and performance, and that goal commitment also has a main effect on performance (Klein et al., 1999b). That study also concluded that while goal commitment has begun to receive empirical attention in response to earlier review articles, additional research on the construct is necessary given its key role in goal setting theory. This is because for goal setting theory to evolve, and to show systematic relationships between goal commitment and prior causal factors and subsequent action (e.g., choice, effort, persistence, and performance), it is imperative that the measures used to assess goal commitment be construct valid and demonstrate appropriate psychometric properties.

As noted earlier, Hollenbeck and his colleagues (Hollenbeck et al., 1989a; Hollenbeck et al., 1989b) developed a seven-item attitudinal self-report measure of goal commitment. It is among the most commonly used measures of goal commitment (Klein et al., 1999a). Despite the popularity of this scale, however, there remains debate over its dimensionality (DeShon & Landis, 1997; Klein et al., 1999b; Tubbs, 1993; 1994; Wright et al., 1994).

Dimensions of the Construct

Goal commitment, as evident in much of the goal setting literature, is viewed as a single or unitary construct. For example, the definition of goal commitment underlying Hollenbeck's goal commitment scale is the determination to try for a goal, and the persistence in pursuing that goal over time. However, Tubbs and his colleagues (Tubbs, 1993; 1994; Tubbs & Dahl, 1991; Tubbs & Ekeberg, 1991) argued that this single-construct interpretation conflicts with theories of motivational choice and decision-making. Tubbs argued that the motivational concepts and measures discussed under the heading of goal commitment do not refer to any single attribute. Instead, he argued, multiple constructs have routinely been discussed and assessed under the heading of goal commitment. These constructs include pre-choice evaluations of potential personal goals, subsequent choice or acceptance of a personal goal, and maintenance intentions of that choice. Tubbs argued that commitment is the outcome of the cognitive evaluation of the goal in terms of likelihood or expectancies of goal attainment and the attractiveness or valence of goal attainment. Once the individual has chosen a personal goal or internalized an assigned or participatively-set goal based on this cognitive evaluation, he or she becomes affectively attached to it. Consequently, the individual is willing to invest effort to attain the goal, and is unwilling to lower the goal when faced with obstacles and setbacks. Pre-choice attitudinal judgments, Tubbs argued, are conceptually distinct from the setting of a personal goal that is based on those judgments. Maintenance is the strength of the intention to adhere to the goal.

Given these conceptual distinctions, Tubbs argued that a single or unitary goal commitment measure such as Hollenbeck's self-report scale cannot adequately address these issues. In other words, if goal commitment is comprised of separate constructs (e.g., initial commitment, and maintenance of commitment) then separate measures should be used to assess it.

In response to Tubbs, Klein and his colleagues (1999a; 1999b) acknowledged that it is possible to make subtle conceptual distinctions among the concepts that he identified, but they pointed out that all of them are motivational choices that are influenced by the same antecedents. For most goal setting purposes, the use of a general, comprehensive measure of goal commitment, they claimed, is adequate. The use of three separate measures violates the principle of parsimony (Klein et al., 1999b). In other words, unless the distinctions outlined by Tubbs and his associates are shown to be empirically useful in the science and practice of goal setting research, a marked separation of the concepts identified by Tubbs is difficult to justify.

Additional concerns regarding Hollenbeck et al.'s self-report measure of goal commitment were articulated by DeShon and Landis (1997). They stated that goal commitment is typically defined as the degree to which the individual considers the goal important, is determined to reach it by expending effort over time, and is willing to abandon or lower the goal when confronted with setbacks or negative feedback. However, only a subset of the items that comprise Hollenbeck et al.'s scale is consistent with this definition (items 4 - 7 in Table 1). In contrast, items 1 thru 3 appear to measure perceptions of goal difficulty and performance expectancies rather than goal commitment.

DeShon and Landis (1997) argued that the inability of researchers to reliably distinguish between the items pertaining to goal difficulty and performance expectancies from the other four items is due to the nature of the task that is used in the majority of goal setting studies. Goal setting is a motivational theory. Consequently, the research tasks have been generally straightforward for the individual so that the effect of a goal on choice, effort, and persistence can be systematically studied. On tasks that are relatively straightforward for the individual, that is, where performance is primarily a function of effort and persistence, a strong relationship between performance expectancies and goal commitment is usually found. Individuals who intend to attain the goal work harder and longer than those with low goal commitment. This increase in effort, in turn, results in high performance, and hence strengthens the effort - performance linkage. In contrast, performance on a task that is complex for the individual is primarily a function of the identification and implementation of task relevant strategies (Locke & Latham, 1990; Winters & Latham, 1996; Wood &

Locke, 1990). Therefore, the connection between increased effort and task performance is weak. DeShon and Landis (1997) hypothesized that it may be easier to distinguish goal difficulty and performance expectancy items from actual goal commitment items on a complex task where performance expectancies are low despite the person's desire to attain the goal. Stated differently, the uni-dimensionality of the Hollenbeck scale will be stronger in studies using relatively straightforward rather than complex tasks. Furthermore, they hypothesized that the magnitude of the effort - performance linkage decreases if individuals receive, on a regular basis, negative feedback indicating that their performance falls short of the goal. In contrast, responses to the four goal commitment items should be relatively stable over time.

Support for these two hypotheses was obtained in three laboratory studies. DeShon and Landis (1997) therefore concluded that, on a complex task, responses to the self-report goal commitment measure are generated by two factors, namely, a goal commitment factor, and the cognitive evaluation of the likelihood of goal achievement, that is, perceptions of self-efficacy. Based on these findings, DeShon and Landis recommended that future assessments of goal commitment should exclude effort - performance items (items 1 thru 3 in Table 1).

Although DeShon and Landis (1997) explicitly stated that task complexity serves as a boundary condition for goal commitment measures, they never manipulated task complexity in any of their studies (Hollenbeck, personal communication, August 19, 1999). Rather, they merely asserted that the tasks used in their studies were more complex than all the other tasks used in the goal setting literature. Their tasks, however, were actually fairly simple relative to many of the tasks that have been studied in the literature. Therefore, the lack of generalizability of Hollenbeck's goal commitment scale over task complexity was never rigorously established prior to Klein et al.'s (1999b) meta-analysis.

A study conducted by Klein et al. (1999b) utilizing meta-analytic techniques and confirmatory factor analysis was conducted in response to DeShon and Landis' (1997) data. The purpose of their meta-analysis was to further address the confusion that exists in the literature regarding what version, if any, of Hollenbeck's attitudinal self-report scale should be used to assess goal commitment. They combined the results of 17 independent samples and 2,918 participants to assess of the dimensionality of Hollenbeck's goal commitment scale. The results of both an exploratory and a confirmatory factor analysis showed that fit of the uni-dimensional model of goal commitment was maximized using a five-item scale consisting of items 1, 4, 5, 6, and 7 (see Table 1). Moreover, differences across studies with respect to goal origin, task complexity, and measurement timing did not provide evidence of multi-dimensionality of the scale. Although DeShon and Landis (1997) recommended removal of the first item (see Table 1) from the self-report scale, Klein and his associates retained it as part of the revised goal commitment scale. The finding that the dimensionality of the revised

Hollenbeck scale was not affected by measurement timing refutes Tubbs' (1993; 1994) argument that conceptual distinctions should be made between initial goal commitment and maintenance of that commitment.

In conclusion, the development of the Hollenbeck et al. attitudinal self-report scale of goal commitment followed a key construct validation principle, namely, that evidence of construct validity is accumulated gradually. The revised self-report scale suggested by Klein and his colleagues retains only five of the original nine items proposed by Hollenbeck. This scale appears to be a robust, psychometrically sound measure of goal commitment. Of the existing goal commitment measures, Klein and Hollenbeck's current scale would seem to be the most promising. Nevertheless, as discussed in the following section, future clarification of the goal commitment construct might contribute to alternate conceptualizations of goal commitment, which, in turn, may necessitate the development of new goal commitment scales.

CONCLUSION AND AREAS FOR FUTURE RESEARCH

This chapter describes the efforts of researchers to develop a construct valid measure of goal commitment. Through systematic research, and adhering to the principles for scale development and validation strategies espoused by Jackson, psychometrically sound measures of goal commitment have been developed. These principles advanced understanding and measurement of goal commitment in the following ways. First, in the past decade there has been an emphasis on the conceptual definition of goal commitment, and the writing of scale items that represent the content domain of the construct. Second, alternate ways of measuring goal commitment have been identified. Goal setting researchers have not limited themselves to using a single-method of measuring goal commitment. Mono-method bias has been avoided. Third, there has been a focus on empirical item selection to establish the internal consistency of the scale, its dimensionality, and validity. In terms of validity, evidence has been obtained that supports both convergent and discriminant validity of goal commitment scales. Fourth, networks of theoretical expectations regarding the links between goal commitment and other critical goal setting variables have been developed.

The following principles for scale development have yet to be implemented. First, as Jackson (1970, 1984) argued, the value of having at hand a large pool of measurement items that are logically related to the definition of the construct cannot be overemphasized. For example, parallel forms of a goal commitment measure may be advantageous when the researcher wishes to undertake a repeated-measures design. A disadvantage of administering the same measurement instrument repeatedly in a relatively short time period is that respondents' memory of previous responses may linger through these intervals. This, in effect, may lead to measurement error; too much stability in tests may indicate that the measure is not sensitive enough to ordinary changes in the construct being measured (Guion, 1965). Thus, the number of goal commitment items should be expanded so that parallel forms of the goal commitment measure can be developed.

Second, Jackson is well known for articulating and examining the effects of different response biases on self-report measures. For example, he has shown how socially desirable responses complicates the interpretation of self-report measures (see Chapter 2 of this volume by Helmes which is devoted to the topic of social desirability as it relates to personality test development). In most contexts it is socially desirable to report that one is committed to goals even when there is little or no commitment to their attainment. Therefore, attitudinal self-report items may, to some extent, be measuring a tendency to respond in a socially desirable fashion. Goal commitment scales have not yet been shown to have discriminant validity with respect to the construct of social desirability. Studying socially desirable responding in relation to goal commitment measurement is an area for future research.

Third, in much of the goal setting research, goal commitment is often a secondary variable (Klein et al., 1999a). That is, goal commitment continues to be measured without specific hypotheses aimed at exploring its nature and role. Statistical relationships between goal commitment and the other variables being studied are frequently not reported. In many cases, goal commitment is measured only as a manipulation check. More elaborate nomological networks, guided by formal theory, should be developed that indicate how goal commitment is related to both its antecedents and consequences. It may be, for example, that individuals are committed to a goal for different reasons. For example, consistent with Meyer and Allen's (1984; 1990; 1998; see Chapter 13 of this volume by Allen & Meyer which discusses the development of their organizational commitment model) organizational commitment construct, goal commitment may take different forms, and the antecedents, consequences, and correlates of each form may be somewhat different. Affective goal commitment may reflect the individual's emotional attachment to and identification with the goal; continuance goal commitment may involve the recognition of costs associated with abandoning the goal; and normative goal commitment may reflect an individual's feelings of obligation to stick with the goal. Although these three forms of goal commitment presumably increase the likelihood that individuals will persist with the goal, the motive for doing so differs (desire, need, and obligation, respectively) and can have implications for individuals' subsequent action. However, Meyer and Allen's findings on organizational commitment have yet to "transfer" to the goal setting literature (Meyer & Herscovitch, in press). There are, of course, additional multi-dimensional models of organizational commitment (e.g., Mayer & Schoorman, 1992; 1998; O'Reilly & Chatman, 1986; Penley & Gould, 1988) that might shed light on how the various antecedents of goal commitment combine and jointly influence its development. Meyer and Herscovitch (in press) argued that differences among these multi-dimensional models of organizational commitment stem largely from the different motives or mind-sets (e.g., emotional attachment, sense of being locked-in, and a belief in and acceptance of goals) involved in their development. Future research should investigate which of these distinguishable dimensions or mind-sets are relevant, that is, should be retained, as a basis for the development of goal commitment. Moreover, given that commitment can take different forms, researchers need to look carefully at the implications of the different dimensions of commitment on subsequent behavior.

REFERENCES

Allen, N.J., & Meyer, J.P. (1990). The measurement and antecedents of affective, continuance, and normative commitment. *Journal of Occupational Psychology, 63,* 1-18.

Bandura, A. (1997). *Self-efficacy: The exercise of control.* New York: W.H. Freeman and Company.

Bargh, J.A., & Chartrand, T.L. (1999). The unbearable automaticity of being. *American Psychologist,* **54,** 462-479.

Campbell, D.T., & Fiske, D.W. (1967). Convergent and discriminant validation by the multitrait-multimethod matrix. In: D.N. Jackson and S. Messick (Eds.), *Problems in human assessment.* New York: McGraw-Hill.

Campion, M.A., & Lord, R.G. (1982). A control systems conceptualization of the goal-setting and changing process. *Organizational Behavior and Human Performance, 30,* 265-287.

Cronbach, L.J., & Meehl, P.E. (1967). Construct validity in psychological tests. In: D.N. Jackson and S. Messick (Eds.), *Problems in human assessment.* New York: McGraw-Hill.

DeShon, R.P., & Landis, R.S. (1997). The dimensionality of the Hollenbeck, Williams, and Klein (1989) measure of goal commitment on complex tasks. *Organizational Behavior and Human Decision Processes,* **70,** 105-116.

Erez, M., & Zidon, I. (1984). Effect of goal acceptance on the relationship of goal difficulty to performance. *Journal of Applied Psychology,* **69,** 69-78.

Fishbein, M., & Ajzen, I. (1975). *Belief, attitude, intention and behavior: An introduction to theory and research.* Reading, MA: Addison Wesley.

Garland, H. (1982). Goal levels and task performance: A compelling replication of some compelling results. *Journal of Applied Psychology,* **67,** 245-248.

Gollwitzer, P.M. (1999). Implementation intentions: Strong effects of simple plans. *American Psychologist,* **54,** 493-503.

Gollwitzer, P.M., & Bargh, J.A. (1996). *The psychology of action: Linking cognition and motivation to behavior.* New York: Guilford Press.

Guion, R.M. (1965). *Personnel testing.* New York: McGraw-Hill Book Company.

Hinsz, V.B., Kalnbach, L.R., & Lorentz, N.R. (1997). Using judgmental anchors to establish challenging self-set goals without jeopardizing commitment. *Organizational Behavior and Human_Decision Processes,* **71,** 287-308.

Hollenbeck, J.R., & Klein, H.J. (1987). Goal commitment and the goal-setting process: Problems, prospects, and proposals for future research. *Journal of Applied Psychology,* **72,** 212-220.

Hollenbeck, J.R., Klein, H.J., O'Leary, A.M., & Wright, P.M. (1989). Investigation of the construct validity of a self-report measure of goal commitment. *Journal of Applied Psychology,* **74,** 951-956.

Hollenbeck, J.R., Williams, C.L., & Klein, H.J. (1989). An empirical examination of the antecedents of commitment to difficult goals. *Journal of Applied Psychology,* **74,** 18-23.

Jackson, D.N. (1970). A sequential system for personality and scale development. In: C.D. Spielberger (Ed.), *Current topics in clinical and community psychology,* **2.,** 61-96 New York: Academic Press.

Jackson, D.N. (1971). The dynamics of structured personality tests: 1971. *Psychological Review,* **78,** 229-248.

Jackson, D.N. (1975). The relative validity of scales prepared by naïve item writers and those based on empirical methods of personality scale construction. *Educational and Psychological_Measurement,* **35,** 361-370.

Jackson, D.N. (1979). Construct validity and personality assessment. In: *Construct validity in psychological measurement. Proceedings of a colloquium on theory and application in education and employment.* Princeton, NJ: U.S. Office of Personnel Management.

Jackson, D.N. (1984). *Personality research form manual* (3rd edition). Port Huron, MI: Research Psychologists Press Inc.

Jackson, D.N. (1990). Quantitative perspectives on the personality - job performance relationship. *The Score*, **13**, 3-6.

Johns, G. (1981). Difference score measures of organizational behavior variables: A critique. *Organizational Behavior and Human Performance*, **27**, 443-463.

Kernan, M.C., & Lord, R.G. (1988). Effects of participation versus assigned goals and feedback in a multi-trial task. *Motivation and Emotion*, **12**, 75-86.

Klein, H.J. (1987). *Reactions to goal setting and feedback: A test of a control theory model of work motivation.* Unpublished doctoral dissertation. Michigan State University, East Lansing.

Klein, H.J., Wesson, M.J., Hollenbeck, J.R., & Alge, B.J. (1999). Goal commitment and the goal setting process: Conceptual clarification and empirical synthesis. *Journal of Applied Psychology.*

Klein, H.J., Wesson, M.J., Hollenbeck, J.R., Wright, P.M., & DeShon, R.P. (1999). The assessment of goal commitment: A measurement model meta-analysis. In: J. Terborg (Chair), *Goal setting, commitment, and performance.* Symposium conducted at the annual meeting of the Academy of Management, August 8 - 11, Chicago, IL.

Latham, G.P., & Lee, T.W. (1986). Goal setting. In: E.A. Locke (Ed.), *Generalizing from laboratory to field settings.* Lexington, MA: Lexington Books.

Latham, G.P., & Locke, E.A. (1991). Self-regulation through goal setting. *Organizational Behavior and Human Decision Processes*, **50**, 212-247.

Lee, C., & Earley, C.P. (1992). Comparative peer evaluations of organizational behavior theories. *Organizational Development Journal*, **10**, 37-42.

Locke, E.A. (1968). Toward a theory of task motivation and incentives. *Organizational Behavior and Human Performance*, **3**, 157-189.

Locke, E.A. (1982). Relation of goal level to performance with a short work period and multiple goal levels. *Journal of Applied Psychology*, **67**, 512-514.

Locke, E.A. (1998). The motivation to work: What we know. In: P. Pintrich and M. Maehr (Eds.), *Advances in motivation and achievement*, **10**.

Locke, E.A., & Latham, G.P. (1984). *Goal setting: A motivational technique that works.* Englewood Cliffs, NJ: Prentice-Hall.

Locke, E.A., & Latham, G.P. (1990). *A theory of goal setting and task performance.* Englewood Cliffs, NJ: Prentice Hall.

Locke, E.A., Latham, G.P., & Erez, M. (1988). The determinants of goal acceptance and commitment. *Academy of Management Review*, **13**, 23-39.

Locke, E.A., & Shaw, K.N. (1984). Atkinson's inverse-U curve and the missing cognitive variables. *Psychological Reports*, **55**, 403-412.

Mayer, R.C., & Schoorman, F.D. (1992). Predicting participation and production outcomes through a two-dimensional model of organizational commitment. *Academy of Management Journal*, **35**, 671-685.

Mayer, R.C., & Schoorman, F.D. (1998). Differentiating antecedents of organizational commitment: A test of March and Simon's model. *Journal of Organizational Behavior*, **19**, 15-28.

Meyer, J.P., & Allen, N.J. (1991). A three component conceptualization of organizational commitment. *Human Resource Management Review*, **1**, 61-89.

Meyer, J.P., & Herscovitch, L. (in press). Commitment in the workplace: Toward a general model. *Human Resource Management Review.*

Meyer, J.P., Irving, P.G., & Allen, N.J. (1998). Examination of the combined effects of work values and early work experiences on organizational commitment. *Journal of Organizational Behavior*, **19**, 29-52.

Miner, J.B. (1984). The validity and usefulness of theories in an emerging organizational science. *Academy of Management Review*, **9**, 296-306.

Naylor, J.C., & Ilgen, D.R. (1984). Goal setting: A theoretical analysis of a motivational technology. In: B.M. Staw and L.L. Cummings (Eds.), *Research in organizational behavior*, **6**. Greenwich, CT: JAI Press.

O'Reilly, C., & Chatman, J. (1988). Organizational commitment and psychological attachment: The effects of compliance, identification, and internalization on prosocial behavior. *Journal of Applied Psychology*, **71**, 492-500.

Penley, L.E., & Gould, S. (1988). Etzioni's model of organizational involvement: A perspective for understanding commitment to organizations. *Journal of Organizational Behavior*, 9, 43-60.

Pinder, C.C. (1998). *Work motivation in organizational behavior*. Upper Saddle River, NJ: Prentice-Hall.

Salancik, G. (1977). Commitment and the control of organizational behavior and belief. In: B.M. Staw and G.R. Salancik (Eds.), *New directions in organizational behavior*. Chicago, IL: St. Claire Press.

Seijts, G.H., & Latham, G.P. (1999a). The relative effect of learning, outcome, and proximal goals on a complex task. In: J. Terborg (Chair), *Goal setting, commitment, and performance*. Symposium conducted at the annual meeting of the Academy of Management, August 8 - 11, Chicago, IL.

Seijts, G.H., & Latham, G.P. (1999b). *The effect of self-set personal and assigned group goal setting on an individual's behavior in small and large groups and group performance in a social_dilemma*. Paper presented at the annual meeting of the American Psychological Association, August 20-24, Boston, Mass.

Seijts, G.H., Meertens, R.M., & Kok, G. (1997). The effects of task importance and publicness on the relation between goal difficulty and performance. *Canadian Journal of Behavioral Science*, 29, 54-62.

Tubbs, M.E. (1993). Commitment as a moderator of the goal-performance relation: A case for clearer construct definition. *Journal of Applied Psychology*, 78, 86-97.

Tubbs, M.E. (1994). Commitment and the role of ability in motivation: Comment on Wright, O'Leary-Kelly, Cortina, Klein and Hollenbeck (1994). *Journal of Applied Psychology*, 79, 804-811.

Tubbs, M.E., & Dahl, J.G. (1991). An empirical comparison of self-report and discrepancy measures of goal commitment. *Journal of Applied Psychology*, 76, 708-716.

Tubbs, M.E., & Ekeberg, S.E. (1991). The role of intentions in work motivation: Implications for goal-setting theory and research. *Academy of Management Review*, 16, 180-199.

Weingart, L.R. (1992). Impact of group goals, task component complexity, effort, and planning on group performance. *Journal of Applied Psychology*, 77, 708-716.

Weingart, L.R., & Weldon, E. (1991). Processes that mediate the relationship between a group goal and group member performance. *Human Performance*, 4, 33-54.

Winters, D., & Latham, G.P. (1996). The effect of learning versus outcome goals on a simple versus a complex task. *Group and Organization Management*, 21, 235-250.

Wood, R.E., & Locke, E.A. (1990). Goal setting and strategy effects on complex tasks. In: B.M. Staw and L.L. Cummings (Eds.), *Research in organizational behavior*, 12. Greenwich, CT: JAI Press.

Wright, P.M. (1987). *Reward contingency as an explanatory variable in the incentive - goal setting relationship*. Unpublished doctoral dissertation. Michigan State University, East Lansing.

Wright, P.M., O'Leary-Kelly, A.M., Cortina, J., Klein, H.J., & Hollenbeck, J.R. (1994). On the meaning and measurement of goal commitment. *Journal of Applied Psychology*, 79, 795-803.

Yukl, G.A., & Latham, G.P. (1978). Interrelationships among employee participation, individual differences, goal difficulty, goal acceptance, goal instrumentality, and performance. *Personnel Psychology*, 31, 305-323.

15 A PERSPECTIVE

Douglas N. Jackson

Since early childhood I have shown an enduring characteristic: I prefer to find things out for myself rather than to accept them on the basis of authority or because they are commonly believed. For example, in high school I perhaps too often challenged my history teacher and the texts we used on points of fact or interpretation. But this approach had some advantages. Our high school guidance counselor advised against my applying to a good university. Ignoring his advice I applied to Cornell University and was accepted. When I wanted to undertake testing to aid me in educational and career planning, this same counselor advised against it. (I suspect he was unwilling to expend the effort.) Instead I spent fifty dollars of my own money (more than six hundred dollars in today's funds) for testing and interpretation at a private agency. I told them that I had been fascinated with chemistry since the time I was ten years old. They advised me that although I was interested in science, I was too much interested in people for them to recommend chemistry. Their advice did not go further than that, although the experience with testing had a lasting influence. I became interested in the tests themselves, and in the manner in which one could make inferences about people based on their test scores. My first essay on testing was at age 18 in freshman English, where we were permitted to choose a topic. Later at Cornell, after I had decided to study psychology in graduate school, I managed to enter a graduate course in testing. But perhaps the most important influence at Cornell on my intellectual development as a psychologist was a seminar entitled "contemporary psychological theory" led by Julian E. Hochberg, who successfully communicated the intellectual excitement of debate and discovery.

Clinical psychology had become enormously popular after World War II. I was attracted to this field and entered the clinical program at Purdue University in 1951. A year later on Julian Hochberg's recommendation I was invited to become Gardner Murphy's research assistant at the Menninger Foundation in Topeka, Kansas. Murphy had just accepted an appointment as director of research there. This experience was a milestone for me. Murphy was a gifted, supportive mentor, who set an example of high standards of communication and productivity, of breadth of interests, and of strong intellectual commitment to research. The intellectual climate at the Menninger Foundation was also an important influence. I admired the depth of knowledge of the European-trained staff psychoanalysts, and of the staff psychologists. Murphy had a steady stream of very distinguished visitors. As his assistant I had an unparalleled opportunity to interact with them. There were also some distinguished speakers invited to the Menninger Foundation. For example, in 1952 Norbert Wiener, with the prescience of a visionary, provided his forecast of the impact of computers on society, as well as of the possibilities for simulating functional and dysfunctional human personality processes by computer. During this period I also attended a talk at the University of Kansas by Hans Bethe, later a Nobel laureate in physics. He spoke of atomic physics and of the "vast sea of ignorance" that was opening before physicists by virtue of primary particles whose life was measured in milliseconds before they transformed into energy. I went away with the idea that the frontiers of knowledge, even in physics, must deal with hypothetical constructs whose existence and nature cannot always be known with certainty and completeness. From this perspective one should not be discouraged by the challenges of studying psychological phenomena.

After completing my Ph.D. in 1955 I returned to the Menninger Foundation as a U.S. Public Health Service postdoctoral fellow, again with Murphy as my sponsor. During that year I worked with Charles Solley, Robert Sommer, and Samuel Messick, then a 24 year-old psychometrician. The collaboration between Messick and me began at that time, lasted for several decades, and resulted in some 26 papers. In addition to our collaboration there was a regular exchange of ideas and criticism. He introduced me to multidimensional scaling and to test theory and factor analysis; I introduced him to response styles, to personality assessment, and to cognitive styles. Although we pooled our efforts in each of these areas, we also had some impact on the other's independent work. For example, Messick wrote a number of important papers on the implications of cognitive styles for education and I applied multidimensional scaling to the understanding of the perception of personality and the trait inferential process, and undertook a number of factor analytic studies.

At the beginning of our collaboration Messick and I took note of the exciting re-conceptualizations of the nature of psychological assessment that were appearing, notably the works of Cronbach & Meehl (1955) , Campbell & Fiske (1959), and Loevinger (1957). The cumulative effect of these and other works was to redefine the validation process as one in which the assessment specialist seeks to evaluate hypotheses about underlying dispositions and processes, a task squarely within the realm of scientific exploration and confirmation. Loevinger's idea that the process of construct validation implies a program of test construction had a special impact on me. It provided an impetus to conceptualize the process of test construction, as well as a basis for evaluating test construction efforts in terms of their conformity with underlying theoretical and structural models.

After my postdoctoral year at the Menninger Foundation I accepted a faculty position at the Pennsylvania State University in clinical psychology, where I met and worked with George Guthrie, Sidney Siegel, and Lee Sechrest. In 1962 I spent a sabbatical year at the Institute for the Study of Human Problems at Stanford University, remaining for a second year to teach in Stanford's department of psychology. Two notable activities while at Stanford were serving as Peter Bentler's dissertation adviser and (almost) completing the Personality Research Form. Nevitt Sanford invited me to join him to lunch with Henry A. Murray, who was visiting Sanford in California. In his earlier years Murray had decided that a major problem confronting personality psychology was the lack of a common language. He contrasted this situation with that of biochemistry, an area in which Murray had worked early in his career. Murray noted that biochemistry had well-established terms and definitions that permitted precise communication, whereas personality psychology did not. He (Murray, 1938) sought to introduce into psychology a set of what are now well-known variables of personality, each with a clear definition. It was on this work that I based the Personality Research Form, and in the process recognized the importance of defining a potential universe of items using more-or-less precise definitions. But in his later years Murray became more of a global theorist, and did not place a high value on rendering personality constructs into psychometric scales. This is a sentiment shared by many in the personality and social psychology areas. I disagree. Many times early in my career I or one of my students wished to investigate some substantive hypothesis about a personality variable. Most of the time there was not adequate instrumentation to undertake the study, leaving us with the choice of employing what we considered less than adequate existing measures, or undertaking the ad hoc development of a new measure for the study. On these grounds I decided that it might be useful to undertake systematically the development of measures of many of the important dimensions of personality, employing techniques that had a grounding in psychometric theory, as well as in personality theory.

After leaving Stanford I joined the faculty of the University of Western Ontario in London, Canada, where I have remained for more than 35 years, with a bit of time off for sabbaticals, including one at the Educational Testing Service, and one at the University of Iowa. My years at Western were and continue to be satisfying. The Canadian winters contribute to productivity, as does the 16-week summer period when regular classes are not in session. My colleagues and students made my work a pleasure.

In the remaining sections I outline a few research topics that have attracted my attention and that of my collaborators. This is not an exhaustive set of topics. For example, I have not included sections on our work in factor analysis, test theory, psychopathology, vocational interest measurement, cognitive styles and intellectual abilities, nor industrial and organizational psychology.

RESPONSE STYLES

For my master's thesis I found a relationship between a measure of the "authoritarian personality" as measured by the California F Scale and a measure of perceptual style. In thinking further about of this finding, I decided it was implausible that social attitudes by themselves could account for such a finding. My hypothesis was that because all of the items were keyed positively in the California F Scale, agree-responding tendencies were tapping a disposition similar to that elicited by the perceptual task. I reversed the items and showed that the tendency to respond "agree" to the original items was positively correlated with a tendency to respond "agree" to the reversals. I thought I had discovered something novel and important about the response process to attitude items. With a background in clinical psychology, I was not aware of prior work in the measurement area on response sets by Cronbach (1946, 1950) and others. Messick and I rectified the situation when we reviewed the literature and sought in a series of papers (e.g., Jackson & Messick, 1958, 1961,1962,1967; Messick & Jackson, 1958) to explicate the implications of general response bias factors. We sought to distinguish the contributions to variance of *content*, as reflected in the putative trait or disposition supposedly measured, and *style*, conceptualized as consistent tendencies associated with a mode of response, which is influenced by the method of measurement, format, wording of an item, or some connotative property of an item, such as its desirability. The term, response set, was reserved for systematic variance independent of item content that was limited to the testing situation and not related to behavior outside of the test situation. [Jackson & Messick (1967) provide more extensive definitions]. There was considerable interest in this formulation, but also it led to controversy. Some psychologists interpreted it as an attack on the whole testing enterprise interpreting our formulation as implying that test scores were nothing but response bias. Some critics argued that since measures showed correlations with external variables, they could not be interpreted as response styles.

Of course, our definition of response styles was based on the idea that they told us something about the non-test behavior of the respondent. This is not a situation for two-valued logic; measures are not solely reflections of content or of style, but a "trait-method composite" (Campbell & Fiske, 1959). Furthermore, it is difficult to improve on Cronbach's (1950) observation that response sets [styles according to our definition] might raise or lower criterion validity, but they always reduce logical [construct] validity. And there is the issue of incremental validity. If one employs a battery of measures to predict a criterion it is well-known that if each scale individually has a fixed validity, the validity of the entire battery will be at a maximum when the correlations between all measures in the battery is zero. But this cannot happen when measures share variance due to large factors, whether the variance is traceable to content, to style, or to a combination of the two. Nor will it do to attempt to remove offending response bias variance by statistical corrections using some variant of the suppressor variable approach. Although this continues to have intuitive appeal Conger and Jackson (1972) showed that suppressor variables are likely to have negligible effects on typical validity coefficients.

Many years ago in an attempt to understand why personality items did not behave like attitude items – agreement with original items does not correlate with agreement with reversed personality items (Rorer, 1965) – I decided that the process of responding to personality items was quite different from that elicited by attitude items. Yea-saying tendencies, which Cronbach referred to as acquiesence, could properly explain a propensity to agree with an attitude item and its reversal, particularly when the item content is of little consequence to the respondent, as is the case with most attitude items. But personality items are of consequence to respondents, if for no other reason than they can be highly evaluative. When respondents are given very little time to respond, they focus primarily on the item's desirability; when more time is given, respondents attend also to content (Trott & Jackson, 1967). The apparent consistency in responding true to original and false to reversed personality items can be understood in terms of the fact that by reversing the direction of wording, one also reverses the desirability of the items. With this as a starting point I formulated a threshold theory of personality responding, a process formulation akin to traditional Thurstonian ideas about responding to attitude item content, but at present best understood as signal detection theory, which had not been developed extensively at the time. These ideas were evaluated by my student, T. B. Rogers (1970) for his dissertation. In one study Rogers undertook a computer simulation in which he employed desirability scale values for each Minnesota Multiphasic Personality Inventory (MMPI) item. He assigned to 200 simulated "respondents" a different threshold for responding desirably to MMPI items. Then Rogers' simulated respondents completed the MMPI. Based on the set of simulated responses Rogers computed MMPI scale scores for each respondent, and separated total scores into true-keyed and false-keyed subscales, He proceeded to intercorrelate and factor analyze these scores. The two largest factors corresponded very closely to factor analytic results from real MMPI data, where there were also two large factors accounting for approximately 75 percent of the common variance. I have published a detailed treatment of the evidence for the threshold theory of personality responding, but in a book of conference proceedings (Jackson, 1986) and not in a main-line journal. Accordingly, authors continue to cite our work of 40 years ago on acquiescence and desirability, rather than the newer and in my view more compelling interpretation of the data.

PERSONALITY SCALE CONSTRUCTION

Early in my career I had a discussion with Milton Rokeach. He stated that he was aware of the limitations of the scales that he and others had produced. He suggested that I devote some time to showing how proper scale construction should be undertaken. After some exploration I undertook the development of a number of personality scales, beginning with those prominent in the personality and social psychological literature, like self-esteem, tolerance, conformity, and complexity. These were later to be incorporated into the Jackson Personality Inventory (1974,1994). Realizing that these scales would not be as acceptable as those from an established system of personality variables, I proceeded first with publication of the Murray variables of personality, somewhat redefined to foster their independence. I learned a great deal in this process, which I summarized in two articles (Jackson, 1970, 1971). Of the principles that I outlined in these articles, perhaps it might be appropriate here to distill them to three.

Of paramount importance in scale construction is to have a good idea about what one is measuring. It is a daunting experience to commit a personality trait name to a scale definition, particularly when there are facets falling within the trait domain. It is also important to identify the opposite of a trait, because established measurement principles require that the dimension be anchored at both poles. In the process of definition it is also important to consider distinct traits that might have some conceptual overlap with the targeted trait. Unless these fall squarely within the trait definition, it is good practice to exclude these from the item pool, but to retain them for measuring distinct traits. This results in sets of scales that intercorrelate less highly than they would otherwise. The process of developing an item pool requires diligence and some hard work, but it does not require extraordinary ability or profound knowledge of personality. In recognition of this, I issued a challenge (Jackson, 1971) proposing that one compare the validity of scales prepared by ordinary people (e.g., undergraduate students) with scales constructed using the most elaborate empirical procedures based on an external criterion. In addressing this challenge Ashton and Goldberg (1973), and later my own study (Jackson, 1975), showed that scales constructed in this way are at least as valid (and usually more so) as are personally scales constructed in more elaborate ways. The critical issue here is that item writers are provided with a definition that they can relate to their own experience.

A second compelling issue in scale construction is the importance of employing the principal of aggregation. The likelihood that an initial item pool of only 10 or 20 items will represent a biased estimate of the hypothetical universe of items is much greater than if one starts with a well-balanced pool of 100 or more. And the final set of items should be sufficiently large and carefully selected to yield reliable scales. But it is not enough simply to correlate each item with its own scale. In recognition of the fact that psychological measures represent trait-method composites, it makes sense to employ multivariate procedures to reduce the impact of extraneous variance. And one should be careful to avoid incorporating systematic irrelevant method variance in the criterion employed for item selection, whether this be an internal consistency criterion or one based on external behavior. It is also a fact that items usually do not measure only one trait but contain components of variance associated with a variety of other traits. This fact is easily understood when one examines a matrix of item and scale correlations, where scales are based on a variety of traits. In recognition of this fact we (Neill & Jackson, 1976) developed an algorithm for minimizing redundancy among scales by selecting items whose variance was maximally associated with their own scale and minimally associated with irrelevant scales, one that employed selection weights based on the relation of scale correlations and correlations between items and both targeted and irrelevant scales. Because minimum redundancy will impact on the incremental validity of scales, such a procedure, if employed with a sufficient number of items, will tend to provide higher aggregated validities for the scales contained in the battery. And scales so constructed are more likely to yield evidence for convergent and discriminant validity. The simple observation that scales should correlate more highly with measures of the same traits assessed by a different methods than with irrelevant traits represented a profound insight on the part of Campbell & Fiske (1959). My only addition to their formulation is the need to recognize that measures constructed without regard for this validational requirement are unlikely to produce evidence meeting it. In recognition of the importance of the distinction between trait-relevant and trait-irrelevant variance contained in a scale, I have argued for the re-formulation of classical reliability theory. What is needed is an index that reflects the reliability of the intended scale variance, while excluding systematic but irrelevant variance.

A third issue in scale construction is the importance of conceptualizing trait measures with sufficient breadth and diversity so as to capture all important facets of the trait dimension. Unfortunately, much of test theory has focused on homogeneity at the expense of scale breadth, as Cronbach (1991) has argued. Unless bandwidth is taken into consideration during scale construction, most item analytic procedures will yield scales that are too specific for their intended purpose.

I have employed these and related principles in scale development for a number of personality and ability measures. It might be useful to list these measures, including two or three that are nearing completion and publication: *Personality Research Form, Jackson Personality Inventory, Basic Personality Inventory* (in collaboration with Edward Helmes, Helmut Hoffmann, Ronald R. Holden, Peter Jaffe, John R. Reddon, W. Carson Smiley, and Paul F. Tremblay), *Survey of Work Styles* (with A. Mavrogannis), *Jackson Vocational Interest Survey, Career Directions Inventory, Ashland Interest Assessment* (with Connie W. Smeekens*), Six Factor Personality Inventory* (with S. V. Paunonen), *Nonverbal Personality Inventory* (with S. V. Paunonen), *Multidimensional Aptitude Battery,* and the *Differential Assessment of Personality Pathology* (with W. J. Livesley). I have had a great deal of help with each of these measures. In fact the number of people who have helped exceed one hundred. I thank each one of them here.

I sometimes wonder whether or not the effort that I and others devote to reviewing the literally thousands of items and dozens of analyses necessary to develop a measure is time well spent. But then I think about the more than 500,000 people who have completed the Jackson Vocational Interest Survey over the years.

The hope that their results have had some impact on their career and life satisfaction gives me some confidence that our extra efforts have been worthwhile when measured in these terms.

THE PERCEPTION OF PERSONALITY

My interest in person perception, trait inference, and the perception of personality is the result of many influences. First, my clinical experience sensitized me to the idea that some clinicians were more perceptive about personality than were others. Second, after undertaking the first study applying multidimensional scaling for the analysis of person perception (Jackson, Messick & Solley, 1957), a number of methodological issues arose such as the degree to which one could map person concepts into a Euclidean space, whether or not distances between persons, traits, or concepts were symmetrical, whether or not measurement procedures can distinguish between central and peripheral traits, and the like. With the support of the U.S. Air Force Office of Scientific Research I completed a review of methodological issues in this type of research (Jackson, 1962). Later we discovered that it was possible to obtain multidimensional distance measures for a variety of different concepts in the same space, including persons; personality traits; attitude and personality items; psychopathological syndromes and behaviors; the same person in different states, such as sober and drunk; and public figures and institutions.

What stood out in our judgmental studies of person perception was the cross-judge stability in the measurements obtained. We would routinely divide judges randomly into two sets and conduct separate multidimensional scaling analyses using independent analytical rotations of axes. The two sets consistently yielded highly congruent results, with correlations between projections on axes usually exceeding .99, and on some occasions .998, values I had not encountered since using physical instruments to gauge the darkness of fingerprints of experimental participants undergoing the fingerprint stain test of palmer sweating, a measure of anxiety. We also found that judges rating the probability that a person known to the judge would endorse a certain personality item was also highly consistent across judges, again usually in the vicinity of .99 for groups of judges (e.g., Rothstein & Jackson, 1980), even occurring when the target person represented a psychopathological syndrome (Reed & Jackson, 1975).

The implication of these findings became evident to me. People share a nomological network of traits and behavior that develops with experience and that is largely valid. We explored this issue in a variety of ways, for example, by considering the links between judges' work suitability ratings of job candidates from recordings of job interviews and empirical findings of the personality attributes of job incumbents. We found in a series of studies (e. g., Jackson, Peacock, & Holden, 1980; Jackson, Peacock, & Smith, 1980; Rothstein & Jackson,

1980; Paunonen, Jackson, & Oberman,1987) that lay judges perhaps know more about the personality of job incumbents than appears in the magazines of psychologists. We (Jackson, MacLennan, Erdle, Holden, Lalonde, & Thompson, 1986) also found that lay people, contrary to "traditional wisdom," had more knowledge of psychopathology than some psychologists credit them with. Our lay experimental participants judged the likely item responses of depressed patients accurately enough so as to yield aggregated personality scale profiles that correlated .90 with the profiles of a large group of actual depressed patients. The group consensus judgments for item ratings had a reliability of .99. Evidence that judges' accuracy was not attributable to base rate or stereotype accuracy was the finding that the profile based on ratings correlated negatively (-.91) with the aggregated profile of normal respondents. The rated profile was also distinct from the profiles of psychiatric patients not falling into the depressed group.

A number of questions arise with findings of this sort. Are there individual differences in judgmental accuracy, or is everyone equally accurate? Regarding accuracy there are indeed individual differences. When one computes a product-moment correlation between individual judgments and the group consensus or a criterion, the central tendency correlation is usually high, typically higher than .80, but there are persons trailing off in the left tail of the distribution down to zero or sometimes lower. One might hypothesize that such persons lacked one component of social intelligence, the ability to infer accurately the behavior of other people when given limited information about the people being judged. Or, when judging the behavior of a person showing psychopathology, the judges showing consistently poorer accuracy could be characterized as lacking clinical judgment skills. Attributing such skills to judges is supported by the fact that we have found evidence that there is consistency in a given judge's level of differential accuracy across persons being rated. A related question is whether or not there are individual differences in the concepts used by judges in rating the personality characteristics. Multidimensional scaling does not impose dimensions on judges, but allows them to emerge from their judgments. Individual differences in concepts are undeniably present in ratings of normal characteristics (Walters & Jackson, 1966), and in ratings of psychopathology (Chan & Jackson, 1982), but they are very small when compared with the powerful consensus judgments.

Another question that arises is whether or not findings such as these arise out of the semantics of the words used in the studies. Mulaik (1964) and D'Andrade (1965) raised this question earlier in the context of factor analyses of trait ratings, arguing that respondents implicitly consulted a kind of dictionary of shared meanings. In its extreme form this semantic overlap hypothesis challenged the notion that findings based on trait ratings had anything at all to do with the actual co-occurrence of behavior, but only told us about the meaning relationships among the words used.

One can address the semantic overlap challenge with at least two lines of evidence. First, one can demonstrate, as we did (Jackson, Chan, & Stricker, 1979) that ratings of co-occurrence of traits, of items representing traits, and of the relation between the two, are strongly associated with the actual correlations of respondents answering personality questionnaires. Of course, one can argue that respondents could also implicitly enter the same hypothetical dictionary, but because the correlations between items and distinct trait measures run the gamut from strongly positive to strongly negative, it is difficult to imagine how respondents could tailor every response so as to generate a space with very consistent multivariate patterns and evidence of external validity based on word meanings that were unrelated to there own characteristic behavior, especially when one recognizes that they are responding to verbal representations of behavior in situations, rather than simple trait names.

Another line of evidence, one that is compelling in our view, is based on results obtained by Paunonen (Paunonen & Jackson, 1978). Paunonen, with the assistance of an artist, devised non-verbal depictions of behavior designed to represent a majority of the personality traits contained in the Personality Research Form. Target persons were described to judges either verbally or nonverbally in the form of simple drawings that represented a central figure engaging in behavior related to the personality trait. The Judge's task was to predict the behavior of target individuals based on the verbal or nonverbal information provided. Judges were randomly assigned to provide this information either in a verbal or nonverbal format. By systematically varying the format of the behavior descriptions and judgments, it was possible to identify the proportion of variance associated with personality content and that associated with the influence of the verbal or non-verbal media. Our results were instructive. More than 88 percent of the reliable variance was associated with relevant personality content, with small factors accounting for the influence of whether the information provided was verbal or nonverbal and the influence of the verbal or nonverbal medium in which they made their judgments. Furthermore, accuracy did not depend upon the use of verbal information. Information provided nonverbally yielded judgments that were similar in accuracy to those made using verbal information. These results are difficult to reconcile with the semantic overlap hypothesis.

If the capacity to make valid predictions about the behavior of other people is a skill developed over time, it should show developmental trends. The availability of the nonverbal materials permitted us to explore developmental progress in trait inferential accuracy. Richard MacLennan (MacLennan & Jackson, 1983) undertook a study of inferential accuracy in four groups of respondents, three groups of children, ages 5-6, 7-8, and 9-11, and a fourth group of adult university students, age 19-22. MacLennan used the same nonverbal materials developed by Paunonen. Our respondents showed consistent developmental trends that increasingly closely approximated what was known about the actual personality types represented in the target persons. Another interesting finding was that as children became older they placed less emphasis on the desirability of behaviors in making inferential judgments.

Knowledge of the processes by which individuals perceive and understand the personality and motives of other people is of crucial importance in understanding human interaction. It is also an extremely important skill in successful human interaction that probably emerged selectively in human evolution as our social environments became increasingly complex. How these processes develop at the individual level and how they relate to the development of social intelligence is largely an unsolved mystery in psychological science. But we can hope that progress is possible, while recognizing that Hans Bethe's observation about a "vast sea of ignorance" applies to this area, as well.

I would like to end on a personal note of gratitude to the distinguished colleagues who have contributed to this volume. I have had the opportunity to read their manuscripts prior to publication and found them both impressive and edifying. To them and to many other colleagues, collaborators, and former graduate students I wish them well in the never-ending venture of attempting to diminish our vast sea of ignorance about human nature.

REFERENCES

Ashton, S. G., & Goldberg, L. R. (1973). In response to Jackson's challenge: The comparative validity of personality scales constructed by the external (empirical) strategy and scales developed intuitively by experts, novices, and laymen. *Journal of Research in Personality*, 7, 1-20.

Campbell, D. T., & Fiske, D. W. (1959). Convergent and discriminant validation by the multitrait-multimethod matrix, *Psychological Bulletin*, 56, 81-105.

Chan, D. W., & Jackson, D. N. (1982). Individual differences in the perception and judgment of psychopathology, *Multivariate Behavioral Research*, 17, 3-32.

Conger, A. J., & Jackson, D. N. (1972). Suppressor variables, prediction, and the interpretation of psychological relationships. *Educational and Psychological Measurement*, 32, 579-599.

Cronbach, L. J. (1946). Response sets and test validity. *Educational and Psychological Measurement*, 6, 475-494.

Cronbach, L. J. (1950). Further evidence on response sets and test design. *Educational and Psychological Measurement*, 9, 149-171.

Cronbach, L. J. (1991). Methodological studies – A personal retrospective. In R. E. Snow & D. E. Wiley (Eds.). *Improving inquiry in social science: A volume in honor of Lee J. Cronbach*. Hillsdale, NJ: Erlbaum, pp. 385-400.

Cronbach, L. J., & Meehl, P. E. (1955). Construct validity in psychological tests. *Psychological Bulletin*, 52, 281-303.

D'Andrade, R. G. (1965). Trait psychology and componential analysis. *American Anthropologist*, 67, 215-228.

Jackson, D. N. (1962). The measurement of perceived personality trait relationships. In N. F. Washburne (Ed.), *Values and groups*. Vol. 2. New York: Pergamon Press, 177-178.

Jackson, D. N. (1970). A sequential system for personality scale development. In C. D. Spielberger (Ed.), *Current topics in clinical and community psychology*. 2. New York: Academic Press, 61-96.

Jackson, D. N. (1971). The dynamics of structured personality tests, *Psychological review*, 78, 229-248.

Jackson, D. N. (1975). The relative validity of scales prepared by naive item writers and those based on empirical method of personality scales construction. *Educational and Psychological Measurement*, 35, 361-370.

Jackson, D. N. (1976). *Jackson Personality Inventory- Manual*. Port Huron, Michigan: Sigma Assessment Systems, Inc.

Jackson, D. N. (1986). The process of responding in personality assessment. In J. S. Wiggins & A. Angleitner (Eds.), *Personality assessment via questionnaires: Current issues in theory and measurement*. New York & Heidelberg: Springer.

Jackson, D. N. (1994). *Jackson Personality Inventory-Revised*. Port Huron, Michigan: Sigma Assessment Systems, Inc.

Jackson, D. N., Chan, D. W., & Stricker, W. J. (1979). Implicit personality theory: Is it illusory? *Journal of Personality*, **47**, 1-10.

Jackson, D. N., MacLennan, R. N., Erdle, S. W. P., Holden, R. R., Lalonde, R. N., & Thompson, G. R. (1986). Clinical judgments of depression. *Journal of Clinical Psychology*, **42**, 136-145.

Jackson, D. N., & Messick, S. (1958). Content and style in personality assessment. *Psychological Bulletin*, **55**, 243-252.

Jackson, D. N., & Messick, S. (1961). Acquiescence and desirability as response determinants on the MMPI. *Educational and Psychological Measurement*, **21**, 771-790.

Jackson, D. N., & Messick, S. (1962). Response styles on the MMPI: Comparison of clinical and normal samples. *Journal of Abnormal Social Psychology*, **65**, pp. 285-299.

Jackson, D. N., & Messick, S. (1967). Response styles and he assessment of psychopathology. In D. N. Jackson & S. Messick (Eds.), *Problems in Human Assessment*, New York: McGraw-Hill, Inc.

Jackson, D. N., & Messick, S., & Solley, C. M. (1957). A multidimensional scaling approach to the perception of personality. *Journal of Psychology*, **44**, 311-318.

Jackson, D. N., Peacock, A. C., & Smith, J. P. (1980). Impressions of personality in the employment interview. *Journal of Personality and Social Psychology*, **39**, 294-307.

Jackson, D. N., Peacock, A. C., & Holden, R.R. (1980). Professional interviewers' trait inferential structures for diverse occupational groups. *Organizational Behavior and Human Performance*, **2**, 1-20.

Loevinger, J. (1957). Objective tests as instruments of psychological theory. *Psychological Reports*, **3**, 635-694.

MacLennan, R. N., & Jackson, D. N. (1985). Accuracy and consistency in the development of social perception. *Developmental Psychology*, **21**, 30 -36.

Messick, S. & Jackson, D. N. (1958). The measurement of authoritarian attitudes. *Educational and Psychological Measurement*, **18**, 241-254.

Mulaik, S. A. (1964). Are personality factor raters' conceptual factors? *Journal of Consulting Psychology*, **28**, 506-511.

Murray, H. A. (1938). *Explorations in personality*, New York: Oxford University Press.

Neill, J. A., & Jackson, D. N. (1976). Minimum redundancy item analysis. *Educational and Psychological Measurement*, **36**, 123-134.

Paunonen, S. V., & Jackson, D. N. (1979). Nonverbal trait inference. *Journal of Personality and Social Psychology*, **37**, 1645-1659.

Paunonen, S. V., & Jackson, D. N., & Oberman, S. M. (1987). Personnel selection decisions: Effects of applicant personality and the letter of reference. *Organizational Behavior and Human decision Processes*, **40**, 96-114.

Reed, P., & Jackson, D. N. (1975). Clinical judgment of psychopathology: A model for inferential accuracy. *Journal of Abnormal Psychology*, **84**, 475-482.

Rogers, T. B. (1971). The process of responding to personality items: Some issues, a theory and some research. *Multivariate Behavioral Research Monographs*, **6 (2)**.

Rorer, L. G. (1965). The great response-style myth. *Psychological Bulletin*, **63**, 129-156.

Rothstein, M., & Jackson, D. N. (1980). Decision making in the employment interview: An experimental approach. *Journal of Applied Psychology*, **65**, 271-283.

Trott, D. M., & Jackson, D. N. (1967). An experimental analysis of acquiescence. *Journal of Experimental Research in Personality*, **2**, 278-288.

Walters, H. A., & Jackson, D. N. (1966). Group and individual regularities in trait inference: A multidimensional scaling analysis. *Multivariate Behavioral Research*, **1**, 145-163.

AUTHOR AND SUBJECT INDEX

16PF,. *See* Sixteen Personality Factors Test

Absolute relative bias, 83-86, 88-90, 94
Accuracy of personality judgements, 217
Acito, F., 59, 69
Ackerman, P.L., 205, 208-209
Acquiescence, 22, 25, 100, 107
Affective commitment, 290, 292, 294
Agahi, E., 205, 211
Ahern, F.M., 205, 210
Ahmed, S.A., 188-189, 193
Ahrens, J.A., 208
Ajzen, I., 318, 330
Albanesi, G., 169
Alge, B.J., 316, 331
Algina, J., 93-94
Allen, J.S., 298, 311
Allen, N.J., 214, 216, 244, 285, 288-292, 294-298, 300, 302, 305, 310, 312, 329-331
Allen, S.J., 46, 49, 51-53, 57, 60, 62, 66, 68-69
Allik, J., 205, 208
Allport, G.W., 204, 208, 253, 262
Alonso, R.A., 117, 120
Alonso, R.C., 288, 310
Alterman, A.I., 163, 167-168
Alutto, J.A., 288, 310-311
Anastasi, A., 215, 235, 244, 251-252, 254, 262
Anderson, R.D., 59, 69
Andres-Pueyo, A., 203, 208
Anokhin, A., 202, 208
Antón, C., 302-304, 311
Appleby, J.D., 267, 283
Arbuckle, J.L., 76, 93
Ariza, M.J., 26, 38
Ash, P., 268-269, 275, 282
Ashforth, B.E., 298, 310
Ashton, M.C., 34, 38, 125, 127, 129, 135-136, 138-139, 235, 241, 243-244, 247, 250, 261-262, 338, 343
Assessment center evaluations, 231, 238
Assessment of personality in the employment interview, 215, 217-218, 220-221
Assigned goal, 302, 316, 320, 322-323
Attitudinal self-report measures, 318, 320-321, 324-325
Attribution, 25-26, 30, 32
Austin, E.J., 205, 208
Austin, G.W., 102, 118

BDI. *See* Beck Depression Inventory.
BPI. *See* Basic Personality Inventory.
BIDR. See Balanced Inventory of Desirable Responding.
Bagby, R.M., 166, 170
Baker, L.A., 201, 206, 208, 210
Balanced Inventory of Desirable Responding, 24
Ball, R., 146, 171
Balla, J.R., 45, 70
Ballard, R., 26, 37
Ban, T.A., 167-168
Bandura, A., 315, 330
Banks, M.H., 299, 312
Bargh, J.A., 316, 318, 330
Barling, J., 299, 311
Barnett, R.W., 197, 208, 210, 212
Baron, J., 205, 208
Barrett, P.T., 200, 202-203, 208-209
Barrick, M.R., 217, 223, 225, 227, 236, 242, 244, 247, 249, 251, 262, 274, 282
Barron, F., 176-177, 192-194
Barthol, R.P., 223, 245
Bartlett test, 46-47
Bartlett, M.S., 42-44, 46-47, 53, 56, 69
BASIC, 52
Basic Personality Inventory, 36, 101-102, 104
Bass, A.R., 15, 19
Bateman, T.S., 286, 311
Bates, T.V., 200, 203, 208
Bayes, P.E., 282
Bazana, P.G., 202, 212
Beane, W.E., 189, 193
Beck Depression Inventory, 145, 166
Beck, A.T., 145-146, 166, 168, 171
Becker, B., 166, 168
Becker, H.S., 287-288, 310
Becker, T. E., 310
Becker, T.E., 289, 300, 310
Beggs, C., 301, 313
Behavior genetics, 201
Bell, M.J., 166-168
Bellantino, N., 208, 211
Bell-Pringle, V.J., 168
Bennett, B., 157, 170
Bennett, R.E., 13, 19-20
Ben-Shakhar, G., 266, 282
Bentein, K., 302, 314

Bentler, P.M., 2, 25, 37, 44-45, 69, 73-74, 76-77, 93-94, 335
Berg, I.A., 21, 37, 99, 118
Bernstein, L.H., 108, 120
Berry, J.W., 126-127, 135, 138
Betancourt, H., 140
Bidirectional relationships, 223-224, 228
Big Five, 125, 128, 136, 223, 225-226, 240-244
Billings, R.S., 289, 300, 310
Billington, R., 166, 168
Bipolarity of personality constructs, 228
Bishop, S.L., 208
Bjorgvinsson, T., 102, 118
Black, J.M., 217, 244
Blashfield, R.K., 145, 166, 168, 170
Blau, G., 296-297, 299, 310
Blinkhorn, S.F., 202, 208, 229, 244
Block, J., 22-23, 25, 27, 37, 125, 138, 155, 168, 196-197, 240-241, 244
Bobbitt, B., 198, 210
Bobocel, D.R., 296, 312
Bogus pipeline, 35
Bollen, K.A., 77, 81-82, 93
Bolton, B., 205, 208
Bonami, M., 302, 314
Bonastre, R.M., 203, 208
Bond, M.H., 130-132, 134, 136, 138-140
Bookstein, F.L., 44, 69
Boomsma, A., 45, 69
Boomsma, D.I., 203, 211
Bootstrap
    non-parametric, 79, 86, 88, 90
    control functions, 80, 86, 88, 90
    regression control, 81, 86, 88, 90
Borman, W.C., 15, 19, 262
Borum, R., 171
Bouchard, T.J., 200, 211
Bowman, M.L., 97, 118
Boyle, G.J., 163-164, 167-168
Braden, W., 202, 210
Brand, C.R., 198, 205, 208-209
Brandon, P.R., 17, 19
Braun, H., 20
Braun, J.R., 234-245
Bray, D.W., 237, 246, 256, 260, 262-263
Brebner, J., 205, 209
Brennan, R.L., 8, 19
Brenner, D.C., 237, 245, 256, 260, 262
Briggs, S.R., 121, 240, 245
Brislin, R.W., 307, 310
Broad versus narrow personality measures, 243
Broca, P., 203, 209
Broverman, D.M., 202, 212
Brown, L., 169
Brown, L.S., 151, 167-168
Brown, R.F., 26, 38, 196
Browne, M.W., 74, 76, 78, 93-94
Bryant, B.R., 151, 169

Buchanan, B., 287, 310
Burisch, M., 226, 250, 262
Burris, L.R., 268, 271, 283
Burt, R.E., 299, 311
Burton, R.V., 278, 282
Butcher, J.N., 95-96, 102, 119, 166, 168, 251-252, 254, 262
Bycio, P., 296, 298, 311
Byrne, D., 27, 37

CPI. See California Psychological Inventory
Caddell, J.M., 166, 170
California Psychological Inventory, 250, 261
Callahan, C., 268, 271, 283
Callister, J.D., 208-209
Camara, W.J., 270, 277, 282
Campbell, D.T., 8, 19, 101, 119, 144, 168, 188, 192, 304, 308, 311, 317, 320, 330, 334, 336, 339, 343
Campbell, J.P., 218, 245
Campion, M.A., 321, 330
Cardon, L.R., 201, 211
Carlson, K.A., 111-113, 119
Carmin, C.N., 197, 212
Carretta, T.R., 208-209
Carroll, J.B., 200, 209, 276, 282
Caruso, D.R., 205, 211
Caryl, P.G., 202, 209
Cascio, W.F., 231, 245
Cashel, M.L., 165, 166, 168
Casella, G., 75, 94
Castaneda, M.B., 296, 311
Cattell, J.M., 176, 192
Cattell, R.B., 42, 45, 47, 49, 53, 56, 59, 69, 130, 138, 176-178, 192-193, 204-205, 209-210, 213-214, 233, 245, 251, 253, 255, 260, 263
Chalke, F., 202, 209
Chambers, J.A., 177, 193
Chan, D.W., 42, 70, 91, 94, 132, 139, 217, 247, 309, 313, 341-344
Chan, W., 74, 91, 94
Chang, E., 302, 311
Chartrand, T.L., 316, 330
Chatman, J., 289, 313, 329, 331
Cherepon, J.A., 167, 169
Cheung, F. M., 138
Chiu, C., 205, 209
Choldin, S., 115, 117, 121
Chou, C.P., 77, 93
Chrisjohn, R.D., 102, 119
Christal, R.E., 241, 248
Christiansen, N.D., 230-231, 233, 236, 245, 252, 254, 263
Church, A.T., 125, 128-136, 138
Clark, D.A., 157, 170
Clark, J.P., 278, 282
Cleary, T.A., 14-15, 19, 157, 169
Cliff, N., 47, 49, 69
Cloninger, C.R., 154, 170, 205, 209

Cognitive abilities, 176
Cognitive ability and job performance, 224
Cole, J.R., 193
Cole, J.W.L., 15, 20
Cole, N.S., 5, 7, 13-15, 19-20, 174
Coleman, D.F., 301, 312
Collins, J., 273, 275, 279-280, 282
Complex task, 327, 332
Component analysis, 41-44, 46, 48, 51, 59-60, 68
Comrey, A.L., 49, 70
Confirmatory factor analysis, 73, 75
Confirmatory research strategies, 224-225, 227, 237
Conforti, K., 167, 171
Conger, A.J., 233, 236, 245, 337, 343
Conn, S.R., 262-263
Conscientiousness, 125, 128, 206-207
Consequences of organizational commitment, 307
Constantini, A., 234, 245
Construct oriented approach to personality assessment, 216, 231
Construct oriented approach to test construction, 31, 99, 118
Construct validation, 4, 5, 91, 108, 123, 130, 133-135, 137, 141-144, 147, 150, 156, 160, 163, 165, 167
Construct validity, 1, 3-10, 12, 14, 16-18, 23, 97, 99-101, 108, 110, 113, 117-118, 120, 124, 133-134, 137-138, 145, 154, 196, 216, 230, 236, 239-240, 281, 288-289, 295, 304, 316-319, 321-322, 328, 330
Content domain, 6-7, 143, 151
Content validity, 32, 100, 106, 150-151, 158
Continuance commitment, 290, 298
Convergent and discriminant validity, 29, 36, 100-102, 107-108, 110, 116-117, 145, 150, 154-156, 162-164, 167, 178, 216, 218-219, 222, 226, 230-231, 244, 252, 328
Cook, T.D., 8, 19
Cooper, C.J., 202, 212
Cooper, C.L., 301, 312
Corrective approaches to faking, 233
Correlation structure, 74
Cortina, J., 317, 332
Costa, P.T., 27, 35, 39, 125, 132, 139, 155, 166-167, 169-170, 241-242, 245, 247, 273, 282
Cota, A.A., 50-53, 57, 60, 69, 70
Cotton, D.H.G., 105, 119
Counterproductivity, 267, 272, 277-279, 281
Covariance structure, 74, 91
Cox, C.M., 176, 193
Crawford, C.B., 50, 69
Crawley, B., 262-263
Creativity, 96
Crino, M.D., 26, 37

Criterion-related validity, 230, 250, 252, 256, 261, 271
Criticisms of personality testing, 229
Cronbach, L.J., 4, 5, 15, 17, 19, 99, 119, 123, 133-134, 138, 143, 151, 163, 169, 215, 245, 290, 311, 319-320, 330, 334, 336-337, 339, 343
Cropanzano, R., 298, 312
Cross-cultural, 123-128, 130-132, 134-138, 303-304, 306-309, 313
Crowne, 2, 21, 23-28, 30, 32, 34-37, 161
Crowne, D.P., 2
Cudeck, R., 74-76, 93
Cull, J.G., 166, 169
Cunningham, M.R., 268, 275, 282

DPI. See Differential Personality Inventory.
Dahl, J.G., 317, 321, 325, 332
Dahlstrom, W.G., 168
Damarin, F., 24, 37
D'Andrade, R.G., 341, 343
Daniels, D., 206, 208-209, 211
Darlington, R.B., 15, 19, 258, 263
Daum, I., 203, 208
Davies, A.D.M., 205, 211
Day, D.A., 252, 254, 263, 296
De Raad, B., 136, 138
Deary, I.J., 205, 208
Decker, P.J., 271, 283
Decker, S.N., 201, 210
DeFries, J.C., 206, 211
del Pilar, G.H., 125, 139
Delhaise, T., 302, 314
Demaree, R.G., 251, 264
den Hartog, D.N., 302-303, 307, 311
Denial, 23, 24, 25, 26, 30-32, 37
Denial scales, 26
Dennis, W., 174, 193
Dependability, 265-268, 278
Depression, 98, 102, 104-110, 113-116, 145-146, 149, 151-152, 160, 166
Derogatis, L.R., 116, 119
Descriptive approaches to faking, 232-234
DeShon, R.P., 317-318, 325-327, 330-331
Desirability, 1, 21-25, 27-38, 100, 107, 114, 131, 155-156
DeVellis, R.F., 108, 119
Diamond, P.M., 171
Dickens, S.E., 166, 170
Difference scores, 321-322
Differential Personality Inventory, 101
Differential Reliability Index, 32, 36
Digman, J.M., 125, 138, 275, 282
Dipboye, R.L., 217, 245
Doan, B.T., 167, 171
Dolan, S., 262, 264
Doll, R.E., 234, 245
Dollinger, S.J., 205, 210

Dominance, 96, 117, 205-206, 229, 237-238, 250, 256-257, 259-260
Donahue, D., 205, 209
Dorais, S., 117, 121
Drasgow, F., 152, 163, 169, 308, 311
Drevdahl, J.E., 176-178, 193
Dreyden, J.I., 205, 211
du Toit, S.H.C., 76, 93
Dubois, P.H., 97, 119
Dugas, J.L., 198, 209
Dunham, R.B., 296-298, 311
Dunnette, M.D., 15, 19, 218, 231, 237, 245-246, 249, 263
Dweck, C.S., 205, 209

EPPS. See Edwards Personal Preference Schedule
Earley, C.P., 315, 331
Eaton, C.A., 41, 56, 69, 132
Eaton, N.K., 231, 246, 249, 263
Eber, H.W., 130, 138, 213-214, 233, 245, 251, 263
Edwards Personal Preference Schedule, 235
Edwards, A.L., 21, 23, 24, 27-30, 32, 34, 36-38, 145, 155, 169, 235, 245, 251, 263
Edwards, J.A., 202, 209
Edwards, M. J., 120
Edwards, W., 171
Efficiency, 16, 161, 280, 323
Efron, B., 76, 80, 93
Egan, V., 205, 209
Eiduson, B.T., 181, 193
Eigenvalues, 45-53, 55, 57, 60, 62, 66, 68
Einhorn, H.J., 15, 19
Ekeberg, S.E., 321, 325, 332
Ekman, P., 265, 282
Ellemers, N., 302-303, 311
Ellingson, J.E., 233, 236, 245
Ellingson, R.J., 202, 209
Ellis, A., 99, 119
Ellis, D.D., 15, 20
Ellis, H., 176, 193
Embretson (Whitely), S., 8, 19
Emery, G., 168
Emic, 125-137
Employment interview, 217, 219-220, 222
Endicott, J., 171
Endler, N.S., 173-175, 193-194
Engstrom, R., 47, 69
Engvik, H., 132, 139
Erdle, S., 341, 344
Erez, M., 316, 330-331
Ertl, J., 202, 209
Etic, 125-131, 134-137
Evans, R.G., 26, 38, 56, 208, 212
Eveleth, D.M., 289, 310
Extraversion, 205, 256-257, 259-260
Eysenck, 35, 176, 190, 193, 200, 202-203, 205, 208-209, 241

Eysenck, H.J., 35, 38, 176, 245
Eysenck, S.B.G., 35, 38
Face validity, 151
Factor analysis, 2, 27, 41-46, 48, 50, 55-56, 59, 68, 70-71, 73-74, 76-77, 81, 91, 102, 114, 130, 132, 184, 188, 197
Faking, 21, 99, 107, 117, 231
Fals-Stewart, W., 165, 169
Fantoni-Salvador, P., 164, 167, 169
Faravelli, C., 169
Faschingbauer, T.R., 101, 119
Faschingbauer, T.S., 95-96
Faulk, D., 208
Faust, D., 147, 169
Fava, J.L., 41-42, 56, 59-60, 68-69, 71, 132
Fear, R.A., 166, 217-218, 245
Feist, G.J., 178, 193
Feiveson, A.H., 60, 70
Fekken, G.C., 27, 38, 50-53, 57, 60, 69-70, 105, 119, 157, 169
Feldman, J.C., 296, 311
Feldt, L.S., 8, 19
Ferguson, G.A., 8, 19
Ferguson, T.S., 79, 93
Feuer, D., 200, 211
Fick, C., 26, 38
Finch, J.F., 32, 40
First, M.B., 120, 171, 204
Fischer, D.G., 26, 38
Fishbein, M., 318, 330
Fiske, D.W., 101, 119, 144, 168, 188, 192, 317, 320, 330, 334, 336, 339, 343
Fjetland, O.K., 168
Flaherty, V.L., 52-53, 57, 60, 62, 66, 70
Flores, J., 163, 170
Flynn, C.F., 208, 210
Foci of commitment, 286, 299
Forced-choice, 34
Ford, R.C., 297, 312
Forsterling, F., 132, 139
FORTRAN, 52, 56, 60
Fraboni, M., 73, 94, 125, 139, 255, 263
Fraser, I.C., 202, 209
Freund, C.G., 302, 304, 311
Friel, J.P., 117, 121
Frijda, N., 127, 138
Fullagar, C., 299, 301, 311
Fullager, C., 311
Furedy, J.J., 266, 282
Furnham, A., 21, 38, 252, 254, 263

"g", 275-276
Gale, A., 202, 209
Galton, F., 97, 176, 193, 203, 209
Garland, H., 315, 330
Gaston, J., 174, 193
Gaugler, B.B., 217, 245
Gellatly, I.R., 238, 245, 252, 254, 256, 263, 297-298, 311-312

Generalizability, 4, 7-9, 17-18, 100, 106, 142, 163
Ghiselli, E.E., 223, 245
Giannitrapani, D., 202, 209
Gibbon, M., 116, 119, 171
Gibertini, M., 208, 211
Gibson, G.J., 205, 208
Gilbert, N.L., 289, 310
Gilbertini, M., 155, 170
Gilder, D., 302, 310-311
Giles, C.L., 171
Gill, W.S., 166, 169
Gilliland, K., 205, 211
Gilliland, S.W., 251, 264
Gleser, G.C., 163, 169
Goal commitment, 317-318, 325
Goal discrepancy measures, 318
Goal setting theory, 315-316, 325
Goff, M., 205, 209
Goffin, R.D., 34, 73, 93-94, 125, 139, 183, 194, 215-216, 229-231, 234, 238, 241, 245-249, 252, 254-256, 262-264, 317
Goldberg, L.R., 98-99, 119, 136, 139, 241, 246, 248, 250, 261-262, 271, 282, 338, 343
Goldberg, R.A., 198, 209
Golder, P.A., 49, 59, 71
Goldinger, L.A., 267, 283
Gollwitzer, P.M., 316, 318, 330
Gonzalez, J.J., 205, 209
González, L., 302-304, 311
Gooding, R.Z., 223, 248
Gordon, E., 11, 12, 19
Gordon, L.V., 235, 246
Gordon, M. E., 311
Gordon, M.E., 299
Gorham, D.R., 166, 170
Gormly, A., 205, 209
Gormly, J., 205, 209
Gorsuch, R.L., 42, 44, 46, 49, 56, 69, 71, 134, 139
Gottfredson, L.S., 15, 19
Gottier, R.F., 217-218, 223-224, 246
Gough, H., 218, 246
Gould, S., 329, 332
Graham, J.R., 168
Grant, D.L., 262
Gray, J.A., 205, 210
Greenstein, D.S., 167, 169
Grenier, J.R., 271, 282
Griffin, M.A., 311
Griffin, R.W., 286, 302-304, 309, 311
Grigoriadis, S., 109-114, 117, 119
Grishenko-Rose, N., 132, 139
Gross, A.B., 301, 311
Gross, A.L., 15, 19
Grube, J.A., 296, 311
Guadagnoli, E., 41, 59-60, 69
Guion, R.M., 217-218, 223-224, 237, 239, 246, 248, 271, 282, 329, 330

Gur, R.C., 24, 27, 32, 38, 40
Guttman, L., 48-49, 69, 71

HPSI. See Holden Psychological Screening Inventory.
Hackett, R.D., 296-298, 311
Hagtvet, K.A., 205, 211
Hahn, J., 302, 311
Haier, R.J., 202, 210
Hakstian, A.R., 45, 47, 59, 69, 169, 205, 210, 269, 273-275, 283
Hamburger, C., 47, 69
Hamilton Depression Rating Scale, 145, 166
Hamilton, M., 145, 166, 169
Hammill, D.D., 151, 169
Hampson, S., 205, 211
Hanson, B.A., 237, 246, 256, 260, 263
Harazin, J.S., 117, 120
Hare, R.D., 166, 169
Harman, H.H., 108, 119
Harpur, T.J., 169
Harrell, M.S., 237, 246, 260, 263
Harrell, T.H., 208, 210, 256
Harrell, T.W., 237, 246, 260, 263
Harris, J.A., 205, 206, 210, 212
Harris, M.M., 268, 271, 274, 282-283
Harrop, J.W., 56, 60, 71
Hartigan, J.A., 15, 19
Hartshorne, H., 27, 38, 278, 282
Hathaway, S.R., 22, 24, 27, 38-39, 98, 101, 119, 166, 169
Hausdorf, P.A., 296, 311
Hayne, C., 145, 170
Hays, R.D., 52, 69
Heapy, N.A., 188-189, 193
Heckhausen, H., 188, 193
Heggestad, E.D., 205, 208
Heller, K.A., 7, 19, 166, 170
Helmes, E., 21, 28, 38, 101, 105, 119-120, 125, 131, 138, 155, 169, 232, 243-244, 246, 329, 339
Helmreich, R.L., 178, 189, 193
Hendrickson A. E., 210
Hendrickson, D.E., 202, 208, 210
Heritability, 200-201
Herrington-Wang, L.E., 171
Herriot, P., 262-263
Herscovitch, L., 295, 300-301, 307, 309, 313, 329, 331
Hetu, M., 208, 210
Heymans, G, 98, 119
Higher-order constructs, 125
Hill, S.A., 117, 120
Hinkin, T.R., 285, 311
Hinrichs, J.R., 262-263
Hinsz, V.B., 323, 330
Ho, H.Z., 201, 210
Hodgson, R.J., 166, 170
Hofstede, G., 304-305, 308, 311

Hogan, J., 273-275, 282
Hogan, R., 23, 38-39, 229, 237, 241, 246, 256, 260, 263, 270, 273, 275, 277-278, 282
Holden Psychological Screening Inventory, 95, 97, 101, 104
Holden, R.R., 27-28, 38, 40, 50-53, 57, 60, 69-70, 95, 97, 101-102, 104-107, 109-114, 117, 119-121, 133, 143, 157, 169, 216-217, 232, 246-247, 339-341, 344
Holland, C. J., 210
Holland, D.C., 205, 210
Hollenbeck, J.R., 316-321, 323-328, 330-332
Hollinger, R.C., 278, 282
Holmes, T.H., 166, 169
Holtzman, W.H., 7, 19
Honaker, L.M., 208, 210
Honesty, 136
Hong, S., 41, 70
Hong, Y., 205, 209
Hopkins, K.D., 242, 246
Horn, J.L., 42, 47, 49-50, 52, 69
Horn, J.M., 205, 212
Hostetter, K., 95-96
Hough, L.M., 225, 231, 233, 241, 245-246, 249, 251, 263
Hourany, L., 132, 139
Howard, A., 237, 246, 256, 260, 263, 313
Howe, H.G., 55, 69
Hrebiniak, L.G., 288, 310-311
Hubbard, R., 46, 49, 51-53, 57, 60, 62, 66, 68-69
Hui, C.H., 303, 307-308, 311
Hulin, C.L., 152, 163, 169, 308, 311
Hung, S.S., 174, 194
Hunt, E., 198, 210
Hunt, M., 192-193
Hunter, J.E., 15, 19, 227, 246-247, 251, 263
Hunter, R.F., 246
Hwang, W., 302, 311
Hynd, G.W., 205, 209

IQ. See Intelligence.
Ilgen, D.R., 317, 331
Implicit personality theory, 222
Implicit theories of trait covariation, 219
Impression formation, 217, 222
Impression management, 27, 29, 37, 165, 232-233
Incremental validity, 230, 238, 257
Inferential accuracy of personality trait covariation, 217
Information matrix, 78, 83
Inspection Time, 199
Integrity, 176, 265-281
Integrity tests, 265-269, 271-279, 281
Intelligence, 1, 7, 96, 135, 143, 163, 174, 176, 181, 195, 197-207
Inter-rater reliability, 220
Irving, P.G., 301, 312, 331

Item Efficiency Index, 31, 33
Item response theory, 152, 163
Iwao, S., 140

JPI. See Jackson Personality Inventory
JPI-R. See Jackson Personality Inventory
Jackson, D.N.,1, 2, 21-22, 24, 27-42, 44, 59, 70-71, 73, 91, 93-97, 99-107, 117, 119-120, 123, 125, 132-133, 136-139, 141-143, 155-156, 167-170, 173-176, 178, 181, 183-196, 198, 205-207, 210-211, 213-214, 216-223, 225, 227-228, 230-236, 238-239, 241, 243-253, 255-256, 260-261, 263-264, 267, 281-282, 285, 294, 299, 310, 312, 317-320, 322, 328-331, 333, 336-344
Jackson D. N. III, 210
Jackson Personality Inventory, 30, 33
Jacobson, L.I., 26, 32, 38-39
Jacquemyns, B., 302, 314
Jaffe, P.G., 102, 118, 120, 339
Jahoda, G., 127, 138
James, L.R., 251, 264
Jamshidian, M., 2, 73, 76, 79, 93-94
Jang, K.L., 205-206, 210, 212
Jaros, S.J., 297, 312
Jaspers, J., 47, 49, 69
Jeanneret, P.R., 239, 247
Jennrich, R.I., 79, 94
Jensen, A.R., 135, 139, 198, 200, 203-204, 210-211
Job performance, 216-219, 222-231, 237-240, 242-244, 249, 252-255, 272-274, 278, 288, 293, 299, 331
John, O.P., 125, 136, 139, 285, 296, 339
Johns, E.F., 255, 264
Johns, G., 322-323, 331
Johnson, J.A., 273, 282
Johnson, R.C., 205, 210, 229, 244
Johnston, N.G., 216, 230-231, 238, 245, 249, 252, 263, 317
Jones, E.E., 35, 39
Jones, J.M., 208, 210
Jones, J.W., 271, 273, 282
Joreskog, K.G., 74-75, 94
Josiassen, R.C., 203, 211

K scale, 27, 34-35
Kaemmer, B., 168
Kaiser rule, 43, 49, 56, 63, 68
Kaiser, H.F., 42-43, 48-49, 56, 63, 65, 68-71
Kalnbach, L.R., 323, 330
Kamp, J.D., 231, 246, 249, 263
Kane, M.T., 10, 19
Kano, Y., 44, 69
Kanter, R.M., 287, 312
Katigbak, M.S., 125, 128-136, 138
Kaut, C.R., 135, 139
Keane, T.M., 166, 170
Keating, D.P., 198, 210

Keinonen, M., 132, 139
Kellas, G., 198, 209
Keller, J.W., 98, 120-121
Kellogg, R.W., 26-27, 38-39
Kelly, E.L., 252, 254, 264
Kernan, M.C., 317, 331
Kerr, P.S., 117, 120
Kesselman, G.A., 239, 247
Kimmons, G., 117, 121
Kinder, A., 249, 264
King, G.A., 237, 248
King, R.E., 208-210
Kirsch, M., 223, 248
Kleijn, W.C., 26, 39
Klein, H.J., 316-319, 325-332
Kleinmuntz, B., 265, 282
Knickerbocker, W.S., 176, 193
Ko, J-W., 302-304, 312
Kok, G., 315, 332
Komocar, J., 308, 311
Konovsky, M.A., 298, 312
Koopman, P., 47, 50, 69, 70
Korman, A.K., 218, 247
Koss, M.P., 162, 170
Kostura, D.D., 205, 211
Kouznetsova, L., 132, 139
Krane, W.R., 93-94
Kranzler, J.H., 197, 200, 210
Kroner, D.G., 232, 246
Krug, S.E., 255, 264
Kurtz, J.E., 167, 170
Kusyzyn, I., 39
Kutcher, M., 168

Ladd, R.T., 251, 264
Lally, M., 198-200, 210-211
Lalonde, R.N., 341, 344
Lamont, L.M., 252, 254, 264
Lance, C.E., 52-53, 57, 60, 62, 66, 70
Landis, R.S., 317-318, 325-327, 330
Landy, F.J., 218, 247
Lane, H.W., 187, 193
Lang, P., 166, 171
Lanier, V.W., 166, 170
Lanigan, C.B., 102, 119
Latham, G.P., 214, 315-316, 318, 320-324,
     326, 331-332
Lautenschlager, G.J., 52-53, 57, 60, 62, 66, 70
Lautenschlager, G.S., 35, 39
Law, K.S., 98, 171, 187, 291, 312
Lawleer, E.E., 245
Lawrence, P.G., 111-113, 120
Lay, C.H., 217, 247
Lebra, T.S., 135, 139
Lee, C., 315, 331
Lee, D.H., 204, 212
Lee, H., 49, 59, 69-70, 335
Lee, K., 136, 138, 298, 302, 304, 312
Lee, M.S., 197, 211

Lee, S., 273-275, 283
Lee, T.W., 315, 331
Lehmann, E.L., 75, 94
Lempert, R., 270, 283
Lennon, R.T., 7, 19
Lennon, T.J., 163-164, 167-168
Leschied, A.W., 102, 118
Leung, K., 130-132, 136, 138-140, 304-306,
     308-309, 314
Leung, L.S., 26, 40
Leung, Y.P., 74, 91, 94
Levin, J., 167, 170
Levin, R.A., 232, 248
Lewis, C., 45, 70
Ley, P., 205, 211
Lin, M.M., 167, 168
Linn, R.L., 14-15, 18-19, 20, 47, 49, 70
Locke, E.A., 214, 315-318, 321-324, 326-327,
     331-332
Loehlin, J.C., 44, 70
Loevinger, J., 8, 17, 20, 99, 120, 123, 133, 139,
     143, 151, 170, 334, 344
Longman, R.S., 50-53, 57, 60, 69-70
Lonner, W.J., 125, 136, 138
Lopez, F.M., 217-218, 239, 247
Loranger, A.W., 166, 170
Lord, F.M., 152, 170
Lord, R.G., 317, 321, 330-331
Lorentz, N.R., 323, 330
Louks, J., 145, 170
Lubich, R.D., 302-304, 307, 312
Lubin, B., 98, 121
Lucker, G.W., 189, 193
Lundstrom, W.J., 252, 254, 264
Luther, N., 265, 283
Lykken, D.T., 200, 211, 265, 282
Lynn, R., 205, 211

MAB,. See Multidimensional Aptitude Battery
MMPI. See Minnesota Multiphasic Personality
     Inventory.
MacCallum, R.C., 41, 70
MacDonald, D.A., 205, 210
MacLennan, R.N., 208, 211, 341-342, 344
Magruder, C.D., 109, 110, 117, 120
Malingering, 37, 146, 156, 161
Maliphant, R., 132, 139
Mangan, G., 203, 208
Mannari, H., 287, 312
Maricauce, A., 26, 38
Markus, K., 17, 20
Marlowe, 2, 23-28, 30, 32, 34-37, 161
Marlowe, D., 25
Marlowe-Crowne scale, 25-27, 30, 32, 35-36
Marsh, H.W., 45, 70, 287, 312
Martin, H.J., 26, 39
Martin, R.P., 205, 209
Martin-Cannici, C., 165, 168
Maser, J.D., 154, 170

Mathieu, J.E., 288, 312
Matthews, G., 205, 211
Matthews, K.A., 178, 193
Maximum likelihood, 42, 44-47, 74, 79
Maximum likelihood factor analysis, 42, 44-45
Maximum likelihood test, 45-47
May, M.A., 278, 282
Mayer, J.D., 205, 211
Mayer, R.C., 289, 312, 329, 331
Mazmanian, D., 117, 120
McArdle, J.J., 44, 70
McCarthy, J.M., 206, 212
McClearn, G.E., 206, 211
McClelland, D.C., 177-178, 188, 193
McCloy, R.A., 231, 246, 249, 263
McCormack, J.K., 208, 210
McCormick, E.J., 239, 247
McCrae, R.R., 27, 35, 39, 125, 132, 136, 139,
    155, 166-167, 169-170, 241-242, 245, 247,
    273, 282
McCusker, C., 140
McDermott, P.A., 167-168
McDonald, R.P., 45, 70, 93-94
McElroy, R.A., 145, 168
McGee, G.W., 297, 312
McGue, M., 200-201, 211
McIntyre, S.H., 237, 246, 256, 260, 263
McKechnie, G.E., 206, 211
McKee, T.E., 282
McKinley, J.C., 22, 38, 98, 101, 119, 166, 169
McLeod, L.D., 120
Mecham, R.C., 239, 247
Meehl, P.E., 24, 27, 39, 99, 119-120, 123, 133-
    134, 138, 143-144, 169-170, 215, 245, 290,
    311, 320, 330, 334, 343
Meertens, R.M., 315, 332
Megargee, E.I., 250, 264
Mehrens, W.A., 17, 20
Mendonca, J.D., 117, 120
Mental abilities. See Cognitive abilities
Mershon, B., 134, 139
Messick, S., 1, 3-5, 7-10, 15-25, 34, 37-39,
    101, 120, 123, 232, 235, 247, 330, 334,
    336, 340, 344
Meta-analysis, 215, 223-228, 242-243, 251-
    252, 261, 271, 274, 288, 296-297, 316,
    325, 327, 331
Method variance, 32, 100, 156, 216, 218, 244
Meyer, J.P., 214, 216, 238, 244-245, 252, 256,
    263, 285, 288-292, 294-298, 300-302, 305,
    307, 309-310, 312-313, 329-331
Mikulay, S.M., 241, 247
Miller, J.L., 232, 248
Miller, L.T., 199, 211
Millham, J., 26, 27, 39
Miner, J.B., 315, 331
Miner, R.A., 147, 169
Minimum Average Partial correlation test, 42-
    43, 54, 56, 62

Minnesota Multiphasic Personality Inventory,
    22, 36, 95, 97-98, 101
Mirowsky, J., 25, 40
Mobley, W.H., 291, 312
Moderators, 223, 251
Montag, I., 167, 170
Montanelli, Jr., R.G., 50, 60, 70
Mook, J., 26, 39
Moorman, R.H., 298, 313
Moos, B.S., 211
Moos, R.H., 206, 211-212
Morey, L.C., 30, 34, 36, 39, 96, 141-143, 145,
    163-168, 170-171, 216, 247
Morf, M.E., 35, 39
Morfitt, R.C., 102, 119
Mori, M., 203, 212
Morrison, D.F., 55, 70
Morrow, P.C., 286, 289, 299-301, 313
Mount, M.K., 217, 223, 225, 227, 236, 242,
    244, 247, 249, 251, 262, 274, 282
Mowday, R.T., 287-288, 294, 313
Muchinsky, P.M., 257, 264
Mueller, C.W., 302, 312
Mulaik, S.A., 44, 70, 251, 264, 341, 344
Multidimensional Aptitude Battery, 96, 195-
    205, 207
Munro, E., 198, 210
Murphy, K., 213-214, 265-269, 271, 273-280,
    282-283, 333, 334
Murray, H.A., 96, 106, 120, 247, 253, 264,
    335, 338, 344
Murray, H.G., 178, 180, 182, 194

Nagoshi, C.T., 205, 210
Naylor, J.C., 317, 331
Neale, M.C., 201, 211
Nederhof, A.J., 34, 39
Need for approval, 2, 23, 25-26
Neill, J.A., 31, 33, 39, 101, 120, 339, 344
Nettelbeck, T., 198-200, 202, 210-212
Newmark, C.S., 95-96, 119
Nicholson, R.A., 23, 38-39
Niehoff, B.P., 298, 313
Noe, R.A., 223, 248
Noguchi, H., 302, 314
Noh, S., 301, 313
Nomological network, 143, 148, 163, 168
Nonlinear constraints, 75-76
Norman, W.T., 233, 241, 247, 249
Normand, J., 270, 283
Normative commitment, 290-291, 293-294,
    298-301, 303, 305, 330
Normlessness, 278-280
Norms, 121, 186
Novick, M.R., 15, 20
Nunnally, J.C., 108, 120, 152, 170

O'Bannon, R.M., 267-269, 273-275, 283
O'Brien, C., 270, 283

O'Dell, L.L. 76, 93
O'Leary, A.M., 330
O'Leary-Kelly, A.M., 316-317, 332
O'Reilly, C., 289, 329, 331
O'Reilly, C.A., 289, 313
O'Sullivan, M., 265, 282
Oberman, S.M., 341, 344
Oberwager, J., 208, 210
Observable behavior, 137, 143
Occupational commitment, 300-301, 308
Odbert, H.S., 253, 262
Odell, P.L., 60, 70
Oldham, J.M., 170
Ones, D.S., 227, 247, 267-268, 271-275, 282-283
Oosterveld, P., 132, 139
Oppenheimer, R., 186, 193
Organ, D.W., 298, 313
Organizational commitment, 285-291, 293-294, 297-302, 307, 309-310, 329, 331
Ornduff, S.R., 165, 171
Orsak, C.L., 296, 313
Osborne, D., 167, 170
Osburn, H.G., 234, 248
Ostendorf, F., 125, 139
Oswald, W.D., 199, 211
Overall, J.E., 67, 117, 166, 170, 207, 301
Ozer, D.J., 106, 120

PAI. *See* Personality Assessment Inventory.
PRF. *See* Personality Research Form.
Pak, S., 302, 311
Parallel Analysis test, 42-44, 49-50, 52-53, 56, 66
Parker, W.D., 125, 139
Parsimony, 167
Parsons, C.K., 152, 163, 169
Participatively-set goals, 320-323
Paul, A., 203, 296, 310, 339
Paulhus, D.L., 2, 22, 24-27, 35, 37, 39, 232-233, 247
Paunonen, S.V., 73, 94-95, 97, 120, 124-125, 127, 129, 132, 134-136, 138-139, 178, 180, 182, 194, 217, 219, 237-238, 243-244, 245, 247-248, 252, 255-256, 263, 304, 307, 313, 339, 341-342, 344
Peabody, D., 248
Peacock, A.C., 59, 71, 183, 193, 217, 247, 340, 344
Peak, H., 8, 20
Pedhazur, E.J., 257-258, 264
Peiro, J.M., 292, 302, 314
Pellett, O., 203, 208
Pelz, D.C., 190-191, 193
Penley, L.E., 329, 332
Performance, 6, 8- 10, 12, 14-15, 17, 46, 49, 53, 56, 58, 60-63, 65-68, 82-83, 138, 174, 183, 188, 190-191, 198

Personality, 1, 2, 8, 21-28, 34, 37, 39, 73, 91, 96, 98-99, 106, 120-121, 123-137, 141, 145, 147-148, 154-158, 162, 167, 173-174, 176-183, 191, 195, 204-207
Personality and job performance, 217, 223-224, 228, 240, 255
Personality assessment in employee selection, 215-216, 224
Personality Assessment Inventory, 34, 36, 96, 142
Personality disorder, 145
    antisocial, 112, 145, 147, 150
    borderline, 147-148
Personality predictors of job performance, 229, 240
Personality Research Form, 28, 32-33, 37, 96, 99, 106, 141, 173, 178, 183, 205
Personality traits, 124-125, 128-130, 133, 176, 178-179, 206
Personnel selection, 217-218, 222-224, 226, 229-234, 236-237, 240, 243-244, 249-250, 252, 254, 261
Perugini, M., 136, 138
Peskin, D.B., 217-218, 248
Petersen, N.S., 15, 20
Peterson, G.W., 157, 170
Petrides, K.V., 200, 208
Philpot, J.W., 299, 311
Pike, K.L., 126, 139
Pinder, C.C., 315, 332
Pinder, R., 262, 263
Piotrowski, C., 98, 120-121
Plomin, R., 206, 209, 211
Ployhart, R.E., 309, 313
Poli, E., 169
Pope, G.A., 117, 121
Popham, W.J., 16-17, 20
Porter, L.W., 69, 287, 313
Power, 23, 45, 57, 58, 60, 62-63, 65, 67-68, 167, 186
Powers, D.E., 20
Predictive hypothesis, 237, 239, 242
Predictive validity, 14-16, 18, 34, 233, 235, 252, 254
Preventive approaches to faking, 234, 236
Price, J.L., 302, 312
Prinzhorn, B., 167, 169
Procidano, M.E., 166, 170
Productivity, 173, 182, 190-192
Promotability, 238, 254, 256-260
Psychopathology, 25, 28, 30-32, 36, 95-98, 101-102, 104, 106-107, 113, 117, 141, 143-144, 146, 148, 153-155, 159, 163
Pullan, M.D., 117, 121

RPM,. *See* Relative Percentile Method
Rachman, S.J., 166, 170
Ragosta, M., 20
Rahe, R.H., 166, 169

Ramanaiah, N.V., 26, 39, 40
Ranieri, W.F., 146, 171
Raymark, P.H., 239, 248
Reaction time, 199
Realo, A., 205, 208
Reddick, R.D., 109-110, 117, 121
Reddon, J.R., 28, 40, 56, 70, 99, 101, 105, 109-113, 115, 117, 119-121, 223, 225, 227-228, 248, 256, 264, 339
Reed, P., 340, 344
Reed, P.C., 217, 248
Reed, T.E., 203, 211
Regression, 14, 35, 44, 50-53, 57, 60, 62, 66-68, 74, 77, 81, 83, 91, 141, 156, 162, 166, 200
Reichers, A.E., 289, 300, 313
Reid, D.B., 24, 26, 39, 270
Reilly, N.P., 296, 313
Reinhardt, V., 171
Reise, S.P., 106, 120
Relative Percentile Method, 238, 256
Reliability, 3, 4, 8, 18, 29, 37, 49, 100, 102, 104-106, 108, 144, 151-152, 163-164, 196
  coefficient alpha, 108, 151
  internal consistency, 29, 100, 106, 108, 131, 133, 144, 151, 163-164
  KR-20, 151
  test-retest, 163-164
Response bias, 22, 31, 100, 107, 252, 336
Response set, 22, 161
Response styles, 21-24, 35, 99, 107, 114, 129, 154-155, 165, 219, 232, 254, 261
Retzlaff, P., 155, 170, 208-209, 211
Revelle, W., 49, 70
Reynolds, W.M., 26, 34, 40
Rhee, K-Y., 302, 312
Riegal, J.W., 190, 193
Rieke, M.L., 262-263
Rijsdijk, F.V., 203, 211
Riley, S., 205, 211
Riordan, C.M., 308, 313
Ritzer, G., 288, 313
Robertson, I.T., 249, 264
Robinson, D.L., 39, 202, 205, 210-211
Rock, D.A., 20
Rocklin, T., 49, 70
Roe, A., 176-177, 193
Roediger, H.L., 174-175, 193
Roemer, R.A., 203, 211
Rogers, R., 163-171
Rogers, T.B., 337, 344
Rogers, W.T., 45, 47, 59, 69
Rolland, J.P., 125, 139
Rorer, L.G., 22-24, 40, 337, 344
Rorschach, 141, 218
Ross, C.E., 25, 40
Rosse, J.G., 232, 248
Roth, E., 199, 211

Rothstein, M.G., 34, 183, 194, 215-218, 220-221, 223, 225, 227-228, 230-231, 237-238, 243-245, 247-249, 252, 254, 256, 263-264, 317, 340, 344
Rouse, S.V., 102, 119
Rovai, E., 174, 194
Royalty, J., 208, 211
Rozeboom, W.W., 44, 70
Rubenfeld, S., 26, 37
Rush, J.C., 237, 248
Rushton, J.P., 96, 173-176, 178, 180, 182, 193-194
Russakoff, L.M., 170
Russell, C.J., 251, 264
Rutherford, M.J., 167, 168
Ryan, A.M., 248, 252, 264, 308, 313

Sackeim, H.A., 24, 27, 32, 38, 40
Sackett, P.R., 15, 20, 233, 245, 252, 264, 268-269, 271, 273-275, 282-283
Saklofske, D.H., 96, 205, 211
Saks, A.M., 298, 310
Salancik, G., 324, 332
Salazar, J.M., 140
Salekin, R.T., 167, 171
Samelson, F., 25, 40
Santy, P.A., 208
Sas, L., 102, 118
Sattler, J.M., 205, 209
Saucier, G., 125, 139
Sawyer, R.L., 15, 20
Schafer, E.W.P., 202, 209
Schill, T., 26, 40
Schinka, J.A., 163, 171
Schizophrenia, 98, 111, 114, 147, 149, 159, 166
Schmidt, F.L., 15, 19, 251, 263, 273-275, 279-280, 282-283
Schmit, M.J., 239, 248
Schmitt, N., 217, 223, 245, 248
Schneider, D.L., 270, 277, 282
Scholl, R.W., 289, 313
Schönemann, P.H., 44, 49, 70, 243, 248
Schoorman, F.D., 289, 312, 329, 331
Schrader, A.D., 234, 248
Schuerger, J.M., 252, 264
Schwab, D.P., 285, 313
Schwartz, M.A., 147, 166, 171
Schwartz, S., 198, 209
Science, 13, 168, 174, 176-177, 183, 186-187, 190-191
Scree test, 44
Screening tests, 95
Sechrest, L.B., 271, 282, 335
Seijts, G.H., 214, 315-316, 320, 323, 332
Self, R.M., 289, 296, 314, 320
Self-deception, 24, 27, 28-29, 37, 165
Self-set goal, 319, 321-323
Selzer, M.L., 166, 171

Sen, A.K., 205, 211
Seo, J.H., 289, 314
Setiadi, B., 140
Sewell, K., 163, 165, 168, 170-171
Shagrass, C., 203, 211
Shapiro, A., 74, 94
Shaw, K.N., 316, 331
Shaw, L., 35, 38
Sheldon, S., 117, 120
Shepard, L.A., 10, 20
Shockley, W., 174, 194
Shore, L.M., 297-298, 313
Shulman, L.S., 8, 20
Siddiqui, N., 167-168
Siess, T.F., 183, 194, 219-221, 248
Sigall, H., 35, 39
Silverman, S.B., 252, 254, 263
Sinha, B.K., 117, 121, 140
Sitarenios, G., 117, 120
Sixteen Personality Factors Test, 130, 143, 214,
    233, 251-257, 259-260, 262
Sjoberg, A., 302-303, 313
Skinner, H.A., 102, 119, 143-143, 166, 171
Slade, L.A., 309, 313
Slavin, R.S., 26, 38
Slovic, P., 99, 119
Smith, C.A., 294, 312
Smith, J., 145, 170, 183, 193, 217, 247, 340,
    344
Solley, C.M., 334, 340, 344
Somers, M.J., 297, 313
Sorbom, D., 75, 77, 94
Spearman, C., 55, 196-197, 199-200, 211
Speechley, M.J., 301, 313
Speed of processing, 200
Spelman, M.S., 205, 211
Spence, J.T., 189, 193
Spielberger, C.D., 38, 70, 120, 166, 170-171,
    330, 343
Spiller, W.E., 299, 311
Spitzer, R.L., 116, 119, 166, 171
St. John, N., 310
Stafford, E.M., 299, 312
Standard errors,
    delta method, 77
    quadratic method, 78
Standardized solution, 74, 77
Stanley, J.C., 242, 246, 295-299, 313
Starzyk, K.B., 117, 120-121
Stebbins, R.A., 288, 313
Stecher, M.D., 232, 248
Steer, R.A., 145-146, 166, 168, 171
Steers, R.M., 287, 313
Steiger, J.H., 44, 70, 75, 94
Stein, S.J., 117, 120
Stelmack, R.M., 202, 212
Sternberg, R.J., 208-209, 212, 276, 283
Stewart, M., 198, 209
Stinglhamber, F., 302, 314

Stough, C., 202, 203, 205, 208-209, 212
Straumanis, J.J., 211
Strelau, J., 205, 210, 212
Stricker, W.J., 217, 247, 342, 344
Strykowski, B.F., 174, 194
Su, W., 15, 19
Subsequent goal change, 318
Suicide, 166
Sulloway, F.J., 176, 194
Susman, V.L., 170
Sverke, M., 302-303, 313
Svoboda, M., 26, 37
Swamanithan, H., 93-94
Swartz, J., 171
Szarota, P., 136, 138
Szucko, J., 265, 282

Takahashi, K., 302, 313-314
Takao, S., 302, 314
Tammany, J.M., 208, 212
Tataryn, D.J., 42, 71
Tatsuoka, M., 130, 138, 213-214, 233, 245,
    251, 263
Taylor, C.W., 176-177, 194
Taylor, E.R., 171
Taylor, K.L., 166, 170
Tellegen, A., 106, 121, 168
Tenopyr, M.L., 17, 20
Teplin, L.A., 166, 171
Terman, L.M., 176-177, 194
Terris, W., 271, 273, 282
Test bias, 156, 157.
Test construction, 1, 2, 5, 13, 17, 22, 31-32, 34-
    36, 95, 97-102, 107, 117, 130, 133-134,
    141, 143, 147, 150-151, 160, 249-251, 267,
    277-278, 329
    construct-based, 30, 36, 96, 99-100, 106-
    107, 117
Test fairness, 4-5, 10-14, 16, 18
Test interpretation, 3-5, 10, 16-18
Tetrick, L.E., 297, 313
Tett, R.P., 217-218, 223-231, 236-237, 239,
    242-243, 247-249, 251-252, 256, 260-262,
    264
Thompson, A.P., 102, 118
Thompson, C.A., 299, 311
Thompson, G.R., 341, 344
Thorndike, R.L., 14, 15, 20
Three-component model of commitment, 306
Tibshirani, R.J., 80, 93
Tomarken, A.J., 167, 170
Topolnytsky, L., 295, 313
Touzard, H., 140
Traditional Values scale, 31
Trait inference, 340
Trapnell, P.D., 166, 171
Travaglione, A., 302-303, 309, 314
Triandis, H.C., 130-132, 140, 303, 305-309,
    311, 314

Trice, H.M., 288, 313
Trickett, E.J., 206, 212
Trott, D.M., 337, 344
Trull, T.J., 167, 171
Trumbo, D.A., 218, 247
Trzebinski, J., 132, 139
Tubbs, M.E., 316-317, 321, 323, 325-326, 328, 332
Tucker, L.R., 45, 47, 70
Tupes, E.C., 241, 248
Turnage, J.J., 257, 264
Turner, R.G., 205, 212
Twin study, 195, 201
Tziner, A., 262, 264

Useda, J.D., 167, 171
Ustad, K., 163, 167, 170-171

Validity of the employment interview, 217
Value orthodoxy scale, 30-31, 260
Values, 3-5, 7, 12-17, 19, 24, 30-31, 266, 287, 289-290
van de Vijver, F., 304, 306, 308-309, 314
van den Heuvel, H., 302, 311
van der Ploeg, H., 26, 39
Vandenberg, R.J., 289, 296, 308, 313-314
Vandenberghe, C., 292, 302-307, 314
Vardi, Y., 287, 314
Velicer, W.F., 2, 41-44, 46-47, 49, 53-56, 59-60, 68-69, 71, 73, 94, 132, 243, 248
Vernon, P.A., 96, 198-207, 209-212
Vernon, P.E., 176, 194
Vidmar, N.J., 132, 139
Viswesvaran, C., 267-268, 271, 273-275, 283
Vocational interests, 1, 181, 183
Vogel, F., 202, 208
Vogel, W., 202, 212
Vogelmann, S.A., 47, 69

WAIS-R. See Wechsler Adult Intelligence Scale - Revised.
Wagner, R.K., 276, 283
Wagner, S.H., 238, 248, 256, 264
Wahler, H.J., 166, 171
Walberg, H., 174, 194
Wallace, J.E., 299-300, 314
Wallbrown, F.H., 197, 211-212
Waller, N.G., 106, 121
Walsh, J.A., 23, 40
Walters, H.A., 341, 344
Walz, P.M., 298, 314
Wanek, J.E., 271, 275, 283
Wang, E.W., 167, 171
Waring, E.M., 117, 121
Warr, P.B., 299, 312
Wasti, S.A., 302, 304-306, 309, 314
Watanabe, N., 302, 314
Waugh, M.H., 166, 170
Wayne, S.J., 2, 41, 68, 298, 313

Wechsler Adult Intelligence Scale, 195
Wechsler, D., 212
Weeks, D.G., 74, 93
Weick, K.E., 218, 245
Weinberg, C.B., 237, 246, 256, 260, 263
Weingart, L.R., 320, 332
Weldon, E., 320, 332
Welsh, G.S., 155, 171
Wertheim, E.G., 237, 248, 256, 260, 264
Wesson, M.J., 316-317, 331
West, S.G., 32, 40
White, M.C., 26, 37
Whitener, E.M., 298, 314
Wickett, J.C., 202-204, 212
Widaman, K.F., 41, 44, 70-71
Widom, C.S., 237, 248, 256, 260, 264
Wiener, Y., 287, 294, 314, 334
Wiersma, E., 98, 119
Wigdor, A.K., 15, 19
Wiggins, G., 9, 20
Wiggins, J. S., 40, 121
Wiggins, J.S., 27-28, 97, 99, 155, 166, 171, 215, 241, 248, 252, 254, 264
Wiggins, O.P., 147, 171
Wiley, D.E., 12, 16, 20, 39, 343
Wilk, S.L., 15, 20
Willerman, L., 205, 212
Williams, C.L., 316, 319, 330
Williams, D., 202, 210
Williams, J.B.W., 116, 119, 171
Willingham, W.W., 5, 7, 10, 12-14, 18, 20
Willis, S.D., 115, 117, 121
Wilson, J.R., 205, 210
Wing, H., 271, 282
Winters, D., 326, 332
Wirth, R.E., 299, 313
Withey, M., 298, 314
Wolpe, J., 166, 171
Wong, C-S., 291, 312
Wood, J.M., 42, 71, 326, 332
Woods, D.M., 234, 246
Woodworth, R.S., 98, 121
Woolley, R.M., 269, 273-275, 283
Wortzel, L.H., 237, 248, 256, 260, 264
Wright, K., 266, 283
Wright, P.M., 316-319, 321-323, 325, 330-332
Wroblewski, V.R., 34, 38, 235, 247

Yang, K.S., 136, 140
Yen, W.M., 18, 20
Yeomans, K.A., 49, 59, 71
Yik, M.S.M., 134, 140
Yuan, K.-H., 74, 93-94
Yukl, G.A., 324, 332
Yung, Y.-F., 76, 94

Zaballero, A.R., 168
Zajac, D., 288, 312
Zaleski, Z., 140

Zeidner, M., 96, 132, 139
Zhang, S., 41, 70
Zidon, I., 316, 330
Zigler, E., 205, 211
Zonderman, A.B., 132, 139

Zuckerman, M., 205, 212, 251-252, 254, 262, 264
Zung Depression Scale, 145
Zwick, W.R., 42-43, 46-47, 49, 53, 56, 59-60, 71